Transcatheter Valve Repair

Transcatheter Valve Repair

Editors

Ziyad M Hijazi MD MPH FACC FSCAI
George M. Eisenberg Professor of Pediatrics and Medicine
Medical Director, University of Chicago Congenital Heart Center
Pritzker School of Medicine
Chicago, IL, USA

Philipp Bonhoeffer MD
Chief of Cardiology and
Director, Cardiac Catheterisation Laboratory
Great Ormond Street Hospital for Children NHS Trust
London, UK

Ted Feldman MD FSCAI FACC
Professor of Medicine
Northwestern University Feinberg Medical School
Director, Cardiac Catheterization Laboratory
Charles R Walgreen Jr. Chair in Interventional Cardiology
Evanston Hospital
Evanston, IL, USA

Carlos E Ruiz MD PhD
Professor, and Chief
Pediatric Cardiology
University of Illinois at Chicago
Chicago, IL, USA

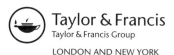
Taylor & Francis
Taylor & Francis Group
LONDON AND NEW YORK

First published in the United Kingdom in 2006
by Taylor & Francis, an imprint of the Taylor & Francis Group,
2 Park Square, Milton Park, Abingdon, Oxon OX14 4RN

Tel.:   +44 (0)20 7017 6000
Fax.:   +44 (0)20 7017 6699
E-mail: info.medicine@tandf.co.uk
Website: http://www.tandf.co.uk/medicine

A CIP record for this book is available from the British Library.

Library of Congress Cataloging-in-Publication Data

Data available on application

ISBN 1-84184-472-1
ISBN 978-1-84184-472-5

Distributed in North and South America by

Taylor & Francis
2000 NW Corporate Blvd
Boca Raton, FL 33431, USA

Within Continental USA
Tel: 800 272 7737; Fax: 800 374 3401
Outside Continental USA
Tel: 561 994 0555; Fax: 561 361 6018
E-mail: orders@crcpress.com

Distributed in the rest of the world by
Thomson Publishing Services
Cheriton House
North Way
Andover, Hampshire SP10 5BE, UK
Tel.: +44 (0)1264 332424
E-mail: salesorder.tandf@thomsonpublishingservices.co.uk

Composition by J&L Composition, Filey, North Yorkshire
Printed and bound in Spain by Grafos SA

Contents

Contributors

Carla Agatiello MD
Interventional Cardiologist
Hospital Italiano
Buenos Aires, Argentina

Ottavio Alfieri MD FETCS
Professor and Chairman of Cardiac Surgery
S.Raffaele University Hospital
Milan, Italy

Junya Ako MD
Stanford University School of Medicine
Division of Cardiovascular Medicine
Stanford, CA, USA

Zahid Amin MD
Medical Director, Cardiac Catheterizations and
Interventions
University of Nebraska/Creighton University
Children's Hospital of Omaha
Omaha, NE, USA

Vasilis Babaliaros MD
Interventional Cardiologist
Charles Nicolle, Hospital
University of Rouen, France

Emile A Bacha MD
Surgical Director
The Congenital Heart Center at the University of
Chicago
The University of Chicago Children's Hospital
Chicago, IL, USA

Steven R Bailey MD FSCAI
Professor of Medicine and Radiology
Janey Briscoe Center for Excellence in
Cardiovascular Research
University of Texas Health Sciences Center at
San Antonio
San Antonio, TX, USA

Fabrice Bauer MD
Interventional Cardiologist
Director, Echocardiography Laboratory
Charles Nicolle Hospital
University of Rouen, France

Ulf H Beler MD PhD
Resident in Pediatrics
University of Illinois
Chicago, IL, USA

Saroja Bharati MD
Director, The Maurice Lev Congenital Heart and
Conduction System Center
The Heart Institute for Children
Advocate Hope Children's Hospital
Palos Heights, IL and
Professor of Pathology
Rush University Medical Center
Chicago, IL, USA

Peter C Block MD
Professor of Medicine/Cardiology
Director of Interventional Cardiology Research
Emory University School of Medicine
Emory University Hospital
Atlanta, GA, USA

Gil Bolotin MD PhD
Visiting Scholar, Section of Cardiothoracic
Surgery
University of Chicago
Chicago, IL, USA

Raoul Bonan MD
Montreal Heart Institute
Montreal, Quebec, Canada

Philipp Bonhoeffer MD
Chief of Cardiology and
Director, Cardiac Catheterisation Laboratory
Great Ormond Street Hospital for Children NHS
Trust
London, UK

Younes Boudjemline MD
Department of Pediatric Cardiology
Hospital Necker for Sick Children
Paris, France

John D Carroll MD
Director, Cardiac Catheterization Lab
University of Colorado Hospital
Denver, CO, USA

Louise Coats MRCP
Department of Cardiology
Great Ormond Street Hospital for Children NHS
Trust
London, UK

Lawrence H Cohn MD
Chief, Division of Cardiac Surgery
Brigham and Women's Hospital
Boston, MA, USA

Jack L Collier MD
Cardiology Fellow
Saint Louis University
St. Louis, MO, USA

Delos M Cosgrove III MD
President and Chief Executive Officer
The Cleveland Clinic Foundation
Cleveland, OH, USA

Alain Cribier MD FACC
Interventional Cardiologist
Service de Cardiologie
Hopital Charles Nicolle
Rouen, France

John E Deanfield FRCP
Cardiothoracic Unit
Institute of Child Health
University College London
London, UK

Stefano DeCastro MD
Associate Chief of Cardiology and
Echocardiography
Professor of Cardiovascular Disease
Department of Cardiovascular and Respiratory
Sciences
Medical School 'La Sapienza'
University of Rome
Rome, Italy

Helene Eltchaninoff MD
Interventional Cardiologist
Director, Catheterization Laboratory
Charles Nicolle Hospital
University of Rouen
Rouen, France

Ted Feldman MD FSCAI FACC
Professor of Medicine
Northwestern University Feinberg Medical
School
Director, Cardiac Catheterization Laboratory
Charles R Walgreen Jr. Chair in Interventional
Cardiology
Evanston Hospital
Evanston, IL, USA

Peter J Fitzgerald MD PhD
Associate Professor of Medicine
Division of Cardiovascular Medicine
Stanford University School of Medicine
Stanford, CA, USA

Mark A Fogel MD FACC FAAP
Associate Professor of Pediatrics and Radiology
Director of Cardiac MRI and Cardiac MRI
Research
The Children's Hospital of Philadelphia
Division of Cardiology
Philadelphia, PA, USA

Francesco Fulvio Faletra MD
Director of Cardiac Imaging
Cardiocentro Ticino
Lugano, Switzerland

Welton M Gersony MD
Department of Pediatric Cardiology
Columbia University Medical Center
New York, NY, USA

A Marc Gillinov MD
Department of Thoracic and Cardiovascular
Surgery
The Cleveland Clinic Foundation
Cleveland, OH, USA

Eberhard Grube MD FACC
Heart Center Siegburg
Siegburg, Germany

Ali HM Hassan MD
Director, Bioinformation Services
Center for Research in Cardiovascular
Interventions
Stanford University School of Medicine
Stanford, CA, USA

William E Hellenbrand MD
Professor of Pediatrics, Columbia University
College of Physicians and Surgeons
Director, Pediatric Cardiac Catheterization
Laboratory
The Children's Hospital of New York
New York, NY, USA

Ziyad M Hijazi MD MPH FACC FSCAI
George M. Eisenberg Professor of Pediatrics and
Medicine
Medical Director, University of Chicago
Congenital Heart Center
Pritzker School of Medicine
Chicago, IL, USA

Yasuhiro Honda MD
Co-Director, Cardiovascular Core Analysis
Laboratory
Division of Cardiovascular Medicine
Stanford University School of Medicine
Stanford, CA, USA

Simon P Hoerstrup MD PhD
Director, Cardiovascular Research
Head, Division of Regenerative Medicine
Clinic for Cardiovascular Surgery and
Department of Surgery
University Hospital and University Zurich
Zurich, Switzerland

Valluvan Jeevanandam MD
Chief, Section of Cardiothoracic Surgery
Professor of Surgery
University of Chicago
Chicago, IL, USA

Joseph D Kay MD
UCHSC: University of Colorado Health Sciences
Center
Denver, CO, USA

Saibal Kar MD FACC FSCAI
Director of Interventional Cardiac Research
Division of Cardiology, Dept of Medicine
Assistant Professor UCLA
Cedars Sinai Medical Center
Los Angeles, CA, USA

Morton J Kern MD
Director, Cardiovascular Research
Pacific Cardiovascular Associates
Costa Mesa, CA, USA

Sachin Khambadkone MD
Cardiac Catheterisation Laboratory
Great Ormond Street Hospital for Children NHS
Trust
London, UK

Bijoy K Khandheria MD
Professor of Medicine and Consultant
Cardiovascular Division
Mayo Clinic College of Medicine
Rochester, MN, USA

Jean-Claude Laborde MD
Unite de Cardiologie Interventionnelle
Clinique Pasteur
Toulouse, France

Roberto M Lang MD
Professor of Medicine
Director, Non invasive Laboratory
Department of Medicine, Section of Cardiology
University of Chicago Hospitals
Chicago, IL, USA

Jack D Lemmon PhD
Principal Product Development Engineer
Medtronic Heart Valves
Minneapolis, MN, USA

Michael J Lim MD
J. Gerard Mudd Cardiac Catheterization
Laboratory
St. Louis University Health Sciences Center
St. Louis, MO, USA

Shannon Mackey-Bojack MD
Jesse E. Edwards Registry of Cardiovascular
Disease
St. Paul, MN, USA

Gerald Ross Marx MD
Department of Cardiology
Boston Children's Hospital
Boston, MA, USA

Vimal Mehta MD DM
Assistant Professor of Cardiology
GB Pant Hospital, New Delhi, India

Deborah Nercolini MD
Interventional Cardiologist
Charles Nicolle Hospital
University of Rouen, France

Natesa G Pandian MD
Associate Professor of Medicine and Radiology
Tufts University School of Medicine
Director, Cardiovascular Imaging and
Hemodynamic Laboratory
Tufts – New England Medical Center
Boston, MA, USA

Ayan R Patel MD
Associate Professor of Medicine and Radiology
Tufts University School of Medicine
Associate Director, Cardiovascular Imaging and
Hemodynamic Laboratory
Tufts – New England Medical Center
Boston, MA, USA

Ronald M Peshock MD
University of Texas Southwestern Medical
Center
Dallas, TX, USA

Emmanuelle Pineau MD
Department of Cardiothoracic Unit
Hospital Necker for Sick Children
Paris, France

Jonathan Rhodes MD
Department of Cardiology
Boston Children's Hospital
Boston, MA, USA

Carlos E Ruiz MD PhD
Professor, and Chief
Pediatric Cardiology
University of Illinois at Chicago
Chicago, IL, USA

Satinder Sandhu MD
Director, Cardiac Catheterization Laboratory
University of Chicago Comer Children's Hospital
Chicago, IL, USA

Susan M Sallach MD
Department of Internal Medicine
University of Texas Southwestern Medical
Center at Dallas
Dallas, TX, USA

Dörthe Schmidt MD
Head, Cardiovascular Tissue Engineering
Research (Divsion of Regenerative Medicine)
Clinic for Cardiovascular Surgery
University Hospital Zurich
Zurich, Switzerland

Partho P Sengupta MD
Assistant Professor of Medicine and Research
Associate
Cardiovascular Division
Mayo Clinic College of Medicine
Rochester, MN, USA

Prediman K Shah MD
Shapell and Webb Chair and
Director, Division of Cardiology and
Atherosclerosis Research Center
Cedars Sinai Medical Center
Professor of Medicine, David Geffen School of
Medicine at UCLA
Los Angeles, CA, USA

Prem S Shekar FRCS
Instructor in Surgery
Harvard Medical School and
Associate Surgeon
Division of Cardiac Surgery
Brigham and Women's Hospital
Boston, MA, USA

Edward G Soltesz MD MPH
Resident in Cardiothoracic Surgery
Brigham and Women's Hospital
Boston, MA, USA

Fred St. Goar MD FACC FSCAI
Director of Interventional Cardiology
Cardiovascular Institute
Mt View, CA, USA

Andrew M Taylor MD MRCP FRCR
Senior Clinical Lecturer in Cardiovascular
Imaging
Cardiothoracic Unit
Institute of Child Health and Great Ormond
Street Hospital for Children
Great Ormond Street
London, UK

Jack Titus MD
Department of Pathology
Children's Hospital of St. Paul
St. Paul, MN, USA

Denis Tixier MD
Service de Chirurgie cardiaque et Vasculaire
Hôpital Foch
Suresnes, France

Alejandro J Torres MD
Assistant Professor of Pediatrics
Section of Pediatric Cardiology, Department of
Pediatrics
Columbia University School of Medicine
New York, NY, USA

Christophe Tron MD
Interventional Cardiologist
Service de Cardiologie
Hôpital Charles Nicolle
Rouen, France

R Parker Ward MD FACC
Assistant Professor of Medicine
Director, Cardiology Clinic
Section of Cardiology
University of Chicago Hospitals
Chicago, IL, USA

Foreword

Before the turn of the 21st century, catheter-based interventional therapies in adults focused on the treatment of coronary and peripheral vascular disease. In parallel, there has been an explosive growth in the interventional management of specific pediatric and adult congenital disorders. The reorientation of our interventional pediatric colleagues on these more 'structural' heart disorders has helped to define a new subspecialty within interventional cardiology – the treatment of non-vascular structural heart disease. Thus, at a time when the world has been waiting for the next interventional revolution beyond drug-eluting stents, this new interventional subspecialty has already captured the imagination of the cardiovascular community. Interventional structural heart disease incorporates the exciting themes of (i) adult and pediatric congenital defect closure (such as ASD, VSD, and PFO closure), (ii) device-based therapies for congestive heart failure, and (iii) transcatheter valve therapies. The current text, *Transcatheter Valve Repair*, represents the first dedicated effort to address the myriad problems and early proposed solutions in the interventional treatment of adult and congenital valve pathologies.

Transcatheter Valve Repair is a unique publication and deserves serious attention, as it definitively encompasses the critical and distinguishing aspects of this newly envisioned therapeutic approach. First, perhaps more than any other subspecialty within interventional cardiology, transcatheter valve therapies require multi-disciplinary engagement, including adult and pediatric interventionalists, cardiac surgeons, non-invasive cardiac imaging specialists, and medical cardiologists with expertise in the pathophysiology,

diagnosis and natural history of specific valve disorders. The current text is not merely a catalogue of novel interventional devices, but rather a compendium of each valve disorder, beginning with disease state definitions, pathology and hemodynamic assessments, diagnostic imaging tools, current surgical therapies, unmet clinical needs, and concluding with a balanced description of current and future transcatheter solutions. This comprehensive approach emphasizes the critical roles of the multi-disciplinary specialists which are contributing to the emerging technologies and procedures.

Second, this new subspecialty is another prime example of the biotechnology revolution in medical device development. The creative applications of new biomaterials, nanotechnology, tissue processing techniques, and catheter-based delivery systems are required to properly engineer this new generation of remotely activated valve repair and replacement technologies. Clearly, we are in the midst of early prototype device and technique development efforts. The devices may appear crude and the techniques uncertain during these early stage efforts. Similarly, with rare exception, we are in the infancy of clinical assessments of these therapies. The necessity of evidence-based medicine clinical trial activities will help to characterize the ultimate clinical utility of these new devices and procedures. Nevertheless, this first edition of *Transcatheter Valve Repair* provides an excellent framework and sets the foundation for the future.

A clarifying image of the structural valve interventionalist resonates throughout this text. Both pediatric and adult interventionalists with a devoted appreciation of valve pathology and hemodynamics, an understanding of non-invasive valve imaging tools, and a flair for new interventional biotechnology devices will form the initial substrate mix. The early intrepid group of practicing clinicians will suffer disappointment and frustration as these devices are iterated and the techniques are refined over the next decade. The senior editors of *Transcatheter Valve Repair* – Drs Hijazi, Bonhoeffer, Feldman, and Ruiz – have already made substantive contributions in this field and lead an impressive author list encompassing all aspects of valve disorder management. In methodical detail each section marches through an exhaustive review of pulmonary, aortic, mitral, and tricuspid valve diseases and therapies.

This text should not only be the required reading for all current interventionalists interested in valvular heart disease, but also should be of great interest to forward-thinking surgeons, medical cardiologists, and cardiology fellows-in-training. As the population ages and we are faced with expanding clinical imperatives to manage our elderly patients with advanced valve disorders, the exploration of lesser-invasive treatments becomes obligatory. Perhaps the greatest achievement of this inaugural text, *Transcatheter Valve Repair*, is to elevate the visibility of an essential new subspecialty which will have an important impact on improved patient care in the future.

Martin B Leon, MD
Professor of Medicine and Associate Director
Center for Interventional Vascular Therapy
Columbia University Medical Center
Chairman, Cardiovascular Research Foundation
New York, NY, USA

Preface

Interest in congenital and structural heart valve disease is increasing. This is evidenced by the number of meetings each year that is dedicated to this field. When Philipp and I talked about the idea of editing a book on this subject (TCT 2003), I must say, we were somewhat skeptical about the project. However, we were determined to pursue the project. We met with Mr Alan Burgess, Senior Publisher at Taylor & Francis Medical Books at the Royal Automobile Club in London (January 2004). We discussed the various aspects of the book and also the timing. Due to the explosion in new technologies for the percutaneous management of valve disease, we all agreed that such a book is badly needed now. We approached Ted and Carlos to join us as editors due to their massive experience in structural heart disease and their pioneering efforts in this field. Both Ted and Carlos have added dimensions that Philipp and I do not have.

Our next task was to choose contributors who are the leaders in their areas of expertise and we believe that we have succeeded in assembling the best.

This book on valvular heart disease is designed to meet the growing needs of cardiologists and other professionals to learn everything they need to know about all cardiac valves in one book. The book initially was thought of as a conduit for understanding the new technologies that are emerging for percutaneous (transcatheter) valve repair/replacement. We realized that in order to get to this step, one needs to learn more about each valve, therefore, chapters in this text chronicle the spectrum of therapy for valve disease, from surgical to percutaneous, and from the diagnosis of patients to the evaluation of the results of novel therapies. First in class approaches describing percutaneous valve replacement by Drs Bonhoeffer and Cribier characterizes the first human applications of catheter based percutaneous prosthetic valve replacement. Second generation aortic valve prostheses have appeared even while the first generation is in its early development, detailed in the description of the self-expanding aortic valve prosthesis by Jean-Claude Laborde and his colleagues.

One needs to realize that all of the percutaneous methods for valve therapy are based on the long history of successful surgical therapy, reflected in the chapters by our distinguished surgeons. While this field is still in its infancy, the future of percutaneous therapy can also be seen on our far horizon. New approaches to prosthetic construction is detailed by Bailey in a chapter on the remarkable properties of nano-synthesized heart valves.

This book is dedicated to the patients who have undergone first in class and novel therapies with percutaneous valve repair and replacement devices. They have both the dire circumstances and individual courage to undergo these procedures. Some have also reaped the remarkable benefits of clinical improvement without the need for a median sternotomy. For example, discharge from the hospital after a 1-night hospital stay among patients treated with Evalve mitral valve repair or with the Bonhoeffer Medtronic percutaneous pulmonic valve reflects some of the most dramatic, early benefits of percutaneous valve therapies.

Ziyad Hijazi
Philip Bonhoeffer

Acknowledgments

I want to thank my assistant Mike Wallig for her dedication and hard work for the book. I want to thank Alan Burgess for believing in me and in supporting the project. This book is dedicated to my parents, wife Marie and son Tarek. Their endless love and support is what keeps me going.

I want to thank Martin B Leon, MD for writing the forward to this book. Marty has been a friend and a mentor for many years and I'm indebted to his generosity and kindness.

ZMH

It is a rare opportunity to be able to contribute to a first book about a new development in Medicine. I would like to thank the many people I have met who have had the open mind and the courage to engage in new ideas and who have inspired me. I have learned a lot from them. I have been lucky to be in the right place, at the right time, with the right people. This helps!

PB

I want to specially thank the many people who have made this work possible. It is not only through their specific support for the endeavors needed to complete this book, but more importantly for the help and forbearance for the large commitment to the broader work necessary to develop all of the new techniques and technology embodied by this text. My wife, Marie, and daughters Tess, Katie, and Julia have tolerated many irregular work hours, and I cannot express enough appreciation for their unwavering support and understanding over so many years. My coworkers at Evanston Hospital, including my physician colleagues Tim Sanborn and Mike Salinger, and the entire Cath Lab and cardiology staff have similarly provided instrumental support. My assistant, Allison Hammer, has helped with great ability to manage the volume of correspondence, writing, and ever-changing scheduling.

TF

The mere fact to participate in the design of a text book, it motivates the authors to an extraordinary level, out of the ordinary, since it truly demands long hours beyond the routine, even when the book is written by many different authors.

The idea of writing a book about the new transcatheter valve interventions was developed while preparing for the First Transcatheter Valve Symposium which was held in London in March 2004, by Dr Ziyad M Hijazi. I am very grateful to have had the opportunity to closely collaborate in this very worthwhile endeavor.

Finally I want to thank my soul mate, wife for thirty-four years, Esperanza and my three children Eva, David and Elizabeth for their constant encouragement and support through the years in all my goals and wishes.

CER

Section 1

The pulmonary valve

Embryology/pathology of the pulmonary valve in both stenosis and regurgitation

Saroja Bharati

This chapter briefly discusses the anatomy/ embryology of the pulmonary valve in both stenosis and regurgitation that will be useful to interventionists in their work.

Pulmonary valve: anatomy

A normally formed pulmonary valve consists of three cusps, two situated posteriorly and the third anteriorly. The posterior cusps extend anterolaterally to some extent to meet the anterior cusp. Thus, the posterior cusps are not entirely situated posteriorly. Likewise, the anterior cusp, although situated in the anterior or parietal wall of the right ventricle, also curves around the right and left sides to meet the posterior cusps. In contrast to the atrioventricular (AV) valves, the semilunar valves have distinct commissures. Normally the sinuses of Valsalva are formed by the valve cusps, the commissures on either side of the cusps, and the wall of the pulmonary trunk. The valve cusps thus have a base, a line of closure, and an edge. The line of closure may be prominent due to increased hemodynamics resulting in thickening, which is also referred to as noduli of Morgagni. The pulmonary valve may present small fenestrations at the commissural level. This may be considered a normal variation.[1]

Embryology

The pulmonary and aortic valves are developed by an undermining process involving the distal bulbar cushions 1–4. This yields the pulmonary right and left posterior cusps (cushions 1 and 3) and the anterior cusp by cushion 2. The aortic right and left anterior cusps are formed by cushions 1 and 3 and the non coronary or the posterior aortic cusp by cushion 4. This occurs during the third stage of development of the heart when the fetus is approximately 4–17 mm long, between the fourth and seventh weeks of gestation. During the same time, there is a differential growth pattern of the entire heart, including the valves, arteries, and veins. It should be noted that specific genes are responsible for the development of the distal bulbar cushions.[1]

Aging of the pulmonary valve

In contrast to the aortic and mitral valves, the valves on the right side of the heart age relatively slowly. This is most likely related to the low-pressure circulation on the right side. Therefore, the pulmonary valve in general shows less thickening in the process of aging.[2] Thus, age-related changes are less predominantly seen on the right side of the heart.

Variations of normal pulmonary valve: unequal size of pulmonary valve cusps

The three cusps may not be of equal size – one may be slightly smaller or larger than the other two. Occasionally, a cusp may extend into the right ventricular myocardium. It is not known whether these anatomic variations have clinical significance.

Isolated valvular pulmonary stenosis

Pathologic anatomy of the pulmonary valve

In general, isolated pulmonary stenosis is at the valvular level and uncommonly may be associated with infundibular pulmonary stenosis. The valve is usually a dome- or diaphragm-shaped structure with attempted formation of three commissures and a central opening. The latter varies in size from minute to small with thickened commissures.[1]

In some, there may be three more or less normally formed cusps with a small central opening. Although in most cases three cusps can be identified, less frequently the valve may be bicuspid or unicuspid and rarely quadricuspid. It is important to note that the valve may comprise three incompletely divided thickened cusps. The thickening may be mild, moderate or marked, and uniform in nature or irregular and nodose throughout (Figure 1.1). Such a valve may not only be stenotic but may also be associated with some degree of regurgitation. Rarely, a part of the cusp may be deficient or absent. Post-stenotic dilatation of the main pulmonary trunk may or may not be present.[1]

Rarely, peripheral pulmonary arterial stenosis may be present either on one or on both pulmonary arteries. The stenosis may be isolated or multiple and variable from one pulmonary artery to the other. When there is peripheral pulmonary arterial stenosis, there may be associated supravalvular aortic stenosis and abnormal calcium metabolism. Rarely, supravalvular pulmonary stenosis may occur with valvular pulmonary stenosis.[1]

Likewise, arrhythmias such as long-QT syndrome may be associated with isolated valvular pulmonary stenosis.[3]

The complex in valvular pulmonary stenosis

The heart is hypertrophied and enlarged, with the apex formed by both ventricles in the majority of hearts and less frequently by the right ventricle. The right ventricle in most cases is hypertrophied and enlarged or only hypertrophied with a smaller than normal chamber. The right atrium is also hypertrophied and enlarged.

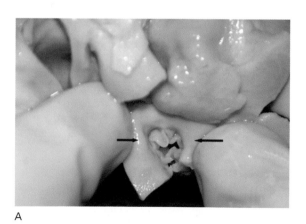

A

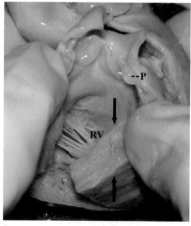

B

Figure 1.1

(A) Irregularly thickened moderately dysplastic pulmonary valve cusps with stenosis and insufficiency in a 4-month-old child who died suddenly. (B) The same heart demonstrating the outflow tract of the right ventricle with tremendous right ventricular hypertrophy. In (A) the arrows point to the dysplastic pulmonary valve; in (B) the arrow points to right ventricular hypertrophy. RV, right ventricle; P, dysplastic pulmonary valve (note the mild to moderate infundibular pulmonary stenosis).

When there is infundibular pulmonary stenosis, there is significant hypertrophy of the septal and parietal band musculature, with anterior deviation of the parietal band. The latter as such may produce infundibular pulmonary stenosis. The infundibular pulmonary narrowing may be immediately below the pulmonary valve, or anywhere below the valve to the apex of the right ventricle.[1] The left side of the heart is usually normal.

Tricuspid valve in isolated pulmonary valvular stenosis

There is a tendency for the tricuspid orifice to be smaller than normal in the majority of the hearts. The septal (medial) and inferior leaflets of the tricuspid valve may be ill defined, with a varying amount of thickening of the valve. The chordae may be abbreviated, with small papillary muscles. Occasionally, accessory orifices within the leaflet may cause insufficiency of the valve.

Although anatomic stenosis of the tricuspid valve may be present, a hemodynamically significant tricuspid stenosis is uncommon. This may in part be related to the presence of an atrial septal defect of a fossa ovalis type, which is present in the majority of the hearts in this anomaly.[1]

Endocardium in pulmonary stenosis

There is diffuse fibroelastosis of the right atrium with focal fibroelastosis of the right ventricle.[1]

Critical pulmonary stenosis in infancy

In some infants, the pulmonary valve, the main pulmonary trunk, and the two pulmonary arteries may be quite small, resembling those of pulmonary atresia with intact ventricular septum. It should be pointed out that these infants have markedly deformed dysplastic pulmonary valves that may be cartilaginous with a small tricuspid annulus and abnormally formed tricuspid val-vular apparatus, tremendous right ventricular hypertrophy, and a very small right ventricle.[1]

Pulmonary stenosis in the older age group

In adults, on the other hand, the valve in isolated valvular pulmonary stenosis may be sclerotic and cartilaginous, resulting in some degree of regurgitation with right ventricular hypertrophy and enlargement (Figure 1.2). In addition, there may be associated coronary artery disease, myocarditis, and/or other acquired diseases such as pulmonary tuberculosis.[1]

The pulmonary valve following interventional procedures in valvular pulmonary stenosis

Although isolated valvular pulmonary stenosis is generally dealt with well by the interventionist today, mild pulmonary insufficiency is seen in

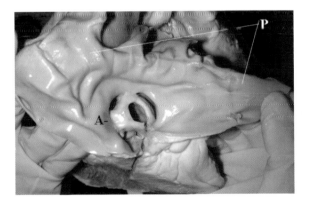

Figure 1.2

Marked pulmonary valvular stenosis with calcification, marked right ventricular hypertrophy, and post-stenotic dilatation of the main pulmonary trunk in a 73-year-old male. P, post-stenotic dilatation of the main pulmonary trunk. A, Marked widening and calcification of the anterior commissure with other two commissures likewise thickened and calcific – note that the valve is fundamentally a diaphragm-like formation with shallow sinuses of Valsalva and a small central opening.

some patients following balloon valvuloplasty. Long-term follow-up will redefine the course of history of pulmonary stenosis following interventional procedures. In general, if the pulmonary valve is dysplastic in nature to start with, balloon valvuloplasty results in insufficiency of the valve.

Likewise, tricuspid stenosis and/or insufficiency may get worse in some patients following interventional procedures involving the pulmonary valve.

Pulmonary valvular regurgitation

Fenestrations in the pulmonary valve

Small fenestrations may result from hemodynamic stress or as a result of previous endocarditis of the pulmonary valve. On the other hand, large fenestrations are usually due to previous infective endocarditis or trauma caused by interventional and/or surgical procedures involving the pulmonary valve. Sometimes interventional procedures may enlarge a small fenestration that may eventually lead to clinically significant pulmonary insufficiency. However, it should be emphasized that small fenestrations may cause mild insufficiency of the pulmonary valve that may not be detected by current technology.

Absent pulmonary valve

In this entity, the absence of the valve may be total or partial (Figure 1.3). An absent pulmonary valve is usually seen in tetralogy of Fallot. Rarely, an isolated absent pulmonary valve may be seen in an otherwise normally formed heart. Absence of the pulmonary valve causes regurgitation to a varying degree. In this entity, there is usually right ventricular enlargement associated with tremendous dilatation of the main pulmonary trunk and the two pulmonary arteries, which may compress the tracheobronchial tree.[1]

In general, in absent pulmonary valve, the annulus is quite small, with either total or partial absence of the pulmonary valve cusps. The valve cusps may be in the form of irregular nodular tissue with no distinct cusp formation. Rarely, absent pulmonary valve may be seen in tricuspid atresia.[1]

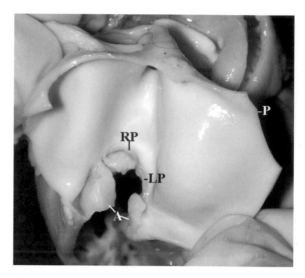

Figure 1.3

Markedly dysplastic, partially absent pulmonary valve with marked pulmonary insufficiency and mild to moderate pulmonary stenosis complex in a 4-month-old child who died suddenly. P, post-stenotic dilatation of the main pulmonary trunk; A, large dysplastic-looking anterior cusp; RP, irregularly thickened smaller right posterior cusp; LP, total absence of the left posterior cusp.

Quadricuspid pulmonary valve

A quadricuspid pulmonary valve may be seen in an otherwise normal heart without any symptoms and may be an incidental finding at autopsy.[1] Although quadricuspid pulmonary valves are generally seen in the older age group, rarely they may be found in children.

In this entity, the valve cusps are usually not of equal size. The fourth cusp, in general, is situated posteriorly and is usually the smallest. However, a quadricuspid pulmonary valve can occur with more or less equally sized valve cusps and may remain asymptomatic for a long period of time. Clinically, there may be mild to moderate regurgitation of the pulmonary valve that may produce volume enlargement of the right ventricle. The valve may be prone to infective endocarditis.

Recently, quadricuspid pulmonary valves have been documented in young, sudden-death victims in an otherwise normally formed heart with or without a history of arrhythmias.[1] They may also be seen in preexcitation,[1] mitral valve prolapse,[1] arrhythmogenic right ventricular dysplasia type of heart,[4] and atypical forms of hypertrophic cardiomyopathy.[5] It is of interest to note that all of the above patients died suddenly.

Pulmonary valve in major cardiac anomalies

The pathologic anatomy of the pulmonary valve when associated with other major cardiac anomalies will be discussed briefly, emphasizing only a few entities. However, it is understood that the pulmonary valve may be stenotic and/or insufficient in other major cardiac anomalies that are not discussed in this chapter. The pathologic anatomy of the pulmonary valve described in the following entities may also be seen, for example, in complete transposition with pulmonary stenosis, corrected transposition, single ventricle, Ebstein's anomaly, and others. Although the pulmonary valve in general is formed normally in major cardiac anomalies, it may be abnormal in some.[1]

Tetralogy of Fallot

In this entity the pulmonary orifice is smaller than normal, with a thickened bicuspid pulmonary valve in 54% of cases. Rarely, the valve may be unicuspid or absent. There are numerous variations in the valve cusps, with or without peripheral pulmonary arterial stenosis. In addition, there may be blood cysts. Rarely, the valve may present infective endocarditis and calcification.[1]

Hypoplastic left heart syndrome

In hypoplastic left heart syndrome, rarely the pulmonary valve may be bicuspid, dysplastic, or quadricuspid. When there is relatively significant stenosis of the pulmonary valve, it is self-evident that a bicuspid or dysplastic pulmonic valve (tri- or quadricuspid) may not be suitable for the stage I Norwood procedure.[1,6]

Common AV orifice

Likewise, rarely, there may be a bicuspid, dysplastic pulmonary valve in common AV orifice (common AV canal), which may result in significant valvular and infundibular pulmonary stenosis.[1]

Congenital polyvalvular disease

In this entity, although all four valves are considerably redundant and nodose, with either stenosis or regurgitation or both, the pulmonary valve shows more redundancy than the other three valves. The valve is referred to as a dysplastic valve. The architecture of the entire valvular apparatus is disorganized both at the gross level and at the light-microscopic level. There is an increase in spongiosa with hypoelastification and disorganization of fibrosa and spongiosa content of the valve. This entity is usually seen in trisomy 13–15 and trisomy 18. However, rarely, congenital polyvalvular disease may be seen in an otherwise-normal child.[1]

Marfan syndrome

It is well known that the aortic and mitral valves are usually affected in this entity. However, in our pathologic material, the pulmonary valve is involved to a varying degree in 26.9% of the cases with pulmonary regurgitation. When the pulmonary valve is affected, it is almost always associated with involvement of the aortic, mitral and tricuspid valves. The valve in general resembles the pulmonary valve previously described in congenital polyvalvular disease at both gross and light-microscopic levels.

Abnormities in fibrillin metabolism have been identified in Marfan syndrome. The relationship of genetic variations of fibrillin to the variations seen in the valves at the gross level and their clinical significance will be further elucidated in the future.[1]

Cardiac tumors

Although tumors of the heart are rare in children and young adults, advances in cardiac imaging techniques have allowed early diagnosis and possible surgical removal. Therefore, this discussion will be limited to one particular tumor, called papillary fibroelastoma, that has an affinity for the pulmonary valve.

Papillary fibroelastomas may occur rarely in children and/or young adults. Grossly, these tumors have multiple papillary fronds attached to the endocardium by a short pedicle. Papillary fibroelastomas may arise anywhere in the heart, but usually from the valvular endocardium. These tumors arise on either the arterial or the ventricular aspect of the pulmonary valve. Occasionally, they are multiple, located on the mitral, aortic, pulmonary, and tricuspid valves.

Histologically, the tumor consists of connective tissue surrounded by a layer of loose connective tissue and covered by hypoelastic endocardial cells. It is unclear whether papillary fibroelastoma is a true tumor or a hematoma. Be that as it may, the child may be asymptomatic if the tumor is small, while if the tumor is large or moderate in size, it may produce moderate to marked pulmonary regurgitation with or without stenosis. Surgical removal is indicated in symptomatic children.

Iatrogenic

Drug abuse

Infective endocarditis of the pulmonary valve may occur following chronic intravenous cocaine addiction. The vegetations destroy the valve to a varying degree, resulting in moderate to marked valvular regurgitation requiring valve replacement. This is usually associated with infective endocarditis of the other valves as well.

The pulmonary valve after corrective surgery for isolated valvular pulmonary stenosis and/or tetralogy of Fallot

Postoperative conditions

In general, following pulmonary valvotomy, the valve cusps are torn to a varying degree, resulting in pulmonary regurgitation (Figure 1.4). The regurgitation may be mild or perhaps moderate, but permits survival to adult life. Occasionally, the valvular regurgitation may be marked. The valve may present irregular thickenings with fenestrations, marked disruption, and discontinuity of the commissures.

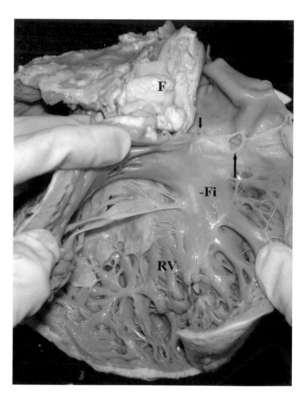

Figure 1.4

Fenestrations of the pulmonary valve following pulmonary valvotomy performed at 2½ years of age in a patient who died suddenly at 24 years of age. Note the tremendous enlargement of the right ventricle (RV). F, fat; Fi, fibroelastosis of the right ventricle. The large arrow points to a large fenestration in the right posterior cusp; the small arrow points to a smaller fenestration in the right posterior cusp at its junction with the anterior cusp.

In tetralogy of Fallot, if the annulus was enlarged during the total surgical corrective procedure, the valve may show thickening to a varying degree. With annular enlargement, there is usually pulmonary regurgitation to a mild to moderate degree, and with time the regurgitation may become significant, resulting in tremendous volume enlargement of the right ventricle.

Banding procedure

Although the banding procedure is no longer performed, the long-standing effects of this procedure on the pulmonary valve are noteworthy. The annulus of the valve remains small and the valve presents considerable increased hemodynamic changes, resulting in valvular pulmonary stenosis.

Pulmonary homograft

Pulmonary homografts are used for total surgical corrections such as those for tetralogy of Fallot, pulmonary atresia with ventricular septal defect, truncus arteriosus, or other conditions where the outflow tract of the right ventricle is reconstructed. Following surgery, in the course of time, pulmonary homograft valves usually exhibit hemodynamic effects. At the gross level, the valve cusps start shrinking to a considerable degree within the first 2 years following surgery. The degenerative changes of the homograft result in varying degrees of pulmonary regurgitation.

References

1. Bharati S, Lev M. The Pathology of Congenital Heart Disease. A Personal Experience With More Than 6,300 Congenitally Malformed Hearts. Armonk, NY: Futura, 1996: Volume I: Chap 6 (29–36), Chap 8 (45–56), Chap 10 (67–134), Chap 36 (553–86), Chap 37 (587–608), Chap 50 (747–56); Volume II: Chap 70 (1189–210), Chap 71 (1211–46), Chap 89 (1429–30), Chap 92 (1445–98).
2. Bharati S, Lev M. Pathologic changes of the conduction system with aging. In: Cardiology in the Elderly, 1994: 152–60.
3. Bharati S, Dreifus L, Bucheleres G, et al. The conduction system in cases with prolonged Q-T interval. J Am Coll Cardiol 1985; 6: 1110–19.
4. Bharati S, Feld A, Bauernfeind R, et al. A case of hypoplasia of the right ventricular myocardium with ventricular tachycardia. Arch Pathol Lab Med 1983; 107: 249–53.
5. Brookfield L, Bharati S, Denes P, et al. Familial sudden death: report of a case and review of the literature. Chest 1988; 94: 989–93.
6. Bharati S, Nordenberg A, Brock RR, Lev M. Hypoplastic left heart syndrome with dysplastic pulmonary valve with stenosis. Pediatr Cardiol 1984; 5: 127–30.

2

Pulmonary regurgitation

Jonathan Rhodes, Gerald Ross Marx

Introduction

Hemodynamically important pulmonary regurgitation rarely exists as an isolated congenital heart defect. However, pulmonary regurgitation is a common, almost invariable consequence of many of the surgical procedures employed to palliate congenital heart defects such as tetralogy of Fallot and pulmonary atresia/intact ventricular septum.[1-4] Significant pulmonary regurgitation also develops in patients who have required implantation of a right ventricular-to-pulmonary arterial conduit (e.g. patients with truncus arteriosus) as the function of the conduit's prosthetic valve tends to deteriorate over time. Indeed, over the past decades, as more and more patients with these congenital heart defects have survived childhood and become adolescents and adults, pulmonary regurgitation has become an increasingly common problem. Although once thought to be a relatively benign condition, the clinical significance and sometimes ominous implications of pulmonary regurgitation have recently come to be recognized and appreciated.[2,5-12]

Physiology

The magnitude of the pulmonary regurgitant volume, as well as the physiologic and clinical consequences of this condition, are determined by a complex interplay between several factors:

- *The size of the regurgitant orifice.* Patients with isolated pulmonary valve stenosis may have a small annulus, despite incompetent valve leaflets. The small annulus is the anatomic site of restriction, and a smaller orifice may limit the magnitude of pulmonary regurgitation. Obviously, a large regurgitant orifice provides little resistance to retrograde flow and can therefore permit a large volume of blood to regurgitate back into the right ventricle. Older patients with tetralogy of Fallot often have undergone surgery in which the pulmonary valve was resected, and a large patch was placed across the annulus. These large patches are frequently constructed from native pericardium and, over time, may become aneurysmally enlarged. Severe regurgitation may develop across this large annular region. In patients with tetralogy of Fallot, the size of the postoperative pulmonary valve diameter has been found to correlate with the severity of pulmonary regurgitation.[13]

- *Pulmonary artery anatomy.* Pulmonary artery stenoses/hypoplasia can impede antegrade pulmonary artery blood flow and raise central pulmonary artery pressure. In the presence of an incompetent pulmonary valve, these factors will increase the severity of pulmonary regurgitation.

- *Pulmonary vascular resistance.* High pulmonary vascular resistance also impedes the flow of blood to the lungs, elevates pulmonary arterial pressure, and exacerbates pulmonary regurgitation.

- *Right ventricular compliance.* Decreased right ventricular compliance is thought by some to decrease the magnitude of pulmonary regurgitation. Decreased compliance causes the right ventricular pressure to rise rapidly during diastole, thereby reducing the gradient for (and hence magnitude of) regurgitant blood flow from the pulmonary artery to the right ventricle.[14]

- *Left ventricular function*. Left ventricular dysfunction, or any left-sided pathology that causes increased pulmonary venous pressures, causes an at least equivalent rise in pulmonary artery pressure and thereby also increases the severity of pulmonary regurgitation.

Hence, in patients with incompetent pulmonary valves, the presence of normal pulmonary artery anatomy, low pulmonary vascular resistance, and low left-sided filling pressures tend to mitigate the severity of pulmonary regurgitation. Under these circumstances, an incompetent pulmonary valve is usually well tolerated, even though a large regurgitant area and 'free' pulmonary regurgitation may be present.

Impact of pulmonary regurgitation upon exercise function

The factors that influence the severity of pulmonary regurgitation (i.e. the pulmonary artery anatomy, pulmonary vascular resistance, and left-sided filling pressures) are particularly important in determining the degree to which an incompetent pulmonary valve may affect an individual's capacity to exercise. Under normal circumstances, exercise is associated with a marked decline in pulmonary vascular resistance. The exercise-induced decline in pulmonary vascular resistance is mediated by dilation of pulmonary arteriolar resistance vessels and by recruitment of pulmonary vascular beds that are normally closed or only partially perfused at rest.[15] Hence, even though pulmonary blood flow may increase four- or fivefold during exercise, the transpulmonary gradient changes little.[16] The fall in pulmonary vascular resistance during exercise promotes forward pulmonary blood flow and, in individuals with incompetent pulmonary valves, decreases the magnitude of pulmonary regurgitation.[17]

However, in some patients, the presence of fixed pulmonary artery stenoses (a condition common among patients with tetralogy of Fallot) negates the beneficial hemodynamic effects of the exercise-related fall in pulmonary vascular resistance.[18,19] In these patients, the stenoses impede the rise in pulmonary blood flow that is normally associated with exercise. Furthermore, the pressure gradient across the stenoses increases and the pressure in the main pulmonary artery, proximal to the stenoses, rises progressively as the intensity of exercise increases. In the presence of an incompetent pulmonary valve, the main pulmonary artery hypertension and the obstruction to pulmonary artery blood flow induced by the pulmonary artery stenoses combine to exacerbate the severity of the pulmonary regurgitation. Hence, in patients with incompetent pulmonary valves, pulmonary artery stenoses impose progressive pressure and volume overload upon the right ventricle during exercise and may dramatically impair the ventricle's ability to increase cardiac output during exercise. A similar pathophysiology will develop in patients with pulmonary vascular obstructive disease, a condition often encountered in patients with tetralogy of Fallot and pulmonary atresia with multiple aortic–pulmonary arterial collaterals.

Exercise is also associated with an increase in ventricular contractility. This in turn is accompanied by the development of a negative pressure within the left ventricle during early diastole secondary to the recoil of series elastic elements.[20] This negative pressure also promotes antegrade blood flow within the pulmonary vascular bed and, along with the fall in pulmonary vascular resistance, tends to mitigate the severity of pulmonary insufficiency during exercise. Impaired left ventricular diastolic function may result in elevated left ventricular end-diastolic pressure, pulmonary venous pressure, and ultimately pulmonary arterial pressure. This in turn would tend to exacerbate the severity of pulmonary regurgitation in a manner analogous to that seen in patients with anatomic pulmonary artery obstruction.

Impact of pulmonary regurgitation upon ventricular function

In patients with significant pulmonary regurgitation, the right ventricle dilates in response to the regurgitant volume load imposed by the incompetent pulmonary valve.[3] In some of these patients, as the right ventricular volume increases, the wall thickness decreases and the right ventricular wall stress increases in accordance with the law of Laplace. These developments may ultimately culminate in right ventricular fibrosis and progressive right ventricular dysfunction,[6] which may eventually become irreversible.[8] The right ventricular dysfunction may also ultimately become associated with left ventricular dysfunction. This phenomenon is thought to be due, at least in part, to altered right/left ventricular interaction. The dilated, volume-overloaded right ventricle causes the ventricular septum to shift posteriorly (towards the left ventricle) during diastole. This abnormal septal configuration can adversely affect both left ventricular filling (diastolic function) and left ventricular systolic function. This left ventricular dysfunction is an ominous development that has been found to be associated with a poor clinical outcome.[6,21]

Clinical findings

Symptoms

Typically, patients with pulmonary regurgitation do not experience symptoms until the cardiovascular system is challenged, for example with physical exertion. Hence, diminished exercise tolerance is the primary symptom associated with severe pulmonary regurgitation. This symptom generally develops in adolescence or young adulthood. Infants and young children usually tolerate pulmonary regurgitation without difficulties and experience normal growth and development. The onset of exercise intolerance is often insidious and, due to a combination of denial and lifestyle adjustments (realizing that they cannot 'keep up with their friends', children and adolescents often develop subtle, self-imposed physical restrictions), may not be appreciated by the patient or his/her family members until the patient is quite limited. Occasionally, long-standing severe pulmonary regurgitation may culminate in right and/ or left ventricular failure, and the symptoms associated with these conditions may develop.

Pulmonary regurgitation and right ventricular dilation have also been found to be associated with an increased risk for arrhythmias. Hence, patients with pulmonary regurgitation may have symptoms of palpitations, fluttering, dizziness, syncope or near-syncope. The most tragic symptom, i.e. sudden death, is also a well-known outcome in postoperative tetralogy of Fallot patients. The risk for sudden death has been found to correlate with magnitude of pulmonary regurgitation, probably on account of the increased incidence of arrhythmias associated with this condition, and the fact that these patients' hemodynamic abnormalities render them less capable of tolerating a rhythm disturbance.[5,9]

Physical examination

On palpation of the precordium, a prominent parasternal heave may be appreciated in patients with significant pulmonary regurgitation and a dilated right ventricle. On auscultation, the pulmonic component of the second heart sound is usually soft or absent. A right-sided S3 gallop is sometimes present. The murmur of pulmonary regurgitation is diastolic decrescendo in nature, and is loudest at the left mid-sternal border. Unless there is associated pulmonary hypertension, the murmur is usually low-pitched. In the presence of significant pulmonary regurgitation, the diastolic murmur is usually easy to appreciate. However, in some patients with significant pulmonary regurgitation, the murmur may be surprisingly soft. This phenomenon may be due to the absence of turbulence across the regurgitant orifice, a posterior orientation of the regurgitant jet, and the thick chest wall present in some older patients. A systolic ejection murmur is also commonly present in the pulmonic area secondary to coexisting pulmonary stenosis and/or increased flow across the pulmonary valve as a consequence of the regurgitant volume. In patients with associated tricuspid regurgitation, a systolic regurgitant murmur may be present at the left lower sternal border as well. In patients with severe pulmonary regurgitation and right ventricular dysfunction, signs of right-sided congestive heart failure, such as hepatosplenomegaly, jugular venous distention, and peripheral edema, may develop. If an interatrial communication is present, cyanosis (especially with exercise) may also develop secondary to right to left shunting that arises as a result of the increased right-sided filling pressures.

Electrocardiography

Patients with right ventricular hypertrophy have increased R-wave amplitude over the right precordium. An rSR' pattern will be seen in patients with significant right ventricular volume overload. If severe regurgitation results in increased right ventricular wall stress, ST–T-wave abnormalities may develop over the right precordial leads. Complete right bundle branch block patterns, due to right ventriculotomies and/or ventricular septal defect closure, are commonly encountered among patients who have had cardiac surgery. In these patients, electrocardiographic parameters for right ventricular hypertrophy are not reliable. In patients with dilated right atria, signs of right enlargement may be detected.

Past studies have noted a link between QRS prolongation >180 ms and malignant arrhythmias/ sudden death in postoperative tetralogy of Fallot patients (Figure 2.1). More recently, this observation has been somewhat revised, with the authors concluding that it is the change in QRS duration over time, and not absolute QRS duration, that is linked to the risk of sudden death.[9,22,23]

Radiography

The right ventricular enlargement that accompanies significant pulmonary regurgitation is reflected by cardiomegaly on a chest X-ray. The cardiomegaly is often best appreciated in the lateral projection, where the dilated right ventricle fills the retrosternal space. In patients with severe pulmonary regurgitation, it may also be possible to appreciate dilation of the central pulmonary

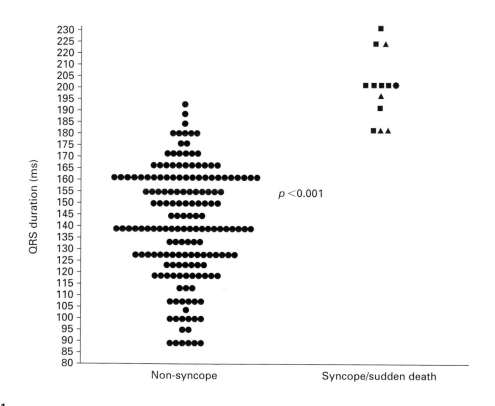

Figure 2.1

Plot of QRS duration in 182 patients with tetralogy of Fallot. The circles depict patients without syncope. The syncopal patients are divided into those with ventricular tachycardia (squares), sudden death (triangles), and atrial flutter (star). (Reproduced from Gatzoulis MA, et al. Circulation 1995; 92: 231–7.[23])

arteries. In patients with pulmonary artery stenoses, decreased vascular markings may be present in areas affected by the stenoses.

Echocardiography

Echocardiographic assessment of the magnitude of pulmonary regurgitation is quite challenging, and no single method has gained universal acceptance. Some laboratories have concluded that pulmonary regurgitation cannot be quantitatively evaluated by Doppler echocardiography and have used the term 'free pulmonary regurgitation' indiscriminately. This is a rather useless term (nothing in life is free). Although exact measurements might be difficult, certain parameters do exist that permit at least semiquantitative and clinically valuable characterizations of pulmonary regurgitation.[24,25]

Some investigators have reported that the ratio of the width of the regurgitation jet's color flow map over the pulmonary valve annulus diameter correlates well with semiquantitative angiography-based estimates of pulmonary regurgitation (Figure 2.2).[26] Others have found that Doppler evidence of holodiastolic retrograde flow in the distal pulmonary arteries indicates the presence of at least moderate pulmonary regurgitation (Figure 2.3). Doppler echocardiography can also be used to obtain quantitative estimates of the pulmonary regurgitant fraction. These estimates are generated by calculating the ratio of the retrograde/antegrade pulmonary artery blood flow velocity–time intervals.[27] The accuracy of this technique requires that the Doppler measurements not be contaminated by systolic pressure jets. Furthermore, this technique assumes a constant pulmonary artery cross-sectional area during systole and diastole. Alternatively, the regurgitant fraction can be

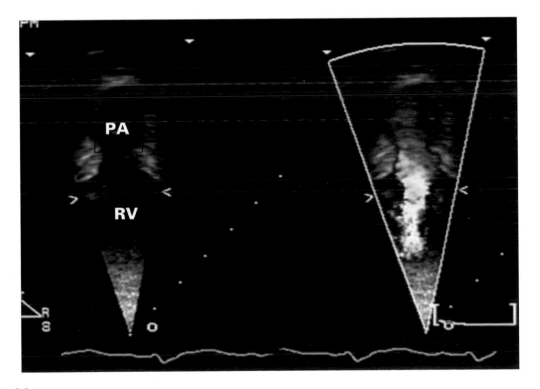

Figure 2.2

Left panel: subcostal coronal view of a dilated right ventricle (RV) and pulmonary artery (PA) from a child with pulmonary regurgitation. Right panel: red color flow jet depicts the pulmonary regurgitant jet.

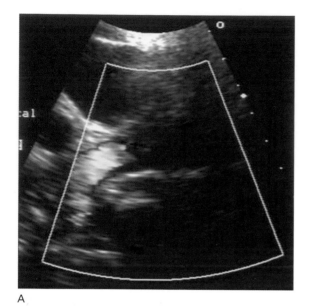
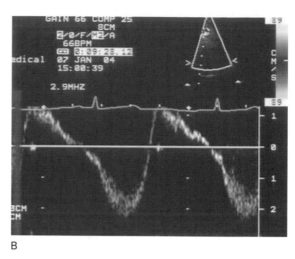

A   B

Figure 2.3

(A) Red color flow in right pulmonary artery demonstrating severe pulmonary regurgitation. (B) Pulse Doppler sample in right pulmonary artery (as shown in A) demonstrating systolic antegrade flow (below baseline) and significant diastolic retrograde flow of significant pulmonary regurgitation (above baseline).

calculated by comparing Doppler estimates of the antegrade aortic and pulmonary blood flows. This technique requires the absence of aortic stenosis or regurgitation, is unreliable in the presence of pulmonic stenosis, and is limited by the fact that small errors in the measurement of the aortic and/or pulmonary diameters are magnified because the cross-sectional area is related to the square of the diameter. Other investigators have reported that the ratio of Doppler-derived pulmonary regurgitation time to total diastole correlates with cardiac magnetic resonance imaging (MRI)-derived estimates of the pulmonary regurgitation fraction.[24] Shorter duration of pulmonary regurgitation was associated with greater severity of pulmonary regurgitation

In infants and young children, echocardiography can also provide important information regarding the interaction between pulmonary regurgitation and other hemodynamic/structural abnormalities. However, echocardiographic analysis tends to become more difficult in older and larger patients, i.e. in those patients in whom pulmonary regurgitation becomes a more significant problem. Compounding the difficulties of imag-

ing the right ventricle in older and larger subjects, many of these patients have had multiple prior thoracic surgical procedures. Their chest walls may therefore be deformed and their lungs hyperexpanded secondary to concomitant lung disease. These difficulties are further complicated by the fact that the right ventricle, pulmonary arteries, and/or right ventricular-to-pulmonary conduits are anterior structures, and echocardiographic imaging in the near-field continues to be problematic. The introduction of harmonic imaging has, by enhancing the signal-to-noise ratio, reduced these imaging problems somewhat. Yet, echocardiography is still challenging in the older operated patient with pulmonary regurgitation.

Perhaps the single most difficult aspect of the echocardiographic assessment of right ventricular function is the quest to optimally measure right ventricular volumes and ejection fraction. The right ventricle consists of three geometrically irregular regions – the inflow, body, and outflow – all of which can contribute significantly to right ventricular function. In the past, measurements of right ventricular volumes and ejection fraction have been based on geometric assumptions of right ventricular shape, which have been difficult to apply even in the normal right ventricle. These assumptions are even less reliable in disease states when the right ventricle becomes dilated and distorted, often with regional systolic wall abnormalities. Additionally, often-present right bundle branch block contributes to the difficulties in assessing right ventricular systolic function.

To date, M-mode echocardiography has commonly been used to estimate right ventricular size. Under two-dimensional guidance, a cursor is placed perpendicular through the right and left ventricles and interventricular septum, allowing measurement of the right ventricular end-diastolic dimension. Since this only provides a one-dimensional assessment of the chamber, regional variations in chamber distortion render this isolated measurement a 'rough' and potentially inaccurate estimate of right ventricular size. Nonetheless, for an individual patient, this methodology can provide worthwhile information regarding changes in right ventricular size over time. It has provided useful information regarding changes in chamber size before and after a surgical or medical intervention, using the patient as his/her own control.[7,11]

Obviously, two-dimensional echocardiography can provide a more comprehensive evaluation of the right ventricular size and function (Figure 2.4). This is especially true in the infant or young child, in whom a comprehensive subcostal exam allows sequential imaging of the inflow, body, and outflow regions of the entire right ventricle. In adult patients, a combined apical four-chamber and short-axis parasternal views allows for qualitative analysis of the right ventricle. Various observers have applied formulas to quantify ventricular volumes from these two-dimensional images.[28,29] However, as mentioned above, these formulas make (often unreliable) assumptions concerning right ventricular shape. Consequently, in clinical practice, calculation of right ventricular volume by two-dimensional echocardiography has not been universally applied.

Recently, three-dimensional echocardiography has been applied to measure right ventricular volume and ejection fraction.[30–33] In the past, this technology relied on obtaining multiple two-dimensional images in a sequential manner, with respiratory and electrocardiographic gating. Some investigators used the technology of free-hand scanning, in which external locators were employed to register the exact location of the various two-dimensional images. Dedicated computer programs would, in essence, compile this two-dimensional information into a singular large digital dataset. Either the entire volume of the right ventricle (volume dataset), or the endocardial and epicardial border (surface reconstruction) was obtained. Researchers then applied either a compilation of polytetrahedrons or a summation of multiple disks method to calculate the ventricular volumes. The application of three-dimensional imaging to calculate ventricular volumes was validated in many in vitro, in vivo, and human clinical studies. Despite these important breakthroughs, this technology was not applied in the clinical arena. Acquisition of the images was too laborious, time-consuming, and difficult, and the quality of the ultimate images was often suboptimal due to respiratory artifacts.

The introduction of real-time three-dimensional echocardiography has been an important advance in the effort to obtain reliable echocardiographically based estimates of right ventricular volumes. A fully sampled matrix array technology allows for the acquisition of the entire right ventricular volume into a singular dataset over four heart beats. In essence, this matrix array

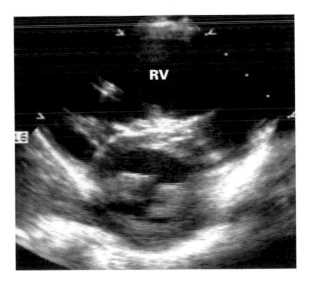

Figure 2.4

Precordial short-axis view demonstrating a markedly dilated right ventricle (RV) in a patient with significant pulmonary regurgitation. The round systolic septal configuration indicates that the right ventricular pressure is less than half systemic.

ultrasound probe has more than 3000 crystal elements, with focus capabilities in both lateral and elevational planes. With real-time scanning, immediate visualization of the heart is seen in three dimensions, albeit in a narrowed sector format. With gating over four heart beats, four sector formats are obtained and then collated into a large-volume dataset (Figure 2.5). In our laboratory, we have been able to scan the entire right ventricle in infants and children with subcostal probe placement. In adolescents and adults, obtaining the entire right ventricle is more problematic, especially when it is markedly dilated. Preliminary experience has shown that optimal right ventricular volume datasets can be obtained in these patients from apical four-chamber views. Using dedicated software, a summation-of-disks method may then applied to measure the ventricular volumes and ejection fraction. With improvements in probe and edge detection technology, this should become a universally accepted method to measure right ventricular volumes, mass, and ejection fraction. Rahman et al[34] found a good correlation between right ventricular volumes measured by three-dimensional echocardiography and MRI in postoperative tetralogy of

Fallot patients. The authors reported a negative correlation between right ventricular size and right ventricular ejection fraction. Additionally, these investigators reported that patients with severe pulmonary regurgitation had lower right ventricular ejection fraction than those with mild to moderate pulmonary regurgitation.

Right ventricular volumes and ejection fraction do not take into account loading conditions and therefore may not accurately reflect right ventricular myocardial function. The Tei myocardial performance index (MPI), however, is a Doppler-derived index of ventricular function that has been reported to be relatively independent of preload, afterload, and heart rate.[35] Moreover, the MPI is not affected by the right ventricular geometry. The MPI is calculated by dividing the isovolumetric contraction time plus the isovolumetric relaxation time by the ejection time. It therefore purportedly is an index of systolic and diastolic function. Among patients after repair of tetralogy of Fallot, individuals with more significant pulmonary regurgitation had higher MPI values than those with mild to moderate regurgitation.[34,36]

The right ventricular dP/dt is another index of right ventricular systolic function that is independent of right ventricular geometry. It can be measured from the slope of the upstroke of the tricuspid regurgitant jet. Using this methodology, Harada et al[37] found that the right ventricular dP/dt of patients with repaired tetralogy of Fallot was lower than that of normal controls and did not increase normally during exercise.

Assessment of left ventricular function is also important in patients with pulmonary regurgitation. Alterations in right ventricular size, function, and pressure will negatively influence both left ventricular systolic and diastolic properties. When the right ventricle is dilated, with right ventricular volume overload, the interventricular septum is flat during diastole. With right ventricular hypertension, the septum will be flat during systole. This finding implies a right ventricular pressure equal to or greater than half systemic. If the ventricular septum bows into the left ventricular cavity during systole, right ventricular pressure is usually equal to or greater than systemic. In an analysis of postoperative tetralogy of Fallot adult patients studied by two-dimensional echocardiography, patients who had sudden cardiac death were more likely to have moderate or severe pulmonary regurgitation, in association with moder-

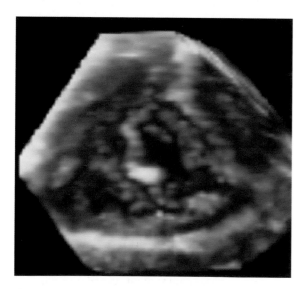

Figure 2.5

Full-volume real-time three-dimensional echocardiogram of a dilated right ventricle.

ate to severe left ventricular dysfunction, and prolongation of the QRS interval.[21]

When the interventricular septal configuration is abnormal secondary to the presence of a dilated/hypertensive right ventricle, echocardiographic assessments of left ventricular function that assume a normal configuration of the left ventricle (e.g. the shortening fraction and two-dimensional echocardiographically based estimates of left ventricular volumes and ejection fraction) are invalid. Under these circumstances, three-dimensional analyses and other indices of left ventricular function that are independent of geometric assumptions or segmental wall motion abnormalities (e.g. the mean dP/dt during isovolumetric contraction[38]) are better suited for determination of left ventricular function.

As previously discussed, the distal pulmonary artery pressure is an important determinant of the magnitude of pulmonary regurgitation. Hence, estimation of pulmonary artery and right ventricular pressure is of paramount importance in the non-invasive evaluation of patients with pulmonary regurgitation. Right ventricular pressure is best estimated by adding the estimated right atrial pressure to the tricuspid regurgitation jet gradient. Some experts have suggested that the absence of pulsatility in the inferior vena cava is consistent with a right atrial pressure $\geqslant 15$ mmHg. As noted above, the right ventricular systolic pressure can also be estimated from the ventricular septal wall position (Figure 2.4). Measurement of the pulmonary regurgitation jet velocity can also provide an estimate of the diastolic pressure differential between the pulmonary artery and right ventricle.

Identification of the severity and location of pulmonary stenoses is also important. This is not difficult for valvar or subvalvar pulmonary outflow tract obstruction. However, accurate assessment of peripheral pulmonary stenosis is exceedingly more difficult. Often these stenoses can best be appreciated by using non-imaging continuous-wave Doppler. However, Doppler often provides a gradient higher than is measured in the catheterization laboratory, or what would be expected on the basis of tricuspid regurgitation jet velocities. Importantly, in the presence of significant pulmonary regurgitation, right-sided systolic gradients will be magnified on account of the increased antegrade stroke volume. Even when the total gradient can be estimated, multiple levels of obstruction may exist in series, and accurate delineation of specific sites of obstruction, and the precise corresponding gradients, may not be possible.

In the past, some experts have claimed that pulmonary regurgitation is not clinically important in the absence of tricuspid regurgitation. Many clinical scenarios have shown this tenet to be untrue. Hence, evaluation of tricuspid valve integrity is important. Rarely, the valves may be congenitally malformed, with either dysplasia or Ebstein's malformation. On the other hand, significant annular enlargement due to pulmonary regurgitation and resultant right ventricular dilation may be the cause of the poor tricuspid valve leaflet coaptation.

Doppler tissue imaging is one of the newest technological advances to be applied to the analysis of right ventricular function. Using set filters, the transducers receive low-velocity, high-amplitude velocity signals of myocardial motion. Myocardial motion from the left ventricle, right ventricle, and septum have been analyzed as indicators of systolic and diastolic function. Vogel et al[39] demonstrated that regional wall abnormalities, detected by echocardiographic Doppler tissue imaging, are associated with prolongation of the electrocardiographic QRS signal. In addition to evaluation of myocardial motion, Doppler tissue imaging can determine the deformation of the myocardium, i.e. as strain, and strain rate. Weidman et al[40] found that postoperative patients with tetralogy of Fallot had lower indices of strain rate and strain than controls. However, neither strain rate nor strain correlated with magnitude of pulmonary regurgitation. The authors hypothesized that while pulmonary regurgitation and right ventricular dilation should increase strain and strain rate, myocardial fibrosis would decrease these indices – hence the competing parameters would normalize the strain rate and strain patterns. Harada et al[37] found the Doppler tissue systolic myocardial velocity of patients with tetralogy of Fallot to be lower than normal at rest and with exercise, and to correlate well with Doppler-derived right ventricular dP/dt.

A patient's right ventricular diastolic function may also have a profound impact upon his/her clinical condition. Controversies and difficulties relating to the assessment of left ventricular diastolic function properties also apply to the right ventricle. Potentially, analysis of Doppler tissue imaging signals may provide clinically valuable insights into right ventricular diastolic properties.

Cardiac MRI, CT and nuclear angiography

Cardiac MRI (Figure 2.6) and cardiac computed tomography (CT) have become the 'gold standards' for measurement of ventricular volumes and ejection fraction in patients with repaired tetralogy of Fallot.[1,41–44] In the absence of other significant regurgitant lesions or residual cardiovascular shunts, these measurements can be used to calculate the pulmonary regurgitant fraction.[17,41,44,45] Phase-contrast cardiac MRI can also be used to generate flow velocity-based estimates of differential pulmonary blood flow and of the pulmonary regurgitant fraction.[17,44,45] The agreement between image-based and phase contrast-based estimates of the pulmonary regurgitant fraction has been found to be excellent. Delayed-enhancement cardiac MRI techniques have also be used to identify areas of right ventricular myocardial fibrosis and/or scarring.[46]

MRI studies have contributed to our understanding of the pathophysiology of pulmonary regurgitation. Niezen et al[43] found that the MRI-based estimates of the magnitude of pulmonary regurgitation correlated with biventricular systolic dysfunction and diminished exercise capacity. Roest et al[17] found that the severity of pulmonary regurgitation at rest correlated strongly with right ventricular end-diastolic volume, and that pulmonary regurgitation tended to decrease during exercise. They also found that the right ventricular ejection fraction of these patients did not increase normally during exercise, whereas their end-diastolic volume tended to increase abnormally. Geva et al[41] found that left and right ventricular dysfunction, but not pulmonary regurgitant fraction or right ventricular diastolic dimensions, were independently associated with impaired clinical status in survivors of tetralogy of Fallot repair. Vliegen et al[42] demonstrated that pulmonary valve replacement improved right ventricular function and symptoms in adults with repaired tetralogy of Fallot.

Assessments of right ventricular size and function can also be obtained using first-pass radionuclear angiography,[6,47] although in many institutions this technology has been supplanted by cardiac MRI. Quantitative radionuclide lung perfusion scans, however, are still quite useful and commonly employed for the detection and quantification of pulmonary artery stenoses.

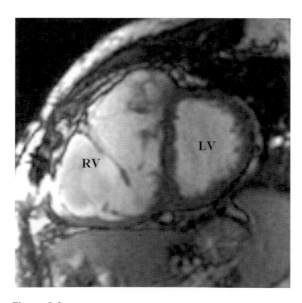

Figure 2.6

Cardiac magnetic resonance imaging of a patient with significant pulmonary regurgitation following repair of tetralogy of Fallot. The right ventricle (RV) is severely dilated. LV, left ventricle.

Exercise tests

Numerous studies have demonstrated that pulmonary regurgitation can have a deleterious impact upon exercise function.[2,8,10,11,18] In general, patients with severe regurgitation have diminished exercise capacity compared with normal subjects and patients with milder degrees of regurgitation. The inability of the right ventricle to increase forward stroke volume appropriately during exercise is usually the primary factor responsible for the patient's poor exercise function.[2] This appears to be especially true when pulmonary regurgitation coexists with branch pulmonary artery stenoses.[2,18] In repaired tetralogy of Fallot patients, ventilation/perfusion mismatch, secondary to coexisting pulmonary artery stenoses, has also been found to cause inefficient ventilation during exercise.[18] Because of the negative synergistic interaction between pulmonary artery stenoses and pulmonary regurgitation, the degree of ventilatory inefficiency during exercise has been found to be a strong correlate of exercise capacity.[18,48] Some studies have demonstrated that exercise function often improves following surgical implantation of a competent pulmonary valve.[10,11]

Cardiac catheterization and angiography

Since the development of improved non-invasive imaging techniques, the primary role of cardiac catheterization and angiography in patients with severe pulmonary regurgitation has been to diagnose and treat residual pulmonary artery stenoses.[49] Successful relief of pulmonary artery stenoses can potentially reduce the severity of pulmonary regurgitation and improve ventilation/perfusion mismatch.[18] In patients with severe pulmonary regurgitation, hemodynamic findings at cardiac catheterization include elevated right-sided filling pressures (especially when right ventricular dysfunction has developed) and equalization of the pulmonary artery and right ventricular end-diastolic pressures. Residual right-sided systolic pressure gradients, secondary to residual stenoses, may also be detected. When left ventricular dysfunction coexists with the right-sided pathology, elevation of left-sided filling pressures is also seen.

Management

When undertaken in young subjects, pulmonary valve replacement has been found to decrease right ventricular dimensions, reduce symptoms, and improve exercise function.[10,11,42] Because of the negative, synergistic interaction between an incompetent pulmonary valve and pulmonary artery stenoses, and because residual pulmonary artery stenoses may promote dysfunction of the new prosthetic valve,[7] optimal outcomes also require an aggressive approach to the palliation of residual stenoses prior to or at the time of pulmonary valve replacement. It must also be noted that the results of pulmonary valve replacement in older subjects have, in some studies, been disappointing, perhaps because the delayed valve

replacement resulted in irreversible right ventricular dysfunction.[8,11] The value of pulmonary valve replacement surgery, under these circumstances, is therefore questionable. These observations have caused some to advocate a more aggressive approach towards patients with severe pulmonary regurgitation, so that restoration of valve function may be undertaken prior to irreversible right ventricular dysfunction.[8,11] However, the function of bioprosthetic valves tends to deteriorates over time, especially in growing children and adolescents. The short-term benefits of pulmonary valve replacement must therefore be weighed against the likely need for additional surgical and/or interventional catheterization procedures. The optimal timing and method of restoring pulmonary valve function are important issues that are yet to be resolved.

A variety of prosthetic valves have been used to restore pulmonary valve function, including aortic homografts, pulmonary homografts, other bioprosthetic valves, and mechanical valves. More recently, success has also been achieved with percutaneous transcatheter deployment of a bovine jugular venous valve mounted within a covered stent.[50,51]

Because of the increased incidence of malignant ventricular arrhythmias in patients with severe pulmonary regurgitation, many centers have advocated resection and/or ablation of potential arryhthmogenic areas at the time of pulmonary valve implantation. In selected patients, the use of an automatic implantable cardiodefibrillator may also be desirable.[5,11,52,53]

References

1. Rebergen SA, Chin JG, Ottenkamp J, et al. Pulmonary regurgitation in the late postoperative follow-up of tetralogy of Fallot. Volumetric quantitation by nuclear magnetic resonance velocity mapping. Circulation 1993; 88: 2257–66.
2. Marx GR, Hicks RW, Allen HD, et al. Noninvasive assessment of hemodynamic responses to exercise in pulmonary regurgitation after operations to correct pulmonary outflow obstruction. Am J Cardiol 1988; 61: 595–601.
3. Graham TP, Jr., Cordell D, Atwood GF, et al. Right ventricular volume characteristics before and after palliative and reparative operation in tetralogy of Fallot. Circulation 1976; 54: 417–23.

4. Jonsson H, Ivert T, Brodin LA. Echocardiographic findings in 83 patients 13–26 years after intracardiac repair of tetralogy of Fallot. Eur Heart J 1995; 16: 1255–63.

5. Harrison DA, Harris L, Siu SC, et al. Sustained ventricular tachycardia in adult patients late after repair of tetralogy of Fallot. J Am Coll Cardiol 1997; 30: 1368–73.

6. Schamberger MS, Hurwitz RA. Course of right and left ventricular function in patients with pulmonary insufficiency after repair of tetralogy of Fallot. Pediatr Cardiol 2000; 21: 244–8.

7. Warner KG, Anderson JE, Fulton DR, et al. Restoration of the pulmonary valve reduces right ventricular volume overload after previous repair of tetralogy of Fallot. Circulation 1993; 88: II-89–II-97.

8. Therrien J, Siu SC, McLaughlin PR, et al. Pulmonary valve replacement in adults late after repair of tetralogy of Fallot: are we operating too late? J Am Coll Cardiol 2000; 36: 1670–5.

9. Gatzoulis MA, Balaji S, Webber SA, et al. Risk factors for arrhythmia and sudden cardiac death late after repair of tetralogy of Fallot: a multicentre study. Lancet 2000; 356: 975–81.

10. Eyskens B, Reybrouck T, Bogaert J, et al. Homograft insertion for pulmonary regurgitation after repair of tetralogy of Fallot improves cardiorespiratory exercise performance. Am J Cardiol 2000; 85: 221–5.

11. Warner KG, O'Brien PK, Rhodes J, et al. Expanding the indications for pulmonary valve replacement after repair of tetralogy of Fallot. Ann Thorac Surg 2003; 76: 1066–72.

12. Harrison DA, Siu SC, Hussain F, et al. Sustained atrial arrhythmias in adult patients late after repair of tetralogy of Fallot. Am J Cardiol 2001; 87: 584–8.

13. Uebing A, Fischer G, Bethge M, et al. Influence of pulmonary annulus diameter on pulmonary regurgitation and right ventricular pressure load after repair of tetralogy of Fallot. Heart 2002; 88: 510–14.

14. Gatzoulis MA, Clark AL, Cullen S, et al. Right ventricular diastolic function 15 to 35 years after repair of tetralogy of Fallot. Restrictive physiology predicts superior exercise performance. Circulation 1995; 91: 1775–81.

15. Linehan JH, Dawson CA. Pulmonary vascular resistance. In: Fishman AP (ed). The Pulmonary Circulation. Philadelphia: University of Pennsylvania Press, 1990: 41–55.

16. Ekelund LG, Holmgren A. Central hemodynamics during exercise. Circ Res 1967; 20/21: I-33–I-43.

17. Roest AAW, Helbing WA, Kunz P, et al. Exercise MR imaging in the assessment of pulmonary regurgitation and biventricular function in patients after tetralogy of Fallot repair. Radiology 2002; 223: 204–11.

18. Rhodes J, Dave A, Pulling MC, et al. Effect of pulmonary artery stenoses on the cardiopulmonary response to exercise following repair of tetralogy of Fallot. Am J Cardiol 1998; 81: 1217–19.

19. Chaturvedi RR, Kilner PJ, White PA, et al. Increased airway pressure and simulated branch pulmonary artery stenosis increase pulmonary regurgitation after repair of tetralogy of Fallot. Real-time analysis with a conductance catheter technique. Circulation 1997; 95: 643–9.

20. Udelson JE, Bacharach SL, Cannon RO III, et al. Minimum left ventricular pressure during beta-adrenergic stimulation in human subjects. Evidence for elastic recoil and diastolic 'suction' in the normal heart. Circulation 1990; 82: 1174–82.

21. Ghai A, Silversides C, Harris L, et al. Left ventricular dysfunction is a risk factor for sudden cardiac death in adults late after repair of tetralogy of Fallot. J Am Coll Cardiol 2002; 40: 1675–80.

22. Berul CI, Hill SL, Geggel, RL, et al. Electrocardiographic markers of late sudden death risk in postoperative tetralogy of Fallot children. J Cardiovasc Electrophysiol 1997; 8: 1349–56 [Erratum: 2000; 11(4): ix].

23. Gatzoulis MA, Till JA, Somerville J, et al. Mechanoelectrical interaction in tetralogy of Fallot. QRS prolongation relates to right ventricular size and predicts malignant ventricular arrhythmias and sudden death. Circulation 1995; 92: 231–7.

24. Weil L, Davlouros PA, Kinler PJ, et al. Doppler-echocardiographic assessment of pulmonary regurgitation in adults with repaired tetralogy of Fallot: comparison with cardiovascular magnetic resonance imaging. Am Heart J 2004; 147: 172.

25. Zoghbi W, Enriquez-Sarano M, Foster E, et al. Recommendations for evaluation of the severity of native valvular regurgitation with two-dimensional and Doppler echocardiography. J Am Soc Echocardiogr 2003; 16: 777–802.

26. Williams RV, Minich L, Shaddy RE. Comparison of Doppler echocardiography with angiography for determining the severity of pulmonary regurgitation. Am J Cardiol 2002; 89: 1438–40.

27. Goldberg SJ, Mendes F, Hurwitz R. Maximal exercise capability of children as a function of specific cardiac defects. Am J Cardiol 1969; 23: 349–53.

28. Hirashi S, Disessa TG, Jarmakani JM, et al. Two-dimensional echocardiographic assessment of right ventricular volume in children with congenital heart disease. Am J Cardiol 1982; 50: 1368–75.

29. Silverman NH, Judson S. Evaluation of right ventricular volume and ejection fraction in children by two-dimensional echocardiography. Pediatr Cardiol 1983; 4: 917–24.

30. Levine RA, Gibson TC, Aretz T. Echocardiographic measurement of right ventricular volume. Circulation 1984; 69: 497–505.

31. Vogel M, White PA, Redington AN. In vitro validation of right ventricular volume measurement by

three-dimensional echocardiography. Br Heart J 1995; 74: 460–3.

32. Vogel M, Gutberlet M, Dittrich S, et al. Comparison of transthoracic three dimensional echocardiography with magnetic resonance imaging in the assessment of right ventricular volume and mass. Heart 1997; 78: 127–30.

33. Papavassilou DP, Park J, Hopkins KL, et al. Three-dimensional echocardiographic measurement of right ventricular volume in children with congenital heart disease validated by magnetic resonance imaging. J Am Soc Echocardiogr 1998; 11: 770–7.

34. Rahman AE, Abdul-Khalig H, Vogel M, et al. Relation between right ventricular enlargement, QRS duration, and right ventricular function in patients with tetralogy of Fallot and pulmonary regurgitation after surgical repair. Heart 2000; 84: 416–20.

35. Eidem BW, O'Leary P, Tei C, et al. Usefulness of the myocardial performance index for assessing right ventricular function in congenital heart disease. Am J Cardiol 2000; 86: 654–8.

36. Rahman AE, Abdul-Khalig H, Vogel M. Value of the new Doppler-derived myocardial performance index for the evaluation of right and left ventricular function following repair of tetralogy of Fallot. Pediatr Cardiol 2002; 23: 502–7.

37. Harada K, Toyono M, Yamamoto F. Assessment of right ventricular function during exercise with quantitative Doppler tissue imaging in children late after repair of tetralogy of Fallot. J Am Soc Echocardiogr 2004; 17: 863–9.

38. Rhodes J, Udelson JE, Marx GR, et al. A new non-invasive method for the estimation of peak dP/dt. Circulation 1993; 88: 2693–9.

39. Vogel M, Songring J, Cullen S, et al. Regional wall motion and abnormalities of electrical depolarization and repolarization in patients after surgical repair of tetralogy of Fallot. Circulation 2001; 103: 1669–773.

40. Weidman WH, Eyskens B, Mertens L, et al. Quantification of regional right and left ventricular function by ultrasonic strain rate and strain indexes after surgical repair of tetralogy of Fallot. Am J Cardiol 2002; 90: 133–8.

41. Geva T, Sandweiss BM, Gauvreau K, et al. Factors associated with impaired clinical status in long-term survivors of tetralogy of Fallot repair evaluated by magnetic resonance imaging. J Am Coll Cardiol 2004; 43: 1074.

42. Vliegen HW, van Straten A, de Roos A, et al. Magnetic resonance imaging to assess the hemodynamic effects of pulmonary valve replacement in adults late after repair of tetralogy of Fallot. Circulation 2002; 106: 1703–7.

43. Niezen RA, Helbing WA, van der Wall EE, et al. Biventricular systolic function and mass studied with MR imaging in children with pulmonary regurgitation after repair for tetralogy of Fallot. Radiology 1996; 201: 135–40.

44. Helbing WA, de Roos A. Clinical applications of cardiac magnetic resonance imaging after repair of tetralogy of Fallot. Pediatr Cardiol 2000; 21: 70–79.

45. Kang I, Redington AN, Benson LN, et al. Differential regurgitation in branch pulmonary arteries after repair of tetralogy of Fallot. Circulation 2003; 107: 2938–43.

46. Valente AM, Idriss SF, Cawley P, et al. Myocardial fibrosis patterns correlate with adverse right ventricular morphology and function in patients with repaired contruncal heart defects. J Am Coll Cardiol 2004; 43(Suppl A): 390A.

47. Hurwiitz RA, Treves S, Kuruc A. Right ventricular and left ventricular ejection fraction in pediatric patients with normal hearts: first-pass radionuclide angiography. Am Heart J 1984; 107: 726–32.

48. Clark AL, Gatzoulis MA, Redington AN. Ventilatory responses to exercise in adults after repair of tetralogy of Fallot. Br Heart J 1995; 73: 445–9.

49. Kreutzer J, Perry SB, Jonas RA, et al. Tetralogy of Fallot with diminutive pulmonary arteries: preoperative pulmonary valve dilation and transcatheter rehabilitation of pulmonary arteries. J Am Coll Cardiol 1996; 17: 1741–7.

50. Boudjemline Y, Khambadkone S, Bonnet D, et al. Non-surgical replacement of the pulmonary valve: from experimental research to human application. Arch Pediatr 2004; 11: 1239–44.

51. Khambadkone S, Bonhoeffer P. Nonsurgical pulmonary valve replacement: why, when, and how? Catheter Cardiovasc Interv 2004; 62: 401–8.

52. Therrien J, Siu SC, Harris L, et al. Impact of pulmonary valve replacement on arrhythmia propensity late after repair of tetralogy of Fallot. Circulation 2001; 103: 2489–94.

53. Saul JP, Alexander ME. Preventing sudden death after repair of tetralogy of Fallot: complex therapy for complex patients. J Cardiovasc Electrophysiol 1999; 10: 1271–87.

3

Assessment of the pulmonary valve with magnetic resonance imaging

Andrew M Taylor

Introduction

Magnetic resonance (MR) is becoming an important imaging modality for the assessment of cardiovascular disease, in both congenital and acquired heart disease.[1] Cardiovascular anatomy can be assessed in three dimensions along with the other structures of the thorax (airways, pulmonary parenchyma, etc.). This places the heart back within the axes of the body, enabling accurate description of cardiac and vascular anatomy in relation to these structures.[2] Furthermore, MR imaging (MRI) currently provides the best available in vivo, quantifiable assessment of both cardiac function[3] and great vessel blood flow.[4] Thus, the anatomic and functional significance of the disease process can be defined using a single non-invasive imaging modality without exposure to X-rays or the nephrotoxic effects of iodinated contrast agents.

The aims of this chapter are:

- to familiarize the reader with the MRI techniques that can be used to assess the right heart and pulmonary arteries
- to summarize the current MR literature on the effects of chronic pulmonary incompetence (with or without pulmonary stenosis)
- to outline a protocol for MR assessment before and after percutaneous pulmonary valve implantation
- to outline the role of computed tomography (CT) in imaging the right heart and pulmonary arteries.

Magnetic resonance imaging

Cardiovascular MR assessment of the pulmonary valve is usually performed in subjects who have undergone surgical intervention to the right ventricular (RV) outflow tract (RVOT) and/or pulmonary trunk (Table 3.1). Echocardiography is the first-line investigation in these subjects, but visualization of the RVOT, pulmonary trunk, and branch pulmonary arteries is often difficult, in particular in older subjects. This is due to the lack of an acoustic window (structures behind the sternum) and changes secondary to multiple operations. Cardiac catheterization is considered the second-line investigation in many centers; however, if access to cardiovascular MR is

---

Table 3.1 Conditions in which assessment of pulmonary valvular or conduit function is necessary

- Repaired tetralogy of Fallot (± transannular patch repair)
- Repaired transposition of the great arteries:
    - Arterial switch operation
- Surgical insertion of a right ventricular-to-pulmonary artery conduit:
    - Pulmonary atresia
    - Common arterial trunk
    - Double-outlet right ventricle
    - Repaired transposition of the great arteries: Rastelli operation
- Repaired aortic valvular disease following the Ross operation
- Following pulmonary valvotomy

available, MRI can provide much of the information of a diagnostic cardiac catheter, with the exception of hemodynamic pressure traces and accurate imaging of coronary artery disease. Thus, three-dimensional (3D) anatomy of the right-sided cardiac and vascular structures can be depicted, and right ventricular and pulmonary valve/conduit function accurately assessed. These parameters, in conjunction with clinical findings, echocardiography, and metabolic exercise testing data can be used to help monitor subjects, define the timing of interventions, and, when intervention is necessary, select the appropriate treatment option – surgery or percutaneous pulmonary valve implantation (PPVI).

RVOT and pulmonary artery anatomy

'Black-blood' imaging

'Black-blood' spin echo imaging was the earliest technique used to image congenital heart disease.[5,6] In this sequence, flowing blood gives no MR signal, while stationary tissue returns an MR signal, allowing excellent delineation between the blood pool and either the vessel wall or myocardium. MR data acquisition is performed during a defined portion of the cardiac cycle to 'freeze' cardiac motion (usually the diastolic diastasis). Most spin echo sequences are now acquired rapidly using fast spin echo imaging algorithms (TSE, TFSE, RARE, SSFSE, and HASTE), which enable images to be acquired in a single breath-hold.[7] The main disadvantage of the 'black-blood' spin echo sequences is that data are acquired in two-dimensional (2D) slices, and skill is required for image acquisition and interpretation. However, although gradient echo sequences (cine imaging and MR angiography (MRA)) are increasingly used in cardiovascular MR (see below), the 'black-blood' spin echo sequence remains important in two situations:

1. 'Black-blood' images are useful for accurate sizing of severe valvular and vascular stenoses. With these lesions, gradient echo sequences are prone to signal loss, due to turbulent flow, while for 'black-blood' imaging

contrast improves when the blood flow velocity is high. 'Black-blood' sequences have been used to successfully image valvular stenosis, conduit stenosis, and baffle obstruction.[8–10] It should be noted, however, that signal loss due to conduit and baffle calcification might lead to underestimation of stenosis.[9]

2. 'Black-blood' images are useful when imaging vessels after metallic stent insertion. The majority of stents are safe to image,[11] but cause marked artifacts on gradient echo sequences secondary to T2* field inhomogeneity. Due to the refocusing pulse, spin echo sequences are not as susceptible to these phenomena, and imaging of the vessel within the stent can be achieved (Figure 3.1).

Two-dimensional 'white-blood' cine imaging

In gradient echo imaging, signal from the blood pool is recovered, and blood appears as white. Data are acquired rapidly with high temporal resolution, enabling acquisition of multiple phases of the cardiac cycle.

More recently, balanced steady-state free precession (balanced-SSFP) sequences have become available (TrueFISP, balanced FFE, FIESTA).[12] These sequences have very short MR parameters, which place high demands on MR hardware. Balanced-SSFP images provide improved blood pool homogeneity throughout the cardiac cycle and faster acquisition times than conventional gradient echo images.[13,14] 2D balanced-SSFP imaging has become widely used in cardiac imaging, and allows qualitative assessment of the cardiac chambers, valvular dysfunction, and dynamic vascular anatomy. Importantly, as information is acquired over the entire cardiac cycle, the dynamic nature of the structure being imaged can be assessed. This is not true for either 'black-blood' spin echo imaging (images acquired at a single point in the cardiac cycle) or MRA (images acquired without ECG gating; see below). This information can be crucial in sizing of the RVOT/pulmonary trunk prior to treatment, as underestimation of the dimension may lead an inappropriate attempt at PPVI.[15]

One disadvantage of gradient echo cine images is that signal loss can occur at sites of stenosis

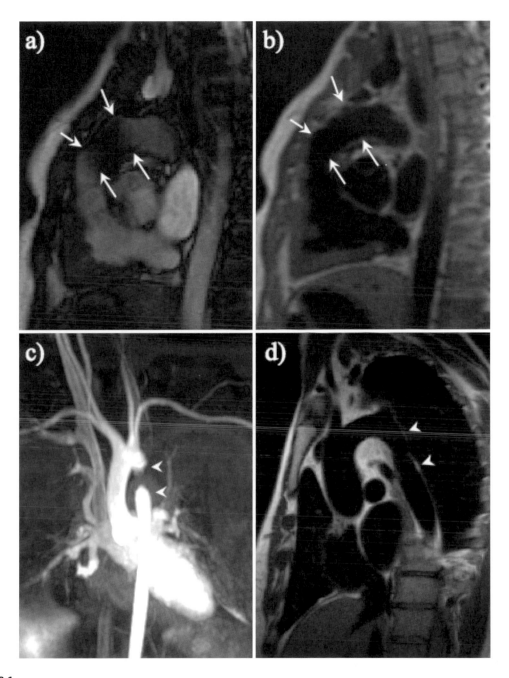

Figure 3.1

(a, b) Oblique sagittal image through the right ventricular outflow tract (RVOT) post percutaneous pulmonary valve implantation (PPVI). In the balanced-SSFP image (diastolic frame, a), the signal artifact secondary to the stent can be seen. In the 'black-blood' spin echo image in the same subject (b), the stent is seen to be widely patent. The arrows identify the extent of the stent. (c) Coronal maximum-intensity projection image from a contrast-enhanced MR angiogram in a subject with an aortic stent (re-coarctation treatment). The appearances are of aortic interruption! (d) 'Black-blood' spin echo images in the same patient as (c), showing a patent stent. The arrowheads identify the extent of the stent.

(secondary to turbulent flow), which can lead to overestimation of narrowings. This is less so with balanced SSFP sequences, which are partially flow-compensated, but care in interpretation is necessary when imaging high-velocity blood flow.

Gadolinium contrast-enhanced MR angiography

Gadolinium contrast-enhanced MRA relies on the T1 shortening effect of dilute gadolinium and has been shown to be useful in delineating thoracic vascular anatomy.[16] A 3D dataset is acquired at the peak of the gadolinium bolus. Timing of the image acquisition is crucial, as most currently available gadolinium contrast agents are first-pass chelates. Sequence design ensures that tissues without gadolinium enhancement are suppressed, leaving contrast-enhanced vessels prominent. Contrast-enhanced MRA images are acquired in a single breath-hold, and have been demonstrated to be accurate at identifying stenotic vessels even in the neonatal population.[17]

The ability of MRI to acquire 3D datasets enables reconstruction of the heart, and in particular the great vessels, in 3D using a number of visualization algorithms (e.g. maximum-intensity projections (MIP) or volume and surface rendering). These 3D reconstructions are more easily interpreted than multiple stacks of 2D images, enabling easier communication of the information between imagers and clinicians (Figure 3.2).[18,19]

The major drawback of contrast-enhanced MRA is that it is usually performed without cardiac synchronization. This has two effects. Firstly, image blurring due to cardiac motion reduces the ability of this technique to visualize intracardiac anatomy.[20] Secondly, the size of the vessel represents an average size over the cardiac cycle. This can lead to underestimation of the maximum systolic dimension of a vessel, which may be crucial for PPVI sizing. For stenoses, data averaging over the cardiac cycle is less of an issue, as motion is less at sites of narrowing (reduced distensibility). A further disadvantage of gadolinium-enhanced MRA is that in the presence of fast-moving turbulent blood, signal dropout can occur, leading to overestimation of stenoses.

Three-dimensional 'white-blood' imaging

One potential method to overcome the disadvantage of lack of cardiac synchronization in MRA, while maintaining the 3D nature of the acquired dataset, is to use a new 3D balanced-SSFP technique.[19,20] With this sequence, axial balanced-SSFP ('white-blood') slices are acquired in multiple 3D chunks over several breath-holds. The entire dataset is then summed to give complete coverage of the heart and great vessels, with near-isotropic resolution (1.0 mm $\times$ 1.0 mm $\times$ 1.3 mm). The simplicity of the technique enables image acquisition to be performed without expert planning. The improved contrast and resolution of the balanced-SSFP technique allows simpler volume rendering based on thresholding techniques. In addition, the almost isotropic dataset allows accurate multiplanar reformatting, which is particularly useful for delineating the complex anatomy of congenital heart disease. Thus, image data can be assessed using slice-by-slice examination, multiplanar reformatting, and 3D reconstruction of the entire cardiac and great vessel volume.

The acquisition is ECG-gated, with a current temporal resolution of 40–80 ms, and it is possible to acquire multiple phases of the cardiac cycle (currently about 10 frames), enabling 4D dataset reconstruction.[21] Thus, theoretically, a 3D reconstruction of the RVOT/pulmonary trunk over multiple phases of the cardiac cycle can be acquired.

Pulmonary valve and homograft function

RVOT and pulmonary valve MRI planes

The imaging planes for the RVOT and assessment of pulmonary flow are outlined in Figure 3.3.[22] The RVOT is visualized by aligning a plane that passes through the pulmonary trunk/conduit and the RV inferiorly from a set of axial images (Figure 3.3a,b). An alternative way to obtain the RVOT view is by aligning a plane that passes through the pulmonary trunk/conduit and descending aorta. This is usually a sagittal, or oblique sagittal plane. A plane perpendicular to

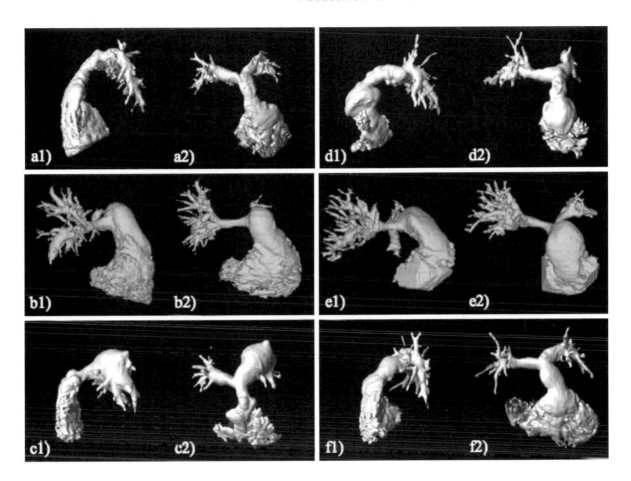

Figure 3.2

Three-dimensional volume-rendered reconstructions of the RVOT in a selection of six subjects: images acquired with contrast-enhanced MR angiography. The reconstructions are viewed from lateral (1) or anterior (2). Note the varying morphologies. Subjects (a), (c), (d), and (f) all underwent successful PPVI. In subjects (b) and (e), marked dilatation of the RVOT and pulmonary trunk was a contraindication to PPVI; surgical repair was performed in these two subjects. Note also the marked left pulmonary artery dilatation in subject (c), and the marked RVOT patch aneurysm in subject (d).

this, in an axial or oblique axial orientation, will give a second view through the RVOT (Figure 3.3d). A plane through the pulmonary trunk/conduit, just above the pulmonary valve, perpendicular to both RVOT views, can be used to assess through-plane pulmonary flow. This plane is used when quantifying pulmonary incompetence (Figure 3.3e).

Pulmonary incompetence

Currently none of the conventional imaging techniques can accurately define valvular regurgitation, and it is here that MRI has particular value. Cardiovascular MR can image the regurgitant jet in any plane, and thus a 3D appreciation of the jet can be acquired. Furthermore, MRI can quantify

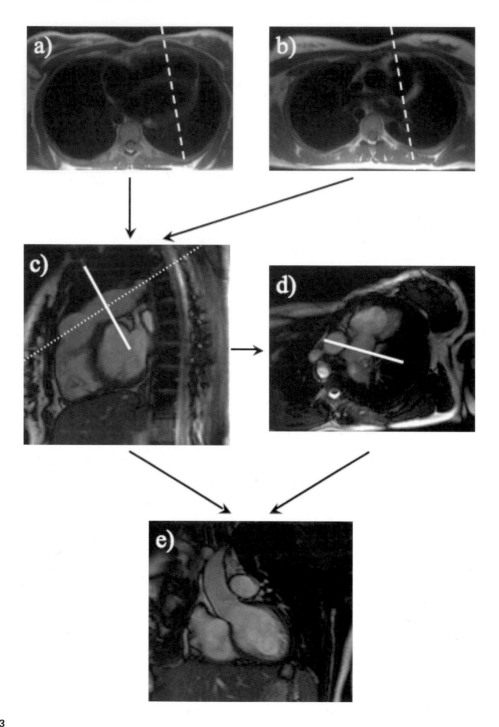

Figure 3.3

Imaging planes for the RVOT. The first RVOT view (c) is prescribed as an oblique plane through the main pulmonary artery and RV on a set of axial images (a, b: dashed lines). The second RVOT plane (d) is prescribed perpendicular to the first RVOT view (c: dotted line). The imaging plane for pulmonary flow assessment (e) is aligned perpendicular to both RVOT views (c, d: solid lines). The imaging plane should be placed just above the pulmonary valve if visible.

the regurgitant volume, either as an absolute value or as the regurgitant fraction. Such a non-invasive quantification of the degree of valvular regurgitation, in combination with information about ventricular function, is of particular clinical relevance for the timing of valve replacement. MR assessment of valvular regurgitation severity can be evaluated using the following techniques:

- qualitative assessment of signal loss on gradient echo MRI
- quantitative assessment by measurement of ventricular volumes
- quantitative assessment by phase-contrast velocity mapping.

In gradient echo cine imaging, dephasing of the proton spins, secondary to turbulent flow, leads to signal loss.[23] Imaging over multiple frames (20–40) enables accurate assessment of the turbulent flow, throughout the cardiac cycle. For regurgitant lesions the signal loss can be graded in a similar way to X-ray angiography: grade 1 = signal loss close to the valve; grade 2 = signal loss extending into the proximal chamber; grade 3 = signal loss filling the whole of the proximal chamber; grade 4 = signal loss in the receiving chamber throughout the relevant half of the cardiac cycle.[24,25] This qualitative method has been validated, but is unable to separate turbulent jets when dual valve disease exists (e.g. aortic regurgitation and mitral stenosis), and there remains poor reproducibility of the technique between centers. In addition, signal loss is very dependent on MR parameters such as echo time (TE), and jet size is easily underestimated when it impinges on the myocardial wall, as has been known from echocardiography for some years.

With the increasing use of balanced-SSFP cine imaging in cardiovascular MR, qualitative assessment of signal loss has become less useful. As outlined above, balanced-SSFP 'white-blood' images are much quicker to acquire, with better endocardial/blood pool definition than conventional gradient echo imaging, but the sequence is designed to be relatively flow-insensitive. This results in reduced visualization of flow disturbance secondary to valvular regurgitation, in particular when regurgitation is mild. Thus, in subjects who are being imaged for other reasons, incidental detection of mild valvular regurgitation may not be apparent on balanced-SSFP cine imaging.

MRI can now be regarded as the best available in vivo technique for the measurement of ventricular volumes (see below).[3] In normal individuals, there is a one-to-one relationship between these stroke volumes. Any discrepancy between the ventricular stroke volumes in a patient with regurgitation will identify the regurgitant volume. The main limitation of this technique, when used alone, is that only patients with a single regurgitant valve can be assessed.

The most accurate quantitative method for assessing great vessel blood flow is to use MR phase-contrast velocity mapping. For velocity mapping, phase information and not magnitude information is displayed. Each point in the imaging plane is encoded with a phase shift that is directly proportional to the velocity at that point.[26,27] Velocity encoding can be applied in any direction (through plane, left-to-right, up-and-down), although for flow quantification, through-plane imaging is used. Stationary material is represented as mid-gray, while increasing velocities in either direction are shown in increasing grades of black or white (Figure 3.4b,c). It is important to define the velocity encode window as close to the peak velocity as possible, to reduce aliasing of peak velocities, while maintaining sensitivity for flow measurements.

Measurement of the spatial mean velocity for all pixels in a region of interest of known area enables the calculation of the instantaneous flow volume at any point in the cardiac cycle. Calculation of the flow volume per heart beat can be made by integrating the instantaneous flow volumes for all frames throughout the cardiac cycle (area under the curve; Figure 3.4d). The pulmonary regurgitant fraction (RF) is given by:

$$RF\ (\%) = \frac{\text{pulmonary retrograde flow (ml/beat)}}{\text{pulmonary forward flow (ml/beat)}} \times 100$$

This technique has been validated in vitro and in vivo, and is extremely accurate and reproducible.[28–30] It now represents the best available in vivo technique for flow measurements. The severity of regurgitation can be defined as follows:[31]

- mild: regurgitant fraction 15–20%
- moderate: regurgitant fraction 20–40%
- severe: regurgitant fraction >40%.

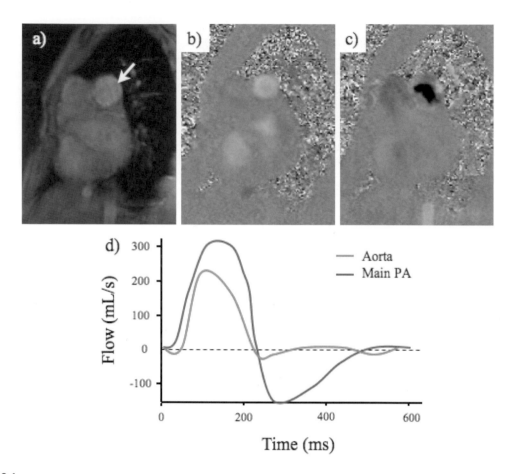

Figure 3.4

MR phase-contrast velocity mapping (TE = 5 ms, velocity encoding window = ± 2.5 m/s). (a) Magnitude image through the pulmonary trunk (arrow; see Figure 3.3 for positioning). (b, c) Velocity image in the same imaging plane during systole (b) and diastole (c). Stationary material is represented as mid-gray while flow towards the lungs is represented by white pixels, and regurgitant flow back into the RV is represented by black pixels. (d) Plot of flow volume versus time. Each point on the graphs represents the blood flow in the pulmonary trunk for each frame of the cardiac cycle. Negative values represent retrograde flow during diastole. Integration of the area under the curve for antegrade and retrograde flow enables calculation of the regurgitant volume per cardiac cycle (ml/beat).

Conventionally, phase-contrast gradient echo images are acquired during shallow respiration over several minutes. Faster imaging can be performed, and it is now possible to acquire real-time phase-contrast data.[32]

Pulmonary valvular or conduit stenosis

The presence of valvular stenosis can be identified by signal loss seen in gradient echo cine images. Velocity mapping may then be used to

establish an accurate peak velocity across the valve to quantify the severity of the stenosis.

Direct measurement from the phase-contrast velocity map enables the measurement of the peak velocity across the valve, and application of the modified Bernoulli equation,

$$\Delta P = 4V^2$$

where *P* is the pressure drop across the stenosis (in mmHg) and *V* is the velocity (in m/s), enables an estimate of the gradient across the valve. The technique is comparable to Doppler echocardiography valvular stenosis measurements and has an in vitro accuracy of 4%.[33] The main advantage of the technique over echocardiography is that the velocity jet can be easily aligned in any direction without the limitation of acoustic windows.

Imaging can be performed through-plane (velocity jet perpendicular to the imaging plane) or in-plane (velocity jet parallel to the imaging plane).[34,35] Both strategies, have their advantages and disadvantages. It is thus best to use a combination of the two strategies, with initial definition of the jet in-plane and quantification with through-plane imaging at the site of maximum velocity on the in-plane image. Selection of the correct velocity encode gradient is essential to maintain sensitivity and accuracy of measurements, while avoiding aliasing. Most scanners now have a fast phase-contrast velocity mapping sequence that can be acquired in approximately 15–20 s. This enables an estimate of the peak velocity to be made before progressing to the more time-consuming conventional phase-contrast velocity mapping sequence.

Right ventricular function

Multislice 2D gradient echo imaging represents the best available in vivo test for ventricular volumetry, as it is not reliant on complex geometric models. The technique has been extensively validated for the assessment of the left ventricle (LV).[36–38] Currently, ventricular function is assessed using balanced-SSFP sequences, which have the benefit of good blood pool/myocardial contrast and relatively fast acquisition times.[39] Although balanced-SSFP sequences allow high-spatiotemporal-resolution imaging of the ventricles, they do require multiple breath-holds. Patients with cardiac disease, in particular children, may not tolerate this. In such cases, the use of respiratory monitoring (respiratory bellows or navigator echoes) may obviate the need for breath-holds, although acquisition times increase significantly. In children less than 8 years of age, general anesthesia can be used to guarantee no patient movement and to allow multiple scans during respiratory suppression.

Accurate quantification of RV volumes, function, and mass is important in the assessment of

the consequence of pulmonary valve disease, congenital heart disease, arrhythmogenic RV dysplasia, and pulmonary hypertension.[40–45] The complex geometry of the RV means that MR volumetric quantification techniques are even more important than for the LV.[46] The value of echocardiography and other imaging techniques that use geometric assumptions to estimate RV function and ejection fraction is limited. Furthermore, due to its complexity, no single imaging plane is well suited for imaging the RV. The short-axis imaging plane used to study the LV, although not ideal, is probably the best method for analyzing the RV (according to the author's personal experience of comparing RV stroke volume calculations with pulmonary artery flow quantification in over 300 children and adults with congenital heart disease) (Figure 3.5). On short-axis images, the interface between right ventricle and right atrium can be difficult to assess, and other strategies such as axial or RV inflow views have been suggested, but these suffer from problems of partial-volume effects of the most inferior slice.[47]

Despite the more complex geometry, the more trabeculated nature, and difficulties of imaging plane analysis, compared with the LV, normal RV volumes, function, and mass can be accurately and reproducibly quantified (Table 3.2).

Stress MRI

Stress MRI can be performed either with exercise (specifically designed MR bicycle) or with dobutamine administration. Dobutamine stress MRI is used to assess LV regional wall motion in subjects with ischemic heart disease. Several large studies have demonstrated the safe application of dobutamine stress MRI.[53] Incremental dobutamine administration enables the definition of regions of the LV that are supplied by significantly stenosed epicardial coronary arteries, or those areas of myocardium that may be hibernating, and recruitable at revascularization. For the right heart, exercise and dobutamine stress have been used as means of assessing global RV function in response to increased workload. An abnormal RV response to stress (either physiologic[54] or pharmacologic[55]) has been demonstrated in patients with tetralogy of Fallot and pulmonary incompetence. In normal subjects, RV ejection fraction

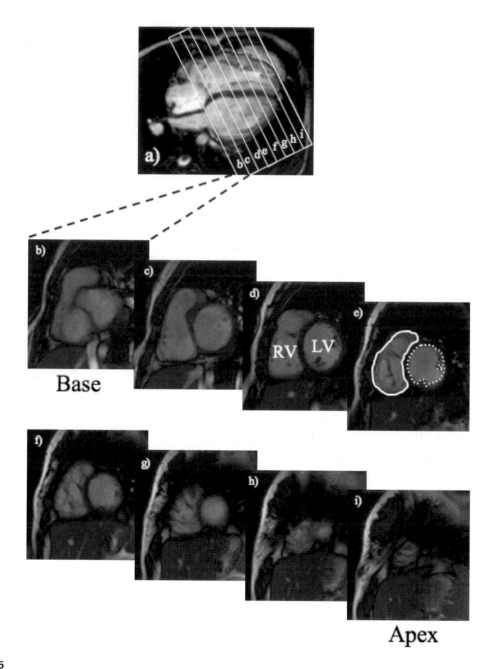

Figure 3.5

Schematic diagram for calculation of right and left ventricular volumes and function. (a) The ventricle is divided into multiple short-axis slices of approximately 6–10 mm thickness, from the atrioventricular valves to the apex on a four-chamber view. Note the dilated RV in this subject. (b–i) Short-axis images from the base to the apex. The volume for each slice (in ml) is given by the area (see e), multiplied by the known slice thickness. These are measured at end-diastole and end-systole. The end-diastolic volume (EDV) and end-systolic volume (ESV) are the sums of all the slice volumes for each ventricle at each respective time point in the cardiac cycle (ml/beat). The stroke volume (SV) = EDV − ESV, the ejection fraction (EF%) = (SV × 100) / EDV, and the cardiac output = SV × heart rate. Mass can also be calculated for each slice by subtracting the endocardial area from the epicardial area (not shown). The sum of these areas is then multiplied by the density of myocardium (1.05 kg/l) to give a measurement in grams.

Table 3.2 RV volumes, function, and mass values in normal adult and pediatric populations, obtained with MRI (values in parentheses are corrected for body surface area)

Study	Number gender	EDV (ml and (ml/m²)	ESV (ml and (ml/m²)	SV (ml and (ml/m²)	EF (%)	Mass (g and g/m²)	CO l/min and l/min/m²
Lorenz et al[48]	47 M	157 (80)	63	95 (48)	60	50 (26)	—
	28 F	106 (67)	40	66 (42)	63	40 (25)	—
Sandstede et al[49]	36	115 (62)	43 (23)	—	64	45 (24)	5.2 (2.8)
Hoeper et al[45]	6	120	47	73	61	44	—
Jauhiainen et al[47]	12	120 (67)	57 (32)	63 (35)	53	38 (26)	—
Alfakih et al[50]	30 M	176	79	98	55	—	—
	30 F	131	52	78	60	—	—
Pediatric							
Helbing et al[51]	22	92 (70)	27 (21)	63 (48)	70	—	—
Lorenz [52]	8	(70)	—	(43)	—	—	(3.2)

EDV, end-diastolic volume; ESV, end-systolic volume; SV, stroke volume; EF, ejection fraction; CO, cardiac output.

increases during stress, while in patients with tetralogy of Fallot, RV function remains unchanged or is reduced during stress.

The responses of subjects with chronic pulmonary incompetence to stress may be able to provide important prognostic indictors to help with the timing of pulmonary valve replacement in this patient population. Further, long-term studies are needed to address these issues.

Pulmonary stenosis/ incompetence: current MRI literature

Late pulmonary incompetence remains an important clinical issue for many patients who have undergone surgery in early childhood for congenital heart disease, whether after augmentation of RV outflow (tetralogy of Fallot repair) or after insertion of an RV-to-pulmonary artery conduit.[56,57]

Initially, pulmonary incompetence was believed to be a relatively benign condition, with few problems associated with RV volume loading.[58,59] However, it has become clear that chronic pulmonary incompetence and RV volume loading can cause RV dysfunction, which can in turn lead to symptoms of reduced exercise tolerance,[60] and increased risk of ventricular tachyarryth-

mias[61] and sudden death.[62,63] This has led to an increasing proportion of patients requiring operative replacement of the incompetent and/or stenosed pulmonary valves and conduits.[64–66]

Surgical repair is currently used to manage symptomatic patients with pulmonary incompetence and/or pulmonary conduit stenosis. Operation is a balance between the operative risk of the procedure,[67] the finite life span of any conduit inserted (about 10 years), and the risk of irreversible RV dysfunction if surgery is performed too late. Some investigators have suggested that RV dysfunction does not improve after operative repair and that treatment is being performed too late.[68]

The accurate quantification of pulmonary incompetence and its effects on the RV with cardiovascular MR should help define the natural history of this condition and the response to treatment.[69–71] Ultimately, this may enable the definition of parameters that can be used to optimize treatment interventions.

Current data from cardiovascular MR assessment of patients with severe pulmonary incompetence have demonstrated elevated RV end-diastolic and end-systolic volumes and reduced RV ejection fraction.[54,55,72] Furthermore, there is increasing evidence that RV function may be irreversibly compromised by such long-term changes.[68] This is exemplified by three findings that have been demonstrated by cardiovascular MR. Firstly, RV ejection fraction has been shown to be significantly lower in patients with both RV pressure and volume overload as compared with RV pressure overload alone.[55] Secondly, an abnormal RV response to stress (either physiologic[54] or pharmacologic[55]) has been demonstrated in patients with tetralogy of Fallot and pulmonary incompetence (as outlined above). And finally, there appears to be no or limited improvement in RV function (ejection fraction at rest) following pulmonary valve replacement.[68,72]

The advent of PPVI[73,74] now provides us with the unique opportunity to study the response of the RV to acute volume and pressure unloading without the confounding effect of cardiopulmonary bypass.

MR assessment pre and post percutaneous pulmonary valve implantation

We have performed PPVI in 66 cases over the last 4 years. This procedure has the potential to overcome many of the disadvantages of surgical valve replacement. In half of these subjects, MRI has been performed before and after PPVI.

MR assessment pre pulmonary valve stent implantation

An MRI protocol for assessing suitability for PPVI is outlined in Table 3.3. The most important current limitation for PPVI is size. If the RVOT/ pulmonary trunk or conduit is too large (the current upper limit of PPVI dimension is 22 mm), then PPVI should not be attempted, as there will be a high risk of stent displacement. This assessment of size is difficult on echocardiography, and cardiovascular MR can be used to avoid diagnostic cardiac catheterization in a number of patients. MR assessment of the RVOT/pulmonary trunk dimensions is best made on the two perpendicular RVOT cine images (Figure 3.3c,d), as it is the maximum (systolic) diameter that is most important. Using only the 'black-blood' spin echo (usually acquired in mid to late diastole) or

the MRA images (non-gated image acquisition), an underestimation of the maximum size of the RVOT/pulmonary trunk may be made. This is particularly true for native tissue that has been treated with transannular patching, which can be extremely dynamic, and can change dimension considerably during the cardiac cycle. Dynamic changes are less pronounced in conduits, but can still be significant and preclude PPVI. If the maximum diameter of the RVOT/pulmonary trunk or conduit is at the upper limit of normal, PPVI may be attempted, but with the use of an accurate sizing balloon prior to actual implantation.

If the RVOT/pulmonary trunk or conduit diameter is too narrow, with marked conduit thickening, PPVI may not be possible, as the dimensions may be too small to enable the implanted pulmonary valve to open, paradoxically worsening the degree of narrowing following PPVI. The minimum diameter at which we have attempted PPVI is 6 mm. In this case, pre-dilatation of the conduit was performed prior to PPVI.

The pre-PPVI MRI is also used to quantify the degree of pulmonary incompetence, the gradient across any stenoses, the RV and LV dimensions and function, the presence of distal pulmonary artery stenoses, and other cardiovascular problems (aortic incompetence, aortic root dilatation, aortic coarctation, airway narrowing, etc.). The complete MRI protocol can be performed in approximately 1 hour.

To date, the majority of patients we have studied for PPVI have been symptomatic, and treatment has been deemed necessary on clinical grounds. In the future, MRI may be able to help select asymptomatic patients, in whom future RV dysfunction may occur, for optimal timing of PPVI or surgical treatment. The amount of pulmonary incompetence and RV dilatation will probably be important factors, but as yet no long-term studies have defined cutoff points for these measurements.

MR assessment post pulmonary valve stent implantation

In our own practice, post-PPVI MRI is performed as part of a research study. The protocol for MRI following PPVI is as for the pre-PPVI assessment, with the exception that MRA is not performed, due to the stent artifact (Figure 3.1c,d). 'Black-

Table 3.3   Prepercutaneous pulmonary valve implantation (PPVI) MRI protocol

Imaging sequence	What to look for
Scouts and reference scans: • Localizers in 3 planes • Parallel imaging reference scans • Rapid axial scout images	• Assess other structures
2D balanced-SSFP cine imaging: • Vertical long axis • 4-chamber view • RVOT in 2 perpendicular planes • LVOT in 2 perpendicular planes	• Assess LV function • Assess RV function, RV/LV interaction (paradoxical septal motion), tricuspid incompetence • Assess stenoses, pulmonary incompetence, RVOT aneurysmal dilatation, pulmonary trunk dimensions, suitability for PPVI? • Assess aortic valve, VSD patch
2D multislice balanced-SSFP cine imaging: • Short-axis planes (10–12 slices to cover both ventricles)	• Assess RV and LV dimensions and function, define severity of RV dilatation
2D 'black-blood' spin echo imaging: • RVOT in 2 perpendicular planes • Branch pulmonary arteries	• Assess stenoses, pulmonary trunk dimensions • Assess branch pulmonary stenoses, bronchial compression
Phase-contrast velocity mapping: • Pulmonary trunk through plane • Aortic root through plane • Vascular stenosis in plane	• Assess pulmonary regurgitant fraction, peak velocity across stenoses • Assess aortic valve function
3D contrast-enhanced MRA of right heart and pulmonary vasculature	• Assess 3D geometry of the RVOT, pulmonary trunk/conduit and branch pulmonary arteries, suitability for PPVI? If there is doubt about maximum dimensions, rely on the maximum dimension on the RVOT cine images

RVOT, right ventricular outflow tract; LVOT, left ventricular outflow tract; LV, left ventricle, RV, right ventricle, VSD, ventricular septal defect.

blood' spin echo imaging across the valve stent is the most useful sequence, as this allows the patency of the PPVI to be defined (Figures 3.1d; 3.6a,b). Pulmonary flow measurements are performed to confirm that the pulmonary valve functions properly (no pulmonary incompetence) and to define any residual peak velocity across the PPVI. The plane for the pulmonary flow measurements is positioned at the distal end of the PPVI to avoid stent artifact (Figure 3.6c,d). Assessment of ventricular indices is also performed to establish the acute affects of PPVI.

Functional response to pulmonary valve stent implantation

We have now performed MR studies in 33 subjects with pulmonary stenosis/incompetence (age 19 ± 8 years) prior to (median 6 days) and soon after (median 6 days) PPVI. All of these subjects had New York Heart Association (NYHA) assessment of symptoms, and a subset of 17 subjects underwent metabolic exercise testing on the same day as MRI. Following PPVI insertion, there were significant reductions in the gradient across

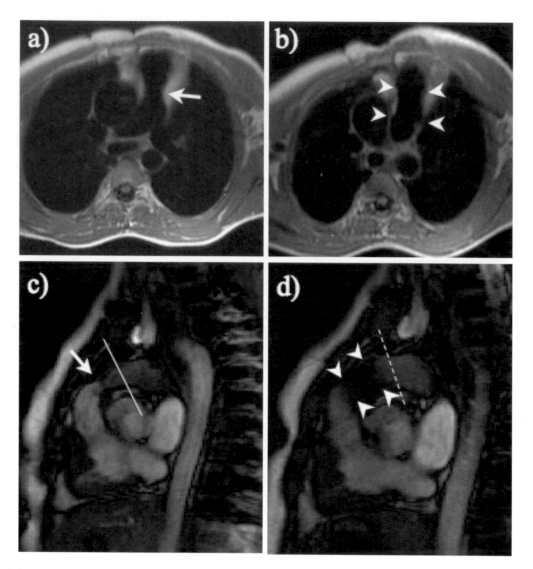

Figure 3.6

(a, b) Axial 'black-blood' spin echo images of the RVOT pre (a) and post (b) PPVI. The narrowing in image (a) (arrow) has been relieved by the PPVI, the extent of which is delineated by the arrowheads in (b). (c, d) Oblique sagittal balanced-SSFP images of the RVOT pre (c) and post (d) PPVI. The tight narrowing in (c) (arrow) appears to have been relieved by the PPVI, the extent of which is delineated by the arrowheads in (d). The internal structure of the stent cannot be seen on balanced-SSFP images due to the prominence of image artifact on this sequence. 'Black-blood' imaging in this subject revealed a widely patent stent (see Figure 3.1b). The dashed and dotted lines on (c) and (d) represent the slice position for pulmonary flow assessment. Note that this position is more distal post PPVI, to avoid stent artifact in the flow measurement.

the pulmonary trunk, pulmonary regurgitant fraction (21 ± 13 vs $3 \pm 4\%$; $p < 0.001$), and RV end-diastolic volume (EDV) ($p < 0.001$), and significant increases in LV EDV ($p < 0.01$) and effective stroke volume ($p < 0.05$). These changes in measurable MR parameters were associated with significant improvements in subjective patient symptoms (NYHA classification 2 vs 1; $p < 0.001$), and metabolic exercise capacity (VO_{2max}; $p < 0.001$) (Figure 3.7).

(a)

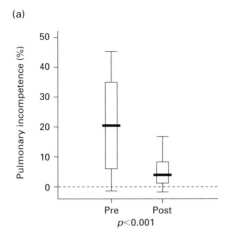

(b)

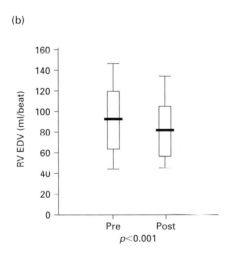

(c)

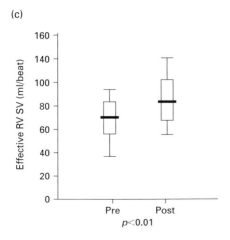

(d)

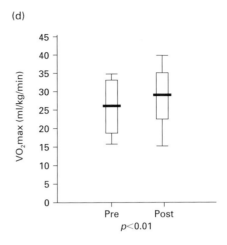

(e)

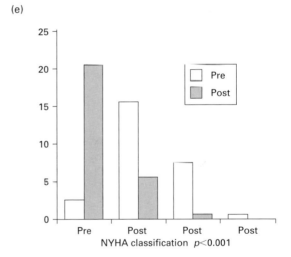

Figure 3.7

Box plots (bold line, mean; box, ± SD; upper/lower limits, maximum/minimum for (a) pulmonary regurgitant fraction, (b) right ventricular (RV) end-diastolic volume (EDV), (c) effective RV stroke volume (SV), and (d) maximal oxygen consumption (VO_{2max}), pre and post PPVI. (e) Numbers of subjects divided according to NYHA classification of symptoms pre and post PPVI. An improvement in the numbers in each category is clearly seen.

There are two possible mechanisms for the improvements in the subject's symptoms following PPVI. Firstly, the increased effective RV stroke volume may lead to an increased pulmonary venous return, increased left atrial filling and LV preload, and hence improved LV filling and LV stroke volume. Secondly, there may be a degree of LV/RV diastolic interaction. The reduction in RV EDV, following reduced pulmonary incompetence, permits an increase in LV filling, and thus LV EDV (as we have observed). This occurs within the constraints of the pericardial space, and, by the Frank–Starling mechanism, results in an increase in stroke volume.

Further long-term follow-up of these subjects will be essential to evaluate the potential for ventricular remodeling and sustained symptomatic relief. We plan to monitor these patients with MRI and functional assessment of exercise capacity in serial studies. Further data collection will allow us to interrogate subsets of patients to elucidate the contribution of RVOT stenosis and incompetence relief to the observed hemodynamics and clinical improvement, refine patient selection for treatment, and optimize timing of PPVI.

Computed tomography

Conventional CT imaging has been used less often in the assessment of congenital heart disease, due to the inability to perform imaging in any plane, the lack of 3D reformatting capabilities, the prolonged imaging time, and the high radiation dose. The development of spiral[75,76] and subsequently multidetector CT (MDCT)[77,78] has overcome many of these issues, so that a volume of data with near-isotropic image resolution can now be acquired over a short period of time (seconds as opposed to minutes). This enables the acquisition of data during a single breath-hold and during the first pass of a contrast bolus, so that images can be reconstructed in any 2D plane or in 3D.

A major advantage of the recent advances in CT technology (16-slice and soon 64-slice MDCT) over MR is the very rapid acquisition time. Imaging can now be performed in a comfortable single breath-hold at the peak of the contrast bolus, reducing the need for general anesthesia and sedation even in very young subjects.[79] Furthermore, MR cannot be used in subjects with

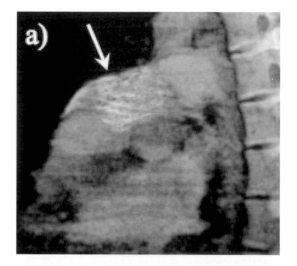

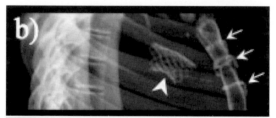

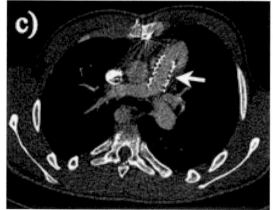

Figure 3.8

(a) Three-dimensional volume-rendered contrast-enhanced multidetector computed tomography (MDCT) viewed from left lateral. There is a percutaneous pulmonary valve stent in situ in the pulmonary trunk (arrow). (b) Pre-contrast 3D volume-rendered MDCT viewed from right lateral. A pulmonary trunk stent is shown (arrowhead). Sternal wires are also clearly seen (arrows). (c) Axial slice from the post-contrast MDCT in the same subject as (b). The pulmonary stent was inserted for conduit stenosis, but led to marked pulmonary incompetence. The stent is widely patent, but the dimensions are sufficient to allow for PPVI, to provide a competence pulmonary valve.

pacemakers, and can be of limited value in subjects with surgical clips and vascular stents, where artifacts may obscure anatomic details. Such constraints do not limit MDCT (Figure 3.8).

There are however, two main disadvantages of MDCT compared with MRI. The first is the risk of future tumorigenesis from exposure to ionizing radiation.[80,81] For individual patients, this can be kept to a minimum by using low-kV, low-mAs acquisitions, with current modulation, and image acquisition over the minimal area of interest.[79] However, for the patient population who will be considered for PPVI, follow-up will be lifelong and the cumulative radiation dose will be high if multiple CT scans are performed. The second disadvantage of current MDCT techniques is that easy quantification of cardiac function (at high heart rates) and arterial flow are not possible compared with cardiac-gated MRI.

To date, we have used CT in only two subjects. The first was performed post PPVI to exclude a peristent leak (Figure 3.8a), and the second in a patient with conduit stenosis treated with previous percutaneous stenting. This latter patient had been left with free pulmonary incompetence, and sizing of the stent was necessary prior to PPVI. The stent size was suitable for PPVI (Figure 3.8b,c). Other indications for cardiovascular CT would include patients with contraindications to MR (permanent pacemaker, intracranial aneurysm clips, etc.) and young subjects in whom general anesthesia for MR is not warranted (CT is performed under sedation).

Conclusion

The recent improvement in non-invasive cross-sectional cardiovascular imaging modalities (MR and CT) has resulted in a change in our approach to the definition of anatomy and physiology in subjects with congenital and acquired heart disease. The precise role of these imaging modalities in assessment of the right heart, pulmonary valve, and pulmonary arteries will evolve over time.

For planning intervention to the RVOT and pulmonary trunk/conduit for stenosis or incompetence, with either transcatheter techniques or surgery, cardiovascular MRI can be used to define intracardiac and great vessel anatomy, and ventricular and valvular function. This approach

reduces the need for diagnostic cardiac catheterization and can provide important data for clinical decision-making. Cardiovascular CT is currently less commonly used due to issues of radiation exposure in a group of patients who will need lifelong follow-up of their clinical condition.

In patients with pulmonary stenosis/incompetence, the optimal timing of intervention remains controversial, and is a balance between the risk of the procedure, the finite life span of any valve or conduit inserted, and the risk of irreversible RV dysfunction if reintervention is performed too late. Although randomized control studies have not been performed, further MR data collection should enable refinement of patient selection for treatment (PPVI vs surgery), and optimize timing of intervention.

Acknowledgments

I would like to acknowledge the following for their help and support with cardiovascular MR. From Great Ormond Street Hospital for Children, London, UK: Professor John Deanfield and Professor Philipp Bonhoeffer of the Cardiothoracic Unit; Dr Cathy Owens, Rod Jones, Wendy Norman, and Clare Thompson of the Department of Radiology; and Dr Angus McEwan of the Anesthetic Department. From the MR Unit, Guy's Hospital, London, UK: Dr Reza Razavi, Dr Vivek Muthurangu, and Dr Sanjeet Hegde.

References

1. Bogaert J, Dymarkowski S, Taylor AM. In: Bogaert J, Dymarkowski S, Taylor AM (eds). Clinical Cardiac MRI. Heidelberg: Springer-Verlag, 2005: 1–549.
2. Anderson RH, Razavi R, Taylor AM. Cardiac anatomy revisited. J Anat 2004; 205: 159–77.
3. Bogaert J. Cardiac function. In: Bogaert J, Dymarkowski S, Taylor AM (eds). Clinical Cardiac MRI. Heidelberg: Springer-Verlag, 2005: 99–141.
4. Mohiaddin RH, Pennell DJ. MR blood flow measurement: clinical applications in the heart and circulation. Cardiol Clin 1998; 16: 161–87.
5. Higgins CB, Byrd BF 3rd, Farmer DW, et al. Magnetic resonance imaging in patients with congenital heart disease. Circulation 1984; 70: 851–60.
6. Fletcher BD, Jacobstein MD, Nelson AD, et al. Gated magnetic resonance imaging of congenital cardiac malformations. Radiology 1984; 150: 137–40.

7. Carr JC, Finn JP. MR imaging of the thoracic aorta. Magn Reson Imaging Clin N Am 2003; 11: 135–48.
8. Greenberg SB, Crisci KL, Koenig P, et al. Magnetic resonance imaging compared with echocardiography in the evaluation of pulmonary artery abnormalities in children with tetralogy of Fallot following palliative and corrective surgery. Pediatr Radiol 1997; 27: 932–5.
9. Martinez JE, Mohiaddin RH, Kilner PJ, et al. Obstruction in extracardiac ventriculopulmonary conduits: value of nuclear magnetic resonance imaging with velocity mapping and Doppler echocardiography. J Am Coll Cardiol 1992; 20: 338–44.
10. Sampson C, Kilner PJ, Hirsch R, et al. Venoatrial pathways after the Mustard operation for transposition of the great arteries: anatomic and functional MR imaging. Radiology 1994; 193: 211–17.
11. Shellock FG, Shellock VJ. Metallic stents: evaluation of MR imaging safety. AJR Am J Roentgenol 1999; 173: 543–7.
12. Zur Y, Wood ML, Neuringer LJ, Motion-insensitive, steady-state free precession imaging. Magn Reson Med 1990; 16: 444–59.
13. Pereles FS, Kapoor V, Carr JC, et al. Usefulness of segmented TrueFISP cardiac pulse sequence in evaluation of congenital and acquired adult cardiac abnormalities, AJR Am J Roentgenol 2001; 177: 1155–60.
14. Barkhausen J, Ruehm SG, Goyen M, et al. MR evaluation of ventricular function: true fast imaging with steady-state precession versus fast low-angle shot cine MR imaging: feasibility study, Radiology 2001; 219: 264–9.
15. Razavi R, Muthurangu V, Hegde SR, et al. Magnetic resonance imaging assessment of percutaneous pulmonary valve-stent implantation. J Cardiovasc Magn Reson 2004; 6: 249 (abst).
16. Prince MR, Grist TM, Debatin JF. 3D contrast MR angiography. Berlin: Springer-Verlag, 1977.
17. Taylor AM, Muthurangu V, Hegde SR, et al. Magnetic resonance imaging for hypoplastic left heart syndrome following the Norwood stage 1 operation. J Cardiovasc Magn Reson 2004; 6: 407 (abst).
18. Razavi R, Hill DLG, Miquel ME, et al. Three-dimensional intracardiac imaging of congenital heart disease. Cardiol Young 2003; 13: 1–5.
19. Sorensen TS, Korperich H, Greil GF, et al. Operator-independent isotropic three-dimensional magnetic resonance imaging for morphology in congenital heart disease: a validation study. Circulation 2004; 110: 163–9.
20. Razavi RS, Hill DL, Muthurangu V, et al. Three-dimensional magnetic resonance imaging of congenital cardiac anomalies. Cardiol Young 2003; 13: 461–5.
21. Miquel ME, Hill DL, Baker EJ, et al. Three- and four-dimensional reconstruction of intra-cardiac anatomy from two-dimensional magnetic resonance images. Int J Cardiovasc Imaging 2003; 19: 239–54.
22. Taylor AM, Bogaert J. Cardiovascular MR imaging planes and segmentation. In: Bogaert J, Dymarkowski S, Taylor AM (eds). Clinical Cardiac MRI. Heidelberg: Springer-Verlag, 2005: 85–98.
23. Evans AJ, Blinder RA, Herfkens RJ, et al. Effects of turbulence on signal intensity in gradient echo images. Invest Radiol 1988; 23: 512–18.
24. Underwood SR, Firmin DN, Mohiaddin RH, et al. Cine magnetic resonance imaging of valvular heart disease. Proc Soc Magn Reson Imaging 1987; 2: 723 (abst).
25. Sechtem U, Pflugfelder PW, White RD, et al. Cine MR imaging: potential for the evaluation of cardiovascular function. AJR Am J Roentgenol 1987; 148: 239–46.
26. Nayler GL, Firmin DN, Longmore DB. Blood flow imaging by cine magnetic resonance. J Comput Assist Tomogr 1986; 10: 715–22.
27. Underwood SR, Firmin DN, Klipstein RH, et al. Magnetic resonance velocity mapping: clinical application of a new technique. Br Heart J 1987; 57: 404–12.
28. Firmin DN, Nayler GL, Klipstein RH, et al. In vivo validation of MR velocity imaging. J Comput Assist Tomogr 1987; 11: 751–6.
29. Meier D, Maier S, Boesiger P. Quantitative flow measurements on phantoms and on blood vessels with MR. Magn Reson Med 1988; 8: 25–34.
30. Bogren HG, Klipstein RH, Firmin DN, et al. Quantification of antegrade and retrograde blood flow in the human aorta by magnetic resonance velocity mapping. Am Heart J 1989; 117: 1214–22.
31. Sechtem U, Pflugfelder PW, Cassidy MM, et al. Mitral and aortic regurgitation: quantification of regurgitant volumes with cine MR imaging. Radiology 1988; 167: 425–30.
32. Korperich H, Gieseke J, Barth P, et al. Flow volume and shunt quantification in pediatric congenital heart disease by real-time magnetic resonance velocity mapping. A validation study. Circulation 2004; 109: 1987–93.
33. Simpson IA, Maciel BC, Moises V, et al. Cine magnetic resonance imaging and color Doppler flow mapping displays of flow velocity, spatial acceleration and jet formation: a comparative in vitro study. Am Heart J 1993; 126: 1165–74.
34. Kilner PJ, Firmin DN, Rees RSO, et al. Valve and great vessel stenosis: assessment with MR jet velocity mapping. Radiology 1991; 178: 229–35.
35. Kilner PJ, Manzara CC, Mohiaddin RH, et al. Magnetic resonance jet velocity mapping in mitral and aortic valve stenosis. Circulation 1993; 87: 1239–48.

36. Bellenger NG, Francis JM, Davies CL, et al. Establishment and performance of a magnetic resonance cardiac function clinic. J Cardiovasc Magn Reson 2000; 2: 15–22.

37. Bellenger NG, Davies LC, Francis JM, et al. Reduction in sample size for studies of remodeling in heart failure by the use of cardiovascular magnetic resonance. J Cardiovasc Magn Reson 2000; 2: 271–8.

38. Grothues F, Smith GC, Moon JC, et al. Comparison of interstudy reproducibility of cardiovascular magnetic resonance with two-dimensional echocardiography in normal subjects and in patients with heart failure or left ventricular hypertrophy. Am J Cardiol 2002; 90: 29–34.

39. Barkhausen J, Goyen M, Ruhm SG, et al. Assessment of ventricular function with single breath-hold real-time steady-state free precession cine MR imaging. AJR Am J Roentgenol 2002; 178: 731–5.

40. Katz J, Whang J, Boxt LM, et al. Estimation of right ventricular mass in normal subjects and in patients with primary pulmonary hypertension by nuclear magnetic resonance imaging. J Am Coll Cardiol 1993; 21: 1475–81.

41. Tardivon AA, Mousseaux E, Brenot F, et al. Quantification of hemodynamics in primary pulmonary hypertension with magnetic resonance imaging. Am J Respir Crit Care Med 1994; 150: 1075–80.

42. Casalino E, Laissy JP, Soyer P, et al. Assessment of right ventricle function and pulmonary artery circulation by cine MRI in patients with AIDS. Chest 1996; 110: 1243–7.

43. Marcus JT, Vonk Noordegraaf A, de Vries PM, et al. MRI evaluation of right ventricular pressure overload in chronic pulmonary disease. J Magn Reson Imaging 1998; 8: 999–1005.

44. Kroft LJM, Simons P, van Laar JM, de Roos A. Patients with pulmonary fibrosis: cardiac function assessed with MR imaging. Radiology 2000; 216: 464–71.

45. Hoeper MM, Tongers J, Leppert A, et al. Evaluation of right ventricular performance with a right ventricular ejection fraction thermodilution catheter and MRI in patients with pulmonary hypertension. Chest 2001; 102: 502–7.

46. Markiewicz W, Sechtem U, Higgins CB. Evaluation of the right ventricle by magnetic resonance imaging. Am Heart J 1987; 113: 8–15.

47. Jauhiainen T, Järvinen VM, Hekali PE. Evaluation of methods for MR imaging of human right ventricular heart volumes and mass. Acta Radiol 2002; 43: 587–92.

48. Lorenz CH, Walker ES, Morgan VL, et al. Normal human right and left ventricular mass, systolic function, and gender differences by cine magnetic resonance imaging, J Cardiovasc Magn Reson 1999; 1: 7–21.

49. Sandstede J, Lipke C, Beer M, et al. Age- and gender specific differences in left and right ventricular cardiac function and mass determined by cine magnetic resonance imaging. Eur Radiol 1999; 10: 438–42.

50. Alfakih K, Plein S, Thiele H, et al. Normal human left and right ventricular dimensions for MRI as assessed by turbo gradient echo and steady-state free precession imaging sequences. J Magn Reson Imaging 2003; 17: 323–9.

51. Helbing WA, Rebergen SA, Maliepaard C, et al. Quantification of right ventricular function with magnetic resonance imaging in children with normal hearts and with congenital heart disease. Am Heart J 1995; 130: 828–37.

52. Lorenz CH. The range of normal values of cardiovascular structures in infants, children and adolescents measured by magnetic resonance imaging. Pediatr Cardiol 2000; 21: 37–46.

53. Wahl A, Gollesch A, Paetsch I, et al. Safety and feasibility of high-dose dobutamine–atropine stress MRI for diagnosis of myocardial ischemia: experience in 1000 consecutive cases. J Cardiovasc Magn Reson 2003; 5: 51 (abst).

54. Roest AAW, Helbing WA, Kunz P, et al. Exercise MR imaging in the assessment of pulmonary regurgitation and biventricular function in patients after tetralogy of Fallot repair. Radiology 2002; 223: 204–11.

55. Tulevski II, Hirsch A, Dodge-Khatami A, et al. Effect of pulmonary valve regurgitation on right ventricular function in patients with chronic right ventricular pressure overload. Am J Cardiol 2003; 92: 113–16.

56. Nollert G, Fischlein T, Bouterwek S, et al. Long-term results of total repair of tetralogy of Fallot in adulthood: 35 years follow-up in 104 patients corrected at the age of 18 or older. Thorac Cardiovasc Surg 1997; 45: 178–81.

57. Wren C, O'Sullivan JJ. Survival with congenital heart disease and need for follow up in adult life. Heart 2001; 85: 438–43.

58. Horneffer PJ, Zahka KG, Rowe SA, et al. Long-term results of total repair of tetralogy of Fallot in childhood. Ann Thorac Surg 1990; 50: 179–83.

59. Rebergen SA, Chin JG, Ottenkamp J, et al. Pulmonary regurgitation in the late postoperative follow-up of tetralogy of Fallot: volumetric quantitation by nuclear magnetic resonance velocity mapping. Circulation 1993; 88: 2257–66.

60. Wessel HU, Paul MH. Exercise studies in tetralogy of Fallot: a review. Pediatr Cardiol 1999; 20: 39–47.

61. Harrison DA, Harris L, Siu SC, et al. Sustained ventricular tachycardia in adult patients late after repair of tetralogy of Fallot. J Am Coll Cardiol 1997; 30: 1368–73.

62. Gatzoulis MA, Till JA, Somerville J, et al. Mechanoelectrical interaction in tetralogy of Fallot: QRS prolongation relates to right ventricular size and predicts malignant ventricular arrhythmias and sudden death. Circulation 1995; 92: 231–7.

63. Gatzoulis MA, Balaji S, Webber SA, et al. Risk factors for arrhythmia and sudden cardiac death late after repair of tetralogy of Fallot: a multicentre study. Lancet 2000; 356: 975–81.

64. Yemets IM, Williams WG, Webb GD, et al. Pulmonary valve replacement late after repair of tetralogy of Fallot. Ann Thorac Surg 1997; 64: 526–30.

65. Oechslin EN, Harrison DA, Harris L, et al. Reoperation in adults with repair of tetralogy of Fallot: indications and outcomes. J Thorac Cardiovasc Surg 1999; 118: 245–51.

66. Hazekamp MG, Kurvers MM, Schoof PH, et al. Pulmonary valve insertion late after repair of Fallot's tetralogy. Eur J Cardiothorac Surg 2001; 19: 667–70.

67. Parr GVS, Kirklin JW, The early risk of re-replacement of aortic valves, Ann Thorac Surg 1997; 23: 319–22.

68. Therrien J, Siu SC, McLaughlin PR, et al. Pulmonary valve replacement in adults late after repair of tetralogy of Fallot: Are we operating too late? J Am Coll Cardiol 2000; 36: 1670–5.

69. Helbing WA, Niezen RA, Le Cessie S, et al. Right ventricular diastolic function in children with pulmonary regurgitation after repair of tetralogy of Fallot: volumetric evaluation by magnetic resonance velocity mapping. J Am Coll Cardiol 1996; 28: 1827–35.

70. Singh GK, Greenberg SB, Yap YS, et al. Right ventricular function and exercise performance late after primary repair of tetralogy of Fallot with transannular patch in infancy. Am J Cardiol 1998; 81: 1378–82.

71. Davlouros PA, Kilner PJ, Hornung TS, et al. Right ventricular function in adults with repaired tetralogy of Fallot assessed with cardiovascular magnetic resonance imaging: detrimental role of right ventricular outflow aneurysm or akinesia and adverse right-to-left ventricular interaction. J Am Coll Cardiol 2002; 40: 2044–52.

72. Vliegen HW, van Straten A, de Roos A, et al. Magnetic resonance imaging to assess the hemodynamic effects of pulmonary valve replacement in adults late after repair of tetralogy of Fallot. Circulation 2002; 106: 1703–7.

73. Bonhoeffer P, Boudjemline Y, Qureshi SA, et al. Percutaneous insertion of the pulmonary valve. J Am Coll Cardiol 2002; 39: 1664–9.

74. Boudjemline Y, Agnoletti G, Bonnet D, et al. Percutaneous pulmonary valve replacement in a large right ventricular outflow tract: an experimental study. J Am Coll Cardiol 2004; 43: 82–7.

75. Westra SJ, Hill JA, Alejos JC, et al. Three-dimensional helical CT of the pulmonary arteries in infants and children with congenital heart disease. AJR Am J Roentgenol 1999; 173: 109–15.

76. Kawano T, Ishii M, Takagi J, et al. Three-dimensional helical computed tomographic angiography in neonates and infants with complex congenital heart disease. Am Heart J 2000; 139: 654–60.

77. Lawler LP, Fishman EK. Multi-detector row CT of thoracic disease with emphasis on 3D volume rendering and CT angiography. Radiographics 2001; 21: 1257–73.

78. Siegel MJ. Multiplanar and three-dimensional multi-detector row CT of thoracic vessels and airways in the pediatric population. Radiology 2003; 229: 641–50.

79. Rossi UG, Owens CM, Sridharan S, et al. Three-dimensional anatomy of the great vessels defined by 16-slice multidetector CT angiography in neonates, infants, children and adolescents with congenital heart disease. Society of Pediatric Radiology 2005; in press (abst).

80. Guidelines on Patient Dose to Promote the Optimisation of Protection for Diagnostic Medical Exposures. National Radiation Protection Board NRPB, 1999; 10: No. 1.

81. ICRP 60. Recommendations of the International Commission on Radiological Protection. Ann ICRP 1990; 21: 1–3.

4

Hemodynamic evaluation of pulmonary valve disease. Part I: pediatric perspectives

Satinder Sandhu, Ziyad M Hijazi

Introduction

The pulmonary valve is derived from the distal part of the bulbis cordis. The anterior leaflet of the pulmonary valve develops from the two endocardial cushions within the truncus arteriosus. The two posterior leaflets are derived from the major truncus cushions after they have fused to form the truncus septum. The pulmonary valve can be stenotic or regurgitant. Pulmonary valve stenosis (PS) accounts for about 90% of right ventricular (RV) outflow tract (RVOT) obstructive lesions. Hemodynamically significant pulmonary regurgitation (PR) is rarely congenital and most often is secondary to RVOT reconstructive surgery in patients with tetralogy of Fallot, double-outlet right ventricle, pulmonary atresia, and truncus arteriosus. In these patients, the presence of PS may exaggerate the progression of PR. The clinical manifestations of pulmonary valve disease are determined by the anatomic site, the severity of obstruction, and the presence of other associated cardiac abnormalities.

RVOT obstruction can be valvar, subvalvar, or supravalvar. Isolated PS can be due to cuspal fusion or stenosis with a hypoplastic annulus. The pathophysiology of PS is impedance to the ejection of blood from the RV. This results in an increase in RV pressure, which may lead to hypertrophy, which is proportional to the degree of obstruction. In neonates with critical PS and in children with severe stenosis, RV diastolic dysfunction will occur, resulting in reduced filling and a decrease in the cardiac output.

Mild PR is well tolerated. In patients with moderate to severe PR, the RV is chronically volume-overloaded, leading to RV dilation, and ultimately may result in RV dysfunction. Significant RV dysfunction over a period of time will lead to left ventricular (LV) systolic dysfunction secondary to ventricular interdependence.

Evaluation

Increased RV pressure or volume overload leads to progressive RV dilation that may result in right heart failure and ventricular dysrrhythmias. Therefore, RV dysfunction is the final consequence in patients with pulmonary valve disease, and may result in increased risk of late morbidity and mortality. Such patients will present with decreased exercise tolerance and syncope.

The hemodynamic evaluation of patients with pulmonary valve disease can be done by both non-invasive and invasive techniques. The non-invasive techniques include echocardiography, magnetic resonance imaging (MRI),[1,2] radionuclide studies, and exercise stress testing. Further hemodynamic and angiographic evaluation can be done by cardiac catheterization.

Echocardiography

The echocardiographic evaluation of pulmonary valve disease can be done using transthoracic two-dimensional (2D), Doppler and M-mode echocardiography. A complete study is done to evaluate for the presence of PS, PR, and associated cardiac defects. In addition, the degrees of pulmonary, tricuspid, mitral, and aortic regurgitation as well as RV dilation and RV and LV systolic function are assessed.

A 2D echocardiogram allows for accurate evaluation of the presence of stenosis and regurgitation. The anatomy of the pulmonary valve can be well defined by echocardiography, as can the site of the regurgitation.

Since severe PS and PR result in RV dilation, it is important to define this by echocardiography. de Ruitjer et al[3] used 2D views to describe the size of the RV compared with the size of the LV. In patients with normal RV size, the ratio of the LV to the RV was 3 : 1 and was assigned the value 0. In patients with a severely dilated RV, the RV size was equal to or even exceeded that of the LV and was assigned the value 2, while anything in between was classified as mildly dilated RV and assigned the value 1. Misbach et al[4] assessed RV dilation from RV inlet measurements, which were made at end-diastole from the apical four-chamber view. RV enlargement was considered mild when the RV inlet measured between 40 and 50 mm, moderate when it was between 50 and 60 mm, and severe when it was >60 mm. LV ejection was classified as normal (LV ejection fraction (LVEF >0.60)), mildly reduced (LVEF = 0.40–0.59), moderately reduced (LVEF = 0.20–0.39), and severely reduced (LVEF <0.20). It has been suggested that LV dilation would eventually affect LV systolic function. The close relationship between LVEF and RVEF suggests unfavorable ventricular–ventricular interaction. Thus, evaluation of LV dimensions and function is as important in these patients as assessment of the right heart. Moderate or severe RV and LV systolic dysfunction, but not regurgitant fraction or RV diastolic dimensions is an important factor associated with poor clinical status of long-term survivors of tetralogy of Fallot repair.

It has been demonstrated that patients with tetralogy of Fallot with restrictive physiology fare better.[5] This is assessed with the help of Doppler echocardiography done at the atrioventricular (AV) valves.

Radionuclide ventriculography

Radionuclide angiography[6,7] is a useful means of identifying RV dysfunction following repair. Estimation of RVEF is limited due to the complex shape and heavy trabeculations of the RV. First-pass radionuclide angiocardiography of the RV is relatively independent of ventricular shape and trabeculations, and is a reliable and objective way for determination of RVEF.

The patient's own blood cells are labeled in vitro with 200 µCi/kg technetium-99m. A rapid bolus is injected into a brachial vein. The RV and LV are imaged in a projection showing maximal septal separation between them. RVEF is estimated by the first-pass technique in a right anterior oblique position for best delineation of the RV. One to three cardiac cycles are evaluated and the average of these cycles is used to define the RV region of interest and estimate the RVEF. Normal RVEF is 0.53±0.06. Values <0.42 are considered abnormal. After obtaining the RVEF by the first-pass technique, the patient is repositioned to allow measurement of the LVEF by equilibrium ventriculography in a left anterior oblique position with a slight caudal tilt. Normal LVEF is 0.68±0.09. Values <0.51 are considered abnormal. Failure of the RV to increase its ejection during exercise may be an early sign of RV dysfunction as seen on a radionuclide study.

Cardiac catheterization

The important hemodynamic parameters obtained during cardiac catheterization in pulmonary valve stenosis include the relationship of the RV pressure to the systemic arterial pressure, the RV end-diastolic pressure, and the cardiac output.

Cardiac output is measured by the Fick technique in patients with PR. A peak-to-peak pressure gradient is measured across the pulmonary valve using an end-hole catheter or a multitrack catheter over a wire. Simultaneous pressures are measured in the RV and descending aorta. The RV end-diastolic pressure is elevated in patients with RV dysfunction.

Right-to-left shunting is present in patients with severe or critical PS and RV dysfunction where an intracardiac defect is present. In patients with moderate to severe PS or in patients with PR, the RV end-diastolic pressure is usually elevated. In patients with severe PR, there is ventricularization of the pulmonary artery diastolic pressure (Figure 4.1). The right atrial pressure tracing in patients with severe PS will show an increased a-wave, whereas in patients with PR, there is a prominent v-wave.

Measurement of pulmonary regurgitant fraction can be done using pressure–volume loops. Such loops can be constructed from measurements of RV volume obtained from biplane angiography and simultaneous pressures measured with a micromanometer.

The LV has an oval-shaped cavity and the LVEF can be easily estimated by echocardiography or angiography in the catheterization laboratory.

Angiography of the RV will illustrate its size and function. In addition, it will also delineate the RVOT and any associated obstruction, as well as the diameter of the pulmonary valve annulus. In patients with tetralogy of Fallot and in those with Rastelli-type repair, it is also important to evaluate for distal pulmonary artery stenosis. Thirty-five percent of patients with tetralogy have branch pulmonary artery stenosis. Pulmonary artery angiography is done to evaluate the branch

pulmonary arteries and to look for central or segmental stenosis. Some patients will have pulmonary artery hypertension, and in these patients it is important to evaluate LV function and also to document the presence or absence of aorto-pulmonary collaterals or a previous palliative aortopulmonary shunt.

Indications for repair/replacement of the pulmonary valve

These comprise:

- symptomatology
- presence of RV dilation: RV size ratio compared with the LV >1 by echocardiogram and MRI
- decreased RVEF: <0.42 by radionuclide study
- decreased LV systolic function
- PS with a peak-to-peak gradient >40 mmHg
- moderate PR.

PS is defined as mild if the gradient is <35 mmHg, moderate if 35–55 mmHg and severe if >55 mmHg. Critical PS is defined as the presence of cyanosis in addition to the stenosis. In addition to the gradient, the cardiac output and RV end-diastolic pressures should also be addressed. A decreased cardiac output would falsely give a low gradient across the valve. In addition, an elevated RV end-diastolic pressure during cardiac catheterization is also a determining factor of the severity of the PS. All patients with a gradient >40 mmHg should be treated with pulmonary valvuloplasty. If the gradient is <40 mmHg, then catheterization findings of decreased cardiac output, elevated RV end-diastolic pressure, and the presence of cyanosis should lead to an intervention. Balloon pulmonary valvuloplasty has excellent results in patients with isolated PS. Patients with dysplastic pulmonary valves or narrowing of the sinotubular junction or those with a hypoplastic annulus do not respond well to balloon valvuloplasty, and surgical repair is indicated.

PR can result from RVOT reconstruction with a transannular patch or as a result of deteriorating conduit or homograft. In patients with severe PR, there is progressive RV dilation, arrhythmias, and sudden death. The Mayo Clinic series[8] reported that in 42 patients with tetralogy of Fallot repair,

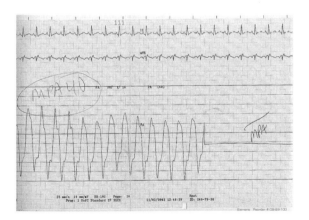

Figure 4.1

Main pulmonary artery tracing of a 4-year-old child with tetralogy of Fallot who underwent complete repair at 3 months of age by the transannular patch technique. There is ventricularization of the main pulmonary artery pressure tracing suggestive of severe pulmonary regurgitation. This patient underwent surgical resurrection of her valve uneventfully.

the indications for pulmonary valve replacement were decreased exercise tolerance (58%), right heart failure (21%), arrhythmias (14%), syncope (10%), and progressive RV dilation (7%). Among patients with tetralogy of Fallot or double-outlet RV where reconstruction[2] is done with a transannular patch, this results in severe RV dilation and PR in 30% of the cases, with a need to replace the pulmonary valve in 10–15%. The presence of right atrial dilation and associated lesions can result in a need for early intervention.

Exercise tolerance

Moderate PR leads to an increase in RV diastolic area, and this has a negative relationship with exercise duration and vital capacity. Moderate PR is associated with decreased breathing reserve during maximal exercise[9] and decreased vital capacity. This indicates that decreased exercise capacity in these patients is related to RV volume loading and ventilatory dysfunction.

Patients with tetralogy of Fallot[10,11] with residual PR have impaired exercise capacity. Resurrection of the pulmonary valve in patients with tetralogy of Fallot[12] leads to a decrease in the RV volume overload and to an improvement in exercise tolerance. Furthermore, the New York Heart Association (NYHA) classification[8] is seen to improve from class III/IV to I/II after the resurrection of the pulmonary valve in patients with PR.

Arrhythmias

Chronic RV volume overload after tetralogy of Fallot repair is related to depressed diastolic function, which on a surface electrocardiogram (ECG) correlates with QRS prolongation. The ECG in patients with RV dysfunction[13] will demonstrate the presence of a QRS duration >150 ms and/or a frontal plane QRS northwest quadrant axis. The risk of symptomatic arrhythmias[14,15] is high when marked RV enlargement and QRS prolongation develop. The presence of either increased RV systolic pressure or RV volume overload leads to an increase in RV systolic wall stress, which may be a nidus for sustained ventricular tachycardia.

RV function

Late pulmonary valve replacement[8,16,17] for PS/PR significantly improves RV function and exercise tolerance and decreases the risk of arrhythmias. MRI measurements demonstrate remarkable hemodynamic improvement of RV function after pulmonary valve replacement in adult patients with PR after total correction of tetralogy of Fallot.

Discussion

Isolated moderate PR is well tolerated for a long period of time in patients with tetralogy of Fallot. However, patients with tetralogy often have other associated anomalies such as residual ventricular septal defect, aortopulmonary collaterals, and distal branch pulmonary artery stenosis, which result in additional volume or pressure overload. The presence of these associated defects will further add to the deterioration of RV function. In patients who are symptomatic, the indication for pulmonary valve replacement is not controversial. However, in an asymptomatic patient with preserved RV function, the optimal timing for pulmonary valve replacement is debatable. Therrien et al[18] reported that in patients with chronic PR following replacement of the pulmonary valve, RV function recovery was compromised in the adult population, and recommended early replacement of the pulmonary valve. Bove et al[16] described a decrease in volume as demonstrated by echocardiography and an improvement in RV function by radionuclide imaging in patients with tetralogy of Fallot following pulmonary valve replacement. The patients in Bove's group were younger, with a mean age of 14.6 years, compared with Therrien's group, where the mean age was 33.9 years at the time of pulmonary valve replacement. This may signify that earlier pulmonary valve replacement in patients with chronic PR may be indicated. Conte et al[19] described their results following homograft placement in patients with PR late after placement of a valveless conduit from the RV to the pulmonary artery. They concluded that patients who did not have improvement in RV function had undergone pulmonary valve replacement an average of 18.7 years following initial repair, compared with an average of 12.6 years in patients who had improvement in RV function following complete repair.

Therefore, we recommend that patients with chronic PR undergo very careful serial evaluation of RV size and function. A progressive increase in RV dimensions should lead to a clinical pathway to rule out any associated defects such as pulmonary artery stenosis, aortopulmonary collaterals, or a hemodynamically significant residual ventricular septal defect that would aggravate the negative hemodynamics of chronic PR. These associated defects must be aggressively corrected, preferably by a transcatheter approach, to prevent further deterioration of RV function. In the presence of a progressive increase in RV dimensions, pulmonary valve replacement should be recommended.

Treatment of a high-risk individual prior to the onset of myocardial dysfunction is the ultimate goal. Currently, there are no clear indications for the treatment of PR. It is our opinion that the presence of moderate PR with a progressive increase in RV dimensions should be sufficient indication for resurrection of the pulmonary valve. Concern regarding deterioration in RV function should be confirmed by MRI to allow optimal timing in the decision-making process tailored to the individual patient.

References

1. Geva T, Sandweiss BM, Gauvreau K, et al. Factors associated with impaired clinical status in long-term survivors of tetralogy of Fallot repair evaluated by magnetic resonance imaging. J Am Coll Cardiol 2004; 43: 1068–74.
2. Singh G, Greenberg B, Yap YS, et al. Right ventricular function and exercise performance late after primary repair of tetralogy of Fallot with the transannular patch in infancy. Am J Cardiol 1998; 81: 1378–82.
3. de Ruijter FTH, Weenink I, Hitchcock FJ, et al. Right ventricular dysfunction and pulmonary valve replacement after correction of tetralogy of Fallot. Ann Thorac Surg 2002; 73: 1794–800.
4. Misbach GA, Turley K, Ebert PA. Pulmonary valve replacement for regurgitation after late repair of tetralogy of Fallot. Ann Thorac Surgery 1997; 64: 526–30.
5. Munkhammar P, Cullen S, Jogi P, et al. Early age at repair prevents restrictive right ventricular physiology after surgery for tetralogy of Fallot. Diastolic RV function after TOF repair in infancy. J Am Coll Cardiol 1998; 32: 1083–7.
6. Bove EL, Byrum CJ, Thomas FD, et al. The influence of pulmonary insufficiency on ventricular function following repair of tetralogy of Fallot. Evaluation using radionuclide ventriculography. J Thorac Cardiovasc Surg 1983; 85: 691–6.
7. Schamberger MS, Hurwitz RA. Course of right and left ventricular function in patients with pulmonary insufficiency after repair of tetralogy of Fallot. Pediatr Cardiol 2000; 21: 244–8.
8. Discigil B, Dearani JA, Puga FJ, et al. Late pulmonary valve replacement after repair of tetralogy of Fallot. J Thorac Cardiovasc Surg 2001; 121: 344–51.
9. Rowe SA, Zahka KG, Manolio TA, et al. Lung function and pulmonary regurgitation limit exercise capacity in postoperative tetralogy of Fallot. J Am Coll Cardiol 1991; 17: 461–6.
10. Wessel HU, Cunningham WJ, Paul MH, et al. Exercise performance in tetralogy of Fallot after intracardiac repair. J Thorac Cardiovasc Surg 1980: 582–93.
11. Carvalho JS, Shinebourne EA, Busst C, et al. Exercise capacity after complete repair of tetralogy of Fallot: deleterious effects of pulmonary regurgitation. Br Heart J 1992; 67: 470–3.
12. Warner KG, Anderson JE, Fulton DR, et al. Restoration of the pulmonary valve reduces right ventricular volume overload after previous repair of tetralogy of Fallot. Circulation 1993; 88: 189–97.
13. Book WM, Parks WJ, Hurst JW. Electrocardiographic predictors of right ventricular volume measured by magnetic resonance imaging late after total repair of tetralogy of Fallot. Clin Cardiol 1999; 22: 740–6.
14. Marie PY, Marcon F, Brunotte F, et al. Right ventricular overload and induced sustained ventricular tachycardia in operatively 'repaired' tetralogy of Fallot. Am J Cardiol 1992; 69: 785–9.
15. Gatzoulis MA, Till JA, Somerville J, Redington AN. Mechanoelectrical interaction in tetralogy of Fallot: QRS prolongation relates to right ventricular size and predicts malignant ventricular arrhythmias and sudden death. Circulation 1995; 92: 231–7.
16. Bove EL, Kavey RE, Byrum CJ, et al. Improved RV function following late pulmonary valve replacement for residual pulmonary insufficiency or stenosis. J Thorac Cardiovasc Surg 1985; 90: 50–5.

17. Vliegen HW, van Straten A, de Roos A, et al. Magnetic resonance imaging to assess the hemo-dynamic effects of pulmonary valve replacement in adults late after repair of tetralogy of Fallot. Circulation 2002; 106: 1703–7.

18. Therrien J, Siu SC, McLaughlin PR, et al. Pulmonary valve replacement in adults late after repair of tetralogy of Fallot: Are we operating too late? J Am Coll Cardiol 2000; 36: 1670–5.

19. Conte S, Jashari R, Eyskens B, et al. Homograft valve insertion for pulmonary regurgitation late after valveless repair of right ventricular outflow tract obstruction. Eur J Cardiothorac Surg 1999; 15: 143–9.

5

Hemodynamic evaluation of pulmonary valve disease. Part II: adult perspectives

Vimal Mehta, Partho P Sengupta, Bijoy K Khandheria

Introduction

The normal pulmonary valve is a semilunar valve with anterior, left, and right leaflets. The area of the pulmonary valve orifice in a normal adult is about 2.0 cm²/m² of body surface area, and there is no systolic pressure gradient across the valve. The texture and function of valve leaflets as well as the diameter of the valve annulus can be adversely affected in a variety of disease states. The initial observations of Edler[1] and Edler and Gustafson[2] on abnormalities of mitral valve motion using high-frequency ultrasound prompted studies of other valves. However, initial echoes from the pulmonary valve were difficult to obtain because of the anatomic position of the valve, the plane of motion with respect to the anterior chest, and a tendency to be obscured by intervening lung during part of the respiratory cycle. Investigators subsequently described alternative methods for obtaining pulmonary valve echoes. Weyman and colleagues[3] first described the M-mode pattern of pulmonary valvular stenosis. The development of two-dimensional sector scanning subsequently allowed real-time tomographic images of cardiac structures.[4] With the pioneering work of Hatle and Angelsen,[5] color flow and continuous-wave Doppler became prime modalities for accurate hemodynamic evaluation of pulmonary valve disease.

Pulmonary valve stenosis

Isolated pulmonary valve stenosis (PS) is a relatively common congenital defect constituting 8–10% of cases of congenital heart disease.[6] The congenital obstruction to right ventricular (RV) outflow is valvular in 90% of patients; in the remainder, it is subvalvular or supravalvular. Among patients with valvular stenosis, up to 15% have dysplastic leaflets, which are thickened, immobile, and composed of myxomatous tissue, sometimes with pulmonary annular hypoplasia; the commissures, however, are not fused. About two-thirds of patients with Noonan syndrome have PS due to dysplastic valves.[7] Very rarely, PS may occur due to acquired causes, for example carcinoid syndrome and rheumatic heart disease, or due to extrinsic compression.

Evaluation of pulmonary stenosis

Two-dimensional echocardiography

Two-dimensional echocardiographic (2D-echo) observations of PS (Figure 5.1) include thickened pulmonary valve cusps that show decreased excursion and dome in systole.[8,9] Typically, the valve annulus is normal in size, and post-stenotic dilatation of the main pulmonary artery and its

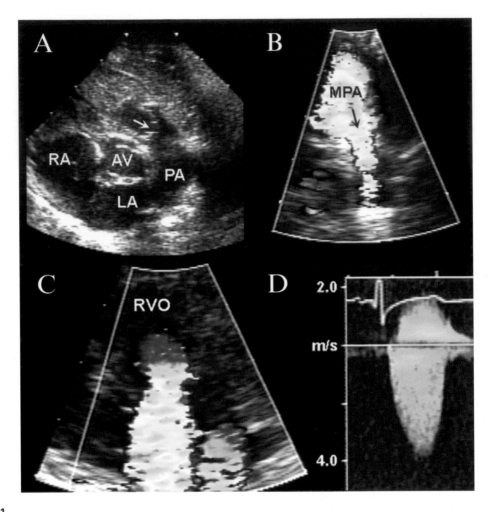

Figure 5.1

2D and Doppler hemodynamic evaluation of pulmonary valve stenosis. (A) Parasternal short-axis view at the level of the aortic valve. Note the thickened and doming pulmonary valve leaflet. (B, C) Suprasternal and subcostal views for aligning the pulmonary valve jet with the Doppler scan line. Note the turbulence at the level of the pulmonary valve. The color envelope expands in the main pulmonary artery due to the presence of post-stenotic dilatation. (D) Continuous-wave Doppler envelope used for measuring peak instantaneous and mean gradients across the pulmonary valve. AV, aortic valve; LA, left atrium; MPA, main pulmonary artery, RA, right atrium, RVO, right ventricular outflow.

branches, especially the left pulmonary artery, is present. Color flow Doppler imaging shows a high-velocity jet directed towards the left pulmonary artery. In contrast to classic valvular PS, patients with a dysplastic pulmonary valve have thickened and immobile leaflets with hypoplasia of the pulmonary valve annulus and absent post-stenotic dilatation of the pulmonary artery. In mild obstruction, cardiac chambers are normal. With severe PS, RV hypertrophy with varying

degrees of infundibular hypertrophy may result. In moderate to severe obstruction, the right atrium may also be dilated, with the atrial septum bulging towards the left atrium. Calcification of the valve is absent in children, but may be present in adults. Large Doppler gradients can be measured in patients with left-to-right shunts such as an atrial septal defect. In such situations, 2D-echo features of PS help in its differentiation of functional from pulmonary valvular stenosis.

However, neither the degree of cusp thickening nor the severity of RV hypertrophy correlates well with the severity of valvular stenosis.

M-mode echocardiography

A large a-wave on the pulmonary valve M-mode echocardiogram suggests PS. Earlier studies reported that the depth of the a-wave is roughly proportional to the peak pressure gradient.[8,9]

Continuous-wave Doppler

Continuous-wave (CW) Doppler is useful for recording the velocity across the stenotic pulmonary valve and helps in estimating the peak instantaneous gradient. Presently, Doppler is the technique of choice to quantify the degree of stenosis. Proper alignment of the Doppler beam with the stenotic jet is essential to quantify the severity correctly, as improper alignment may underestimate the severity of stenosis (Figure 5.1). For this, color Doppler may be helpful in localizing the direction of the stenotic jet, whereupon the CW Doppler beam may be applied. For most patients, adequate alignment of the CW Doppler beam with the stenotic jet can be achieved in the parasternal short-axis view. Some patients may require Doppler interrogation one intercostal space lower, especially those with superiorly directed jets. In children, the subcostal approach may provide optimal beam alignment and thereby detection of maximal jet velocity. The peak velocity measured across the RV outflow tract (RVOT) is used to calculate the pressure gradient, using the modified Bernoulli equation $p = 4V^2$ (where p is the peak instantaneous pressure gradient in mmHg across the obstructed RVOT and V is the peak flow velocity in m/s distal to the obstructive orifice).[10–12] Several studies have demonstrated that the Doppler-predicted systolic gradients correlate highly significantly with gradients measured by manometry at cardiac catheterization.[10–12]

Examination of infundibular stenosis is more difficult than that of valvular stenosis and may require atypical transducer locations to detect the maximal jet. The subcostal plane usually offers the best information in patients with infundibular

stenosis. In cases where both valvular and infundibular stenosis are present, two Doppler signals superimposed upon each other may be recorded. In these, the contribution of each to the overall severity of stenosis can be determined, as the Doppler signal of infundibular stenosis is typically late-peaking because of the dynamic nature of obstruction. Also in these cases where both valvular and infundibular stenosis are present, the presence of serial obstructions may result in apparent overestimation of the degree of severity by CW Doppler as compared with catheterization-derived pressure gradient. This occurs because the phenomenon of pressure recovery distal to the initial stenosis (infundibular stenosis) results in underestimation of the peak-to-peak gradient by the catheter withdrawal technique during catheterization in this situation.[13]

Contrast echocardiography

Contrast echocardiography with agitated saline contrast often detects the presence of right-to-left shunting through a patent foramen ovale. This occurs as a result of right atrial pressure exceeding left atrial pressure. Its detection is important for two reasons: firstly, right-to-left shunting results in systemic arterial desaturation, and in severe long-standing cases may result in manifest central cyanosis and clubbing; secondly, it may result in paradoxical embolism.

Integrative approach to assessment of pulmonary stenosis

The presence or absence of symptoms, and the prognosis, are influenced by the severity of stenosis, RV systolic function, and the competence of the tricuspid valve. In children and young adults, the probability of 25-year survival is 96%. Patients with an initial transpulmonary gradient <25 mmHg do not experience an increase in gradient. Less than 20% of patients initially managed medically subsequently require a valvotomy, and only 4% of operated patients require a second operation. In contrast, patients with moderately-severe or severe stenosis (gradient ≥50 mmHg) require relief of the severity of stenosis, since only 40% of such patients remain free of any intervention 10 years after the initial diagnosis.[14]

When the valve becomes stenotic, the RV systolic pressure increases and a systolic pressure gradient occurs between the RV and the pulmonary artery. PS is considered mild if the valve area is >1.0 cm^2/m^2, the peak transvalvular gradient is <50 mmHg, or the peak RV systolic pressure is <75 mmHg. PS is considered moderate if the valve area is 0.5–1.0 cm^2/m^2, the peak transvalvular gradient is 50–79 mmHg, or the RV systolic pressure is 75–100 mmHg. Severe PS is characterized by a valve area <0.5 cm^2/m^2, a peak transvalvular gradient ≥80 mmHg, or a RV systolic pressure >100 mmHg.[14,15]

Cardiac catheterization is presently rarely used to establish or preclude other diagnostic possibilities. The usual indication for catheterization is therapeutic balloon valvuloplasty.[15] In selected cases, cardiac catheterization may additionally help in localizing the site of obstruction, evaluating its severity, and documenting the coexistence of additional cardiac malformations.

Balloon pulmonary valvuloplasty for pulmonary stenosis

Since its description in 1982,[16] percutaneous balloon pulmonary valvuloplasty (BPV) has shown excellent early and midterm results in infants and children in earlier series and subsequently also in adults.[17–19] Presently, BPV has become the procedure of choice for isolated PS in both children and adults. In patients with severe or long-standing valvular obstruction, secondary infundibular hypertrophy may occur and may result in incomplete resolution of gradient following BPV. This, however, regresses over a period of time, resulting in a further decrease in transvalvular gradient.[19]

Pulmonary valvuloplasty is indicated in symptomatic patients and those with a transpulmonary valve gradient >50 mmHg for a patient with normal cardiac output (Table 5.1). In critical PS, the transpulmonary valve gradient may be significantly higher or lower than 50 mmHg, depending on cardiac output and RV function, especially in the newborn.[20,21] Patients with moderate PS have an excellent prognosis with either medical or interventional therapy. Interventional therapy is usually recommended, since most patients with

Table 5.1 Indications for pulmonary balloon valvuloplasty[20]

Indication	Class
Patients with exertional dyspnea, angina, syncope, or presyncope	I
Asymptomatic patients with normal cardiac output (estimated clinically or determined by catheterization):	
RV-to-PA peak gradient >50 mmHg	I
RV-to-PA peak gradient 40–49 mmHg	IIa
RV-to-PA peak gradient 30–39 mmHg	IIb
RV-to-PA peak gradient <30 mmHg	III

RV, right ventricular; PA, pulmonary artery.

moderate PS eventually have symptoms requiring such therapy. Relief of valvular stenosis can be accomplished easily and safely with BPV, and a delay in intervention offers no advantage.

The role of BPV in patients with a dysplastic pulmonary valve is debated, and, depending upon the site and on the diameter of the pulmonary annulus, smaller balloons may be required, resulting in suboptimal result.

Pulmonary stenosis: special situations

Pulmonary stenosis in the newborn

The clinical presentation in a newborn with PS depends on the severity of obstruction and the maturity of the RV, infundibulum, tricuspid valve, and pulmonary arteries and the patency of the ductus arteriosus. Newborns with severe PS with pinhole orifice present with manifestations resembling pulmonary atresia and intact ventricular septum. 2D-echo and color Doppler examination help in establishing the diagnosis and in assessing the severity of stenosis and the degree of RV hypoplasia.[22–24] BPV is the therapeutic procedure of choice in newborns with severe PS with mobile doming valve and relatively well-developed RV. Surgical pulmonary valvotomy and systemic-to-pulmonary arterial shunt may be necessary in infants with underdeveloped RV. Those with valve dysplasia or annular hypoplasia also require surgical valvotomy. Adequate relief of obstruction has been reported to result in growth of the RV in those with underdeveloped RV cavity.[23]

Pulmonary stenosis in pregnancy

Isolated PS is rarely a significant impediment to a successful pregnancy. This lesion can be approached with percutaneous BPV under echocardiographic guidance when necessary.

Pulmonary regurgitation

The most common cause of pulmonary regurgitation (PR) is dilatation of the valve ring secondary to pulmonary hypertension.[25] The pulmonary valve is anatomically normal in these cases. Dilatation of the valve ring may also be seen in patients with Marfan syndrome. PR may also result from iatrogenic causes – for example as a consequence of BPV or surgical repair of tetralogy of Fallot. Other rare causes include infective endocarditis, carcinoid syndrome (Figure 5.2), chest trauma, and rheumatic heart disease. Absent pulmonary valve syndrome is an extreme form of congenital pulmonary valve dysplasia that is often seen with tetralogy of Fallot and leads to severe PR.

Pulmonary regurgitation with normal pulmonary artery pressures

Two-dimensional echocardiography

Mild pulmonary regurgitation can be physiologic and must be distinguished from pathologic regurgitation. The pulmonary valve is normal in these cases and opens as three separate mobile leaflets that coapt during diastole. The evaluation of the size and function of the RV in the absence of pulmonary hypertension provides a measure of PR and adaptation of the RV to the volume-overload state. Evaluation of the RVOT and pulmonary valve by 2D-echo is possible from the parasternal and subcostal views. RV volume overload often causes paradoxical interventricular septal wall motion, which appears as flattening of the septum during diastole.

Color flow Doppler imaging

Color flow imaging with Doppler interrogation establishes the depth, width, duration, and peak velocity of the diastolic jet of PR (Table 5.2). A diastolic jet in the RVOT, beginning at the line of

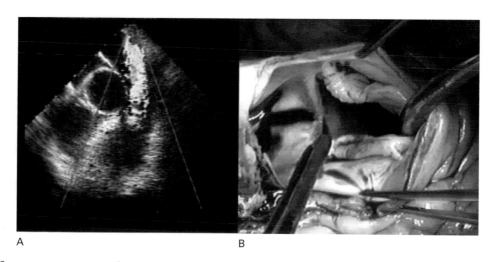

A   B

Figure 5.2

Carcinoid disease affecting the pulmonary valve. (A) Color flow across the pulmonary valve, showing severe pulmonary valve regurgitation. (B) Findings of the pulmonary valve during surgery. Note the leaflet thickening and retraction, which are hallmarks of carcinoid valve lesions.

Table 5.2   Echocardiographic and Doppler parameters used in grading severity of pulmonary regurgitation (PR)[26]

Parameter	Mild	Moderate	Severe
Pulmonary valve	Normal	Normal or abnormal	Abnormal
RV size	Normal[a,b]	Normal or dilated	Dilated
Jet size by color Doppler[b,c]	Thin (usually <10 mm in length) with a narrow origin	Intermediate	Usually large, with a wide origin; may be brief in duration
Jet density and deceleration rate – CW[b,d]	Soft; slow deceleration	Dense; variable deceleration	Dense; steep deceleration, early termination of diastolic flow
Pulmonary systolic flow compared with systemic flow – PW[e]	Slightly increased	Intermediate	Greatly increased

CW, continuous-wave Doppler; PW, pulsed-wave Doppler; RA, right atrium; RF, regurgitant fraction; RV, right ventricle.
[a] Unless there are other reasons for RV enlargement. Normal 2D measurements from the apical four-chamber view; RV mediolateral end-diastolic dimension ⩽4.3 cm, RV end-diastolic area ⩽35.5 cm^2.
[b] Exception: acute PR
[c] At a Nyquist limit of 50–60 cm/s.
[d] Steep deceleration is not specific for severe PR.
[e] Cut-off values for regurgitant volume and fraction are not well validated.

leaflet coaptation and directed towards the RV, is diagnostic of PR. Color Doppler jet depth, extent, and duration can provide an estimate of the severity of pulmonary regurgitation, but are influenced by regurgitant volume as well as by the gradient between the pulmonary artery and the RV. In severe free PR, where equalization of diastolic pulmonary artery and RV pressures occurs early in diastole, the color jet area can be brief and misleading. Regurgitant jets seen in normal pulmonary valves are usually very small, and originate centrally from the pulmonary leaflet coaptation site. Initial studies attempted to quantify PR by measuring jet length. Jets ⩽10 mm in length are considered trivial, while larger jets are more commonly associated with significant heart disease.[26] However, jet depth is dependent on regurgitant volume as well as on the pressure gradient between the pulmonary artery and the RV, and is therefore not a very reliable index of severity. The planimetered jet areas, indexed for body surface area, have been used to quantify the severity of PR,[26] but because of a high degree of variability and overlap among different grades of regurgitation, they are not used. Multiple views such as the parasternal short-axis view and the subcostal view may be necessary to adequately quantify PR. The vena contracta width can also be

used to evaluate the severity of PR by color Doppler,[27] similar to other regurgitant lesions; however, it has not been validated in larger trials. The large width of the vena contracta suggests severe regurgitation.

Continuous-wave Doppler

CW Doppler is frequently used to measure the end-diastolic velocity of PR and thus estimate pulmonary artery end-diastolic pressure (Figure 5.3). Regurgitation that persists throughout diastole suggests the presence of pulmonary hypertension, whereas regurgitation that diminishes earlier in diastole suggests normal pulmonary artery pressures. In the absence of pulmonary artery hypertension, a slow deceleration rate of the PR jet suggests mild PR, whereas a steep deceleration suggests severe PR, resulting in early equalization of diastolic pressures.[28] The density of the CW Doppler signal also provides a qualitative measure of regurgitation. A pulmonary pressure half-time <100 ms calculated from the CW Doppler profile of the PR jet has been reported to be a good and reproducible indicator of hemodynamically significant regurgitation.[29]

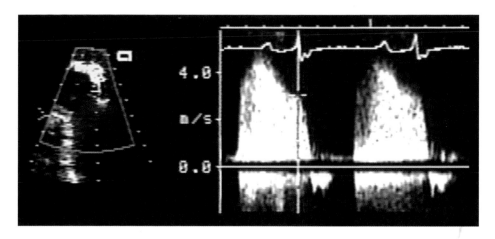

Figure 5.3

Continuous-wave Doppler across a regurgitant pulmonary valve. Velocities obtained at end-diastole are used for estimating the pulmonary artery end-diastolic pressure.

Pulsed-wave Doppler

PR can also be graded with the help of pulsed Doppler study of the RVOT.[30] Pulsed Doppler assessments of the forward and reverse flows in the pulmonary artery have been used to calculate regurgitant volume and regurgitant fraction. The ratio of reverse to forward velocity time integral can be used to estimate the regurgitant fraction, assuming the diameter of the pulmonary artery to be constant. Although differences in regurgitation fraction have been reported among groups with varying severity of PR, there is a considerable overlap. Therefore, this method is not routinely used. Furthermore, this method is not valid in patients with associated PS stenosis because of post-stenotic turbulent flow.

Pulmonary regurgitation with pulmonary artery hypertension

M-mode echocardiography

M-mode echocardiography can show RV hypertrophy and dilatation. Interventricular septal motion is usually paradoxical because of volume overload. Absence of a-wave suggests pulmonary artery hypertension and is the result of elevated pulmonary artery end-diastolic pressure.

However, as RV failure supervenes, the a-wave may reappear as the atrial component of the RV diastolic component is increased.[31] Thus, the presence of a normal-sized a-wave does not exclude pulmonary hypertension, especially when RV failure is suspected. Mid-systolic notching of the posterior leaflet is also suggestive of pulmonary hypertension. Systolic time intervals derived from M-mode echocardiography have been used to estimate pulmonary artery pressure. The RV pre-ejection period lengthens and the RV ejection time shortens with earlier closure of the pulmonary valve with pulmonary hypertension. The RV pre-ejection period-to-RV ejection time ratio increases with pulmonary hypertension.[32]

Doppler estimation of RV and PA pressures

Doppler echocardiography detects the pressure abnormalities by determining a pressure drop or pressure gradient. In the presence of tricuspid regurgitation, a systolic pressure gradient exists between the right ventricle and the right atrium. With knowledge of the gradient across the tricuspid valve, the right atrial pressure is added so as to determine the RV systolic pressure. The right atrial pressure can be estimated clinically by judging the jugular venous pressure at the bedside. An estimate of the right atrial pressure can also be used for simplification, the estimated range being 10–14 mmHg. Doppler echocardiography can also determine the pulmonary artery diastolic pressure in the presence of pulmonary regurgitation, where the end-diastolic pulmonary regurgitant velocity can be measured. This measurement provides the pressure gradient between the pulmonary artery and the right ventricle at end-diastole. Combining this pressure with the RV diastolic pressure or right atrial pressure provides a measurement of the pulmonary artery diastolic pressure.

Doppler tracings of the pulmonary artery velocity can also provide an assessment of pulmonary artery pressure. The acceleration time is the time between the onset of systolic pulmonary artery flow to the peak flow. Normally, peak flow velocity across the pulmonary valve (acceleration time) is achieved within 140 ms of systole. With pulmonary hypertension, the peak flow velocity is reached more rapidly. The shortened acceleration time is linearly inversely proportional to the severity of pulmonary hypertension.[33]

Pulmonary regurgitation: special situations

Pulmonary regurgitation secondary to repair of tetralogy of Fallot

PR is a common sequela of surgical repair of tetralogy of Fallot. PR is usually well tolerated in childhood. However, long-term studies have demonstrated that PR leads to progressive RV dilatation and, with time, to RV dysfunction, exercise intolerance, propensity for development of arrhythmias, and sudden cardiac death.[34] Evaluation of the pulmonary valve, RVOT morphology (especially for the presence of hypokinetic and akinetic areas), and presence and severity of PR, as well as estimation of pulmonary artery systolic and diastolic pressure, can be done with echocardiography.

Tissue Doppler imaging (TDI) can provide information on regional systolic function and thus help in detection of RV dysfunction due to chronic RV volume overload secondary to PR. Following repair of tetralogy of Fallot, abnormal systolic and diastolic myocardial velocities determined by TDI

of the RV free wall are common, and are more prevalent in patients with abnormally long QRS duration and QRS and JT dispersion on electrocardiogram (ECG).[35]

RV strain (ε) and strain rate (SR), where ε is defined as the change or deformation in distance between any two points and SR is defined as the change in velocity between these two points divided by the change in length, are new and promising indices of ventricular function and are independent of geometric constraints, making them potentially useful for evaluation of the RV.[36] In patients with repaired tetralogy of Fallot with significant PR, systolic and diastolic RV SR and ε have been reported to be decreased in the RV free wall.[37]

Pulmonary valve replacement for pulmonary regurgitation

In general, patients should be considered for pulmonary valve replacement (PVR) when moderate to severe or severe PR with progressive RV dilatation is present, irrespective of the presence of overt symptoms (such as shortness of breath).[38] The perioperative risk is higher in patients with established RV dysfunction at the time of pulmonary valve implantation. Delaying surgery in such patients can result in irreversible RV dysfunction. PVR for PR is usually required in about 15% of patients with repaired tetralogy of Fallot.[37] In general, bioprosthetic valves are preferred because of the tendency for mechanical valve thrombosis in this position. Optimal timing of pulmonary valve implantation is essential for preserving RV function. A combination of clinical signs (new-onset tricuspid regurgitation murmur) with an enlarging cardiothoracic ratio, further QRS prolongation, echocardiographic RV dilatation, and/or increasing RV end-systolic volumes (exceeding normal values) constitute reasons for elective PVR.

The life-span of pulmonary valve prostheses in adult patients ranges between 15 and 30 years. Bioprosthetic valves (homograft or porcine) have a lower complication rate compared with mechanical prostheses and are the valves of choice for PVR. Patients with severe RV dilatation and a large akinetic or aneurysmal region in the RVOT should be considered for additional pulmonary infundibuloplasty.[39] The reported 10-year survival rate after PVR is 86–95%.[40] With timely PVR, the functional class improves after valve replacement, along with reduction of RV size (by about 30%) and improvement of RV ejection fraction, whereas when PVR is performed late, RV recovery is incomplete. Unfortunately, recurrence of PR after PVR can occur and is associated with a late increase in RV volume.[41]

Conclusions and future directions

Color flow and CW Doppler have become the prime modalities for accurate hemodynamic evaluation of pulmonary valve disease. Doppler-predicted systolic gradients show excellent correlation with gradients measured at cardiac catheterization. Currently, pulmonary valvuloplasty is indicated in symptomatic patients and those in whom the transpulmonary valve gradient is >50 mmHg in the presence of a normal cardiac output. In contrast to PS, PR is seen more commonly and can be detected in otherwise-normal hearts. PR, however, assumes clinical significance particularly following surgical or percutaneous relief of PS and repair of tetralogy of Fallot, since PR is often moderate to severe in these situations and results in progressive RV dilatation. Color Doppler is the best initial screening modality, followed by CW Doppler of the pulmonary and tricuspid regurgitation jet, which facilitates further quantification of PR. Optimal timing of PVR is crucial for preserving RV function. Although surgical PVR can be performed with a very low mortality, the life span of the prosthetic conduits is limited. Percutaneous implantation of a valve has recently emerged as an alternative safe strategy that can be offered without the requirements for repetitive surgeries.[42] Many adult patients who have marked aneurysmal dilatation of the RVOT are not currently eligible for this procedure. However, despite the technical challenges and the issue of valve durability, this is an important advance that will impact the prognosis of patients with PR in future.

References

1. Edler I. Ultrasound cardiogram in mitral valve disease. Acta Chir Scand 1956; 111: 230–1.

2. Edler I, Gustafson A. Ultrasound cardiogram in mitral stenosis. Acta Med Scand 1957; 159: 85–90.

3. Weyman AE, Dillon JC, Feigenbaum H, Chang S. Echocardiographic patterns of pulmonary valve motion in valvular pulmonary stenosis. Am J Cardiol 1974; 34: 644–51.

4. Tajik AJ, Seward JB, Hagler DJ, et al. Two-dimensional real-time ultrasonic imaging of the heart and great vessels: technique, image orientation, structure identification and validation. Mayo Clinic Proc 1978; 53: 271–303.

5. Hatle L, Angelsen B. Doppler Ultrasound in Cardiology: Physical Principles and Clinical Applications, 2nd edn. Philadelphia: Lea and Febiger, 1985.

6. Hoffman JI, Christianson R. Congenital heart disease in a cohort of 19,502 births with long-term follow-up. Am J Cardiol 1978; 42: 641–7.

7. Pearl W. Cardiovascular anomalies in Noonan's syndrome. Chest 1977; 71: 677–9.

8. Heger JJ, Weyman AE. A review of M-mode and cross-sectional echocardiographic findings of the pulmonary valve. J Clin Ultrasound 1979; 7: 98–107.

9. Weyman AE. Pulmonary valve echo motion in clinical practice. Am J Med 1977; 62: 843–55.

10. Johnson GL, Kwan OL, Handshoe S, et al. Accuracy of combined two-dimensional echocardiography and continuous wave Doppler recordings in the estimation of pressure gradient in right ventricular outlet obstruction. J Am Coll Cardiol 1984; 3: 1013–18.

11. Valdes-Cruz LM, Horowitz S, Sahn DJ, et al. Validation of a Doppler echocardiographic method for calculating severity of discrete stenotic obstructions in a canine preparation with a pulmonary artery band. Circulation 1984; 69: 1177.

12. Frantz EG, Silverman NH. Doppler ultrasound evaluation of valvar pulmonary stenosis from multiple transducer positions in children requiring pulmonary valvuloplasty. Am J Cardiol 1988; 61: 844–9.

13. Goldberg SJ. The principles of pressure drop in long segment stenosis. Herz 1986; 11: 291–5.

14. Hayes CJ, Gersony WM, Driscoll DJ, et al. Second natural history study of congenital heart defects: results of treatment of patients with pulmonary valve stenosis. Circulation 1993; 87(Suppl I): I-28–I-37.

15. Almeda FQ, Kavinsky CJ, Pophal SG, Klein LW. Pulmonic valvular stenosis in adults: diagnosis and treatment. Catheter Cardiovasc Interv 2003; 60: 546–57.

16. Kan JS, White RI Jr, Mitchell SE, Gardner TJ. Percutaneous balloon valvuloplasty: a new method for treating congenital pulmonary valve stenosis. N Engl J Med 1982; 307: 540–2.

17. Rao PS, Fawzy ME, Solymar L, Mardini MK. Long-term results of balloon pulmonary valvuloplasty of valvar pulmonic stenosis. Am Heart J 1988; 115: 1291–6.

18. Sadr-Ameli MA, Sheikholeslami F, Firoozi I, Azarnik H. Late results of balloon pulmonary valvuloplasty in adults. Am J Cardiol 1998; 82: 398–400.

19. Fawzy ME, Awad M, Galal O, et al. Long-term results of pulmonary balloon valvulotomy in adult patients. J Heart Valve Dis 2001; 10: 812–18.

20. Bonow RO, Carabello B, de Leon Jr AC, et al. Guidelines for the management of patients with valvular heart disease. Circulation 1998; 98: 1949–84.

21. Allen HD, Beekman RH III, Garson A Jr, et al. Pediatric therapeutic cardiac catheterization: a statement for healthcare professionals from the Council on Cardiovascular Disease in the Young, American Heart Association. Circulation 1998; 97: 609–25.

22. Stumper O, Piechaud JF, Bonhoeffer P, et al. Pulmonary balloon valvuloplasty in the palliation of complex cyanotic congenital heart disease. Heart 1996; 76: 363–6.

23. Kovalchin JP, Forbes TJ, Nihill MR, Geva T. Echocardiographic determinants of clinical course in infants with critical and severe pulmonary valve stenosis. J Am Coll Cardiol 1997; 29: 1095–101.

24. Rome JJ. Balloon pulmonary valvuloplasty. Pediatr Cardiol 1998; 19: 18.

25. Farber HW, Loscalzo J. Pulmonary arterial hypertension. N Engl J Med 2004; 351: 1655–65.

26. Zoghbi WA, Enriquez-Sarano M, Foster E, et al. Recommendations for evaluation of the severity of native valvular regurgitation with two-dimensional and Doppler echocardiography. J Am Soc Echocardiogr 2003; 16: 777–802.

27. Tweddell JS, Pelech AN, Frommelt PC, et al. Factors affecting longevity of homograft valves used in right ventricular outflow tract reconstruction for congenital heart disease. Circulation 2000; 102: III130–III135.

28. Li W, Davlouros PA, Kilner PJ, et al. Doppler-echocardiographic assessment of pulmonary regurgitation in adults with repaired tetralogy of Fallot: comparison with cardiovascular magnetic resonance imaging. Am Heart J 2004; 147: 165–72.

29. Silversides CK, Veldtman GR, Crossin J, et al. Pressure half-time predicts hemodynamically significant pulmonary regurgitation in adult patients with repaired tetralogy of Fallot. J Am Soc Echocardiogr 2003; 16: 1057–62.

30. Goldberg SJ, Allen HD. Quantitative assessment by Doppler echocardiography of pulmonary or aortic regurgitation. Am J Cardiol 1985; 56: 131–5.

31. Nanda NC, Gramiak R, Robinson TI, et al. Echocardiographic evaluation of pulmonary hypertension. Circulation 1974; 50: 575.

32. Riggs T, Hirschfeld S, Borkat G, et al. Assessment of pulmonary vascular bed by echocardiographic right ventricular systolic time intervals. Circulation 1978; 57: 939.

33. Graettinger WF, Greene ER, Voyles WF. Doppler predictions of pulmonary artery pressure, flow and resistance in adults. Am Heart J 1987; 113: 1426.

34. Gatzoulis MA, Balaji S, Webber SA, et al. Risk factors for arrhythmia and sudden cardiac death late after repair of tetralogy of Fallot: a multicentre study. Lancet 2000; 356: 975–81.

35. Vogel M, Sponring J, Cullen S, et al. Regional wall motion and abnormalities of electrical depolarization and repolarization in patients after surgical repair of tetralogy of Fallot. Circulation 2001; 103: 1669–73.

36. Frigiola A, Redington AN, Cullen S, Vogel M. Pulmonary regurgitation is an important determinant of right ventricular contractile dysfunction in patients with surgically repaired tetralogy of Fallot. Circulation 2004; 110(Suppl II): II-153–II-157.

37. Solarz DE, Witt SA, Glascock BJ et al. Right ventricular strain rate and strain analysis in patients with repaired tetralogy of Fallot: possible intraventricular septal compensation. J Am Soc Echocardiogr 2004; 17: 388–44.

38. Therrien J, Siu SC, Harris L, et al. Impact of pulmonary valve replacement on arrhythmia propensity late after repair of tetralogy of Fallot. Circulation 2001; 103: 2489–94.

39. d'Udekem d'Acoz Y, Pasquet A, Van Caenegem O, et al. Reoperation for severe right ventricular dilatation after tetralogy of Fallot repair: pulmonary infundibuloplasty should be added to homograft implantation. J Heart Valve Dis 2004; 13: 307–12.

40. Yemets IM, Williams WG, Webb GD, et al. Pulmonary valve replacement late after repair of tetralogy of Fallot. Ann Thorac Surg 1997; 64: 526–30.

41. Straten AV, Vliegen HW, Hazekamp MG, et al. Right ventricular function after pulmonary valve replacement in patients with tetralogy of Fallot. Radiology 2004; 233: 824–9.

42. Khambadkone S, Bonhoeffer P. Nonsurgical pulmonary valve replacement: Why, when and how? Catheter Cardiovasc Interv 2004; 62: 401–8.

6

Impact of emerging technologies in cardiology and cardiothoracic surgery: Percutaneous pulmonary valve implantation

Sachin Khambadkone, Louise Coats, Welton M Gersony, John E Deanfield

Introduction

In the last two decades, there have been enormous advances in transcatheter treatment of many cardiovascular disorders, and progress in this field shows no sign of slowing.[1] The pioneering introduction of balloon atrial septostomy by Rashkind and colleagues has been followed by a range of procedures that have enabled occlusion of intracardiac and extracardiac shunts, balloon valvotomy and angioplasty, stent implantation, and radiofrequency opening of atretic valves.[2]

The first significant definitive treatment of valvar pulmonary stenosis by interventional techniques was reported a quarter of a century ago. Prior to the introduction of pulmonary balloon valvuloplasty, surgical treatment was always required for patients with severe obstruction. Initially, blind pulmonary valvotomy (the Brock procedure) was utilized, but with the advent of improved bypass techniques for infants, open-heart repair was far more definitive, and could also eliminate when necessary any associated infundibular obstruction. Such treatment for even the most severe pulmonary valve stenosis at any age has been remarkably successful, and few procedures are as close to the goal of 'curative' than balloon valvuloplasty for pulmonary stenosis. For the vast majority of patients, the mild pulmonary valve insufficiency or residual stenosis does not require reintervention. The utilization of catheterization interventional treatment for postoperative patients with severe pulmonary insufficiency after tetralogy repair in general has not been possible, and surgery has been required. The timing for reoperation for significant pulmonary regurgitation in patients who have had right ventricular outflow patch repairs remains controversial. However, as these patients reach adolescence and adulthood, the need to address the markedly dilated right ventricle in many of them has become apparent, although the timing of such procedures is still somewhat controversial. Until recently, surgical intervention for replacement of a pulmonary valve or conduit has been the only choice.

New approaches for patients with this condition are evolving. Percutaneous pulmonary valve implantation has become the most exciting new development in interventional catheterization, with the ability to deal not only with stenosis but also regurgitation of cardiac valves. Several groups have worked on the development of a compressible heart valve, which could be deployed percutaneously on a customized delivery system. Bonhoeffer and colleagues[3] reported the first successful clinical implantation of a cardiac valve in a stenotic and regurgitant right ventricle to pulmonary artery conduit in a 12-year-old patient who had previously undergone repair of tetralogy of Fallot.[3] This has led to a clinical program that has produced hemodynamic improvements comparable to the results of surgery and that may reduce the lifetime 'reoperation' burden in many patients.

In this chapter, we will consider the potential impact of percutaneous pulmonary valve implantation on medical and surgical management of congenital heart disease involving the right ventricular outflow tract. The indications and current limitations of this approach are discussed, together with opportunities to expand the population of suitable patients. We also review the factors that will influence the integration of percutaneous valve implantation with a surgical strategy to provide optimal management of congenital heart defects. Due to anatomic and hemodynamic suitability as well as ease of access, the clinical percutaneous valve program was deliberately begun with the pulmonary valve. However, valve implantation by interventional catheterization has exciting potential for the treatment of other cardiac valves, particularly aortic valve stenosis and regurgitation, and may well have a major expanded impact on clinical practice in congenital and acquired valve disease.

Indications and timing of intervention in congenital heart disease involving pulmonary stenosis

Improved survival after treatment of congenital heart disease in infancy and childhood has resulted in a new population of adolescents and adults with a range of complex cardiac malformations that frequently require reintervention in later life.[4] Pulmonary regurgitation, with or without stenosis, is the most common residual lesion after surgical repair of defects involving the right ventricular outflow tract, such as tetralogy of Fallot and pulmonary atresia. This may result from repair without preservation of valve function (e.g. valvotomy, valvectomy, or transannular patch insertion) or from insertion of biological or prosthetic valves directly or within conduits that do not have growth potential and degenerate during childhood.[5]

Early surgical practice for repair of tetralogy of Fallot emphasized the importance of relief of right ventricular outflow tract obstruction. The pulmonary regurgitation that often resulted from surgery was considered benign and well tolerated. With longer follow-up, it is now clear that this is not the case in a substantial proportion of patients. Right ventricular dilatation as a consequence of chronic pulmonary regurgitation has been associated with electromechanical changes such as QRS prolongation, risk of malignant ventricular arrhythmia, and sudden death, as well as tricuspid regurgitation with right atrial dilatation and supraventricular arrhythmia.[6] Decline in right ventricular function leads to impaired exercise tolerance and symptoms.[7,8] The presence of additional lesions, such as branch pulmonary artery stenosis and ventricular septal defect, accelerates decline in right ventricular function in the presence of pulmonary insufficiency. Residual or recurrent right ventricular outflow tract obstruction may also be an issue. As a result, surgical pulmonary valve replacement has been performed increasingly frequently in adults, especially after 'correction' of tetralogy of Fallot or repairs involving a right ventricle to pulmonary artery conduit. It is now the commonest indication for reoperation in many adult congenital cardiac programs,[4] although definitive indications may not always be clear.

At surgery, a biological pulmonary valve is usually implanted, as other valve types have been associated with higher early and late complications. A homograft is the most common choice, but even these are prone to calcification and degeneration.[9] Although the mortality for surgical pulmonary valve replacement is low, these operations may be associated with considerable morbidity. As implanted valves are known to deteriorate even in adults, patients face the unattractive prospect of multiple surgical procedures during their lifetime.[10] In current practice, therefore, pulmonary valve surgery has only been recommended for patients with symptoms and significant pulmonary regurgitation or associated lesions, or in asymptomatic patients with marked right ventricular dilatation and/or dysfunction. It is, however, hard to assess symptoms in this population, and the optimal timing of reintervention for preservation or restoration of right ventricular function is not known. Recent evidence indicates that right ventricular function does not improve significantly in many older patients, even after successful implantation of a competent non-stenotic pulmonary valve. As a result, it has been suggested that earlier intervention may be required to prevent irreversible decline in myocardial function.[11] This parallels the shift in practice that has occurred in the management of aortic regurgitation. Understanding of the optimal indications and timing for pulmonary valve intervention in pulmonary stenosis, pulmonary regurgitation, and combined lesions will require a prospective clinical study of randomized cohorts. Availability, however, of a safe, simple, technique for percutaneous pulmonary valve insertion with lower morbidity and excellent patient acceptance is likely to make a major impact on the timing and approach to reintervention in patients with right ventricular outflow tract dysfunction.

Percutaneous pulmonary valve program

The design and development of the bovine jugular venous valve stent that has been developed and employed by Bonhoeffer and associates are described elsewhere.[12] Including the initial series from France, percutaneous pulmonary valve insertion has been performed in 58 patients as of September 2004. Their median age was 16 years (range 9–43 years) and the median weight was 56 kg (range 25–110 kg). Approximately two thirds of the cohort had variants of tetralogy of Fallot. Most (79%) had a homograft between the right ventricle and pulmonary artery and only three patients had a native right ventricular outflow tract that had been augmented by a pericardial or homograft patch. After valve implantation, there was a significant reduction in right ventricular systolic pressure (64.4±17.2 to 50.4±14 mmHg; p <0.0005) and in outflow gradient (33±24.6 to 19.5±15.3 mmHg; p <0.0005) without change in systemic arterial pressure. Pulmonary artery diastolic pressure rose from 9.9±3.7 to 13.5±5.3 mmHg (p <0.005), with a fall in right ventricular end-diastolic pressure (11.5±3.7 to 10.5±4.2 mmHg; p = 0.05). None of the patients had more than trivial to mild pulmonary regurgitation. There has been no procedural or late mortality, but residual or progressive narrowing has occurred in a small percentage. Many of these have been stent/valve-related problems, early in

the experience, resulting from a loss of apposition of the venous wall to the stent. This has been resolved by suturing the entire venous wall to the stent. It is noteworthy that percutaneous pulmonary valve implantation does not preclude performance of further procedures distal to the device, such as stent implantation in the branch pulmonary arteries. Percutaneous pulmonary valve implantation has resulted in early improvement in cardiopulmonary exercise performance, reduction in right ventricular end-diastolic volume, and, interestingly, increases in left-ventricular end-diastolic and stroke volumes, with reduction in pulmonary regurgitation.

Patient selection/current limitations

The current device has been used predominantly in valved conduits (between 16 and 22 mm), which provide a good 'environment' for anchoring a valve stent, but this represents a small proportion of the patients who may require intervention. There are many patients with pulmonary valve problems who have outflow tracts larger than 22 mm, right ventricular outflow tract aneurysms, and dilated pulmonary arteries with a hyperdynamic circulation as a result of severe pulmonary regurgitation. In such patients, right ventricular outflow tract size or morphology precludes implantation of the current valve stent and it will be a major challenge to extend percutaneous pulmonary valve implantation to this wider clinical spectrum of patients. Boudjemline and colleagues[13] have recently described the development of an 'infundibular reducer' stent, which has been implanted in larger native right ventricular outflow tracts in experimental models. The jugular venous valve stent can be implanted within the 'infundibular reducer', either as a one-stage or a two-stage procedure. This approach shows great promise and a clinical program using the device will begin shortly.

The morphology of the right ventricular outflow tract is highly variable, and improved imaging is required for case selection and valve stent development. Three-dimensional reconstruction by magnetic resonance imaging has been used to produce polymer-based casts of the right ventricular outflow tract from individual patients.

This is a stage in the development of a mathematical modeling program that will permit virtual implantation of different valve stent designs into outflow tracts of variable size, shape, and wall characteristics.

Comparison with surgery

The impact of percutaneous pulmonary valve implantation on the management of residual or recurrent right ventricular outflow tract abnormalities will depend on the longevity of the valve stent and the early, medium, and late results compared with surgery. There is little doubt that the jugular venous valve in the stent will deteriorate with time, probably in a manner similar to experience with other biological valves implanted surgically. There is a further risk of metal fatigue, stent fractures, and interactions between the stent and other contiguous implants. It is very encouraging that repeated valve stent implantation is possible with successful experience of a valve stent placement within a previous valve stent ('Russian doll' concept).

In addition to insertion of a functioning pulmonary valve, surgery provides the opportunity to perform other procedures. These include treatment of residual lesions such as ventricular septal defect or tricuspid regurgitation as well as 'remodeling' of the right ventricular outflow tract. In patients with an aneurysm or right ventricular outflow tract patch, excision of the patch together with infundibuloplasty aims to improve the distorted right ventricular geometry and reduce cavity size.[14] Furthermore, electrophysiologic interventions can be performed at surgery in patients who have arrhythmia substrates. The additional value of the surgical 'infundibular resurrection' strategy over relief of uncomplicated pulmonary regurgitation and pulmonary stenosis by percutaneous valve implantation remains unknown.

Comparison of the results of percutaneous pulmonary valve implantation with those of surgery remains challenging. Firstly, the range of patients that can be treated by the two approaches is markedly different. Secondly, assessment of the right ventricle remains problematic due to its complex geometry, its irregular cavity, and an abnormal wall motion pattern in these patients.

Cardiac magnetic resonance and Doppler tissue imaging have been invaluable, but comparison remains difficult. How, for example, can post-procedure ventricular volumes be compared appropriately if significant right ventricular outflow tract resection is carried out at surgery? The Great Ormond Street Hospital for Sick Children has reported a clinical outcome comparison of percutaneous pulmonary valve insertion with surgery in unrandomized, contemporary, parallel groups of patients. The comparison showed that both approaches were safe, with acceptable levels of morbidity.[15] There was a predictable difference in patient characteristics between the two treatment groups; for example, only 11.4% of the percutaneous pulmonary valve patients had a transannular patch or native outflow tract, compared with 60% of the surgical group.

Ethical and practical issues in the introduction of percutaneous valve implantation

Formal clinical trials will need to be undertaken once the percutaneous pulmonary valve design is at a mature stage with wider clinical applicability. Design and conduct of such trials are challenging for a number of ethical and practical reasons common to the introduction of new untested treatment approaches into clinical practice.

Selection of patients and informed consent are important issues, as is the choice of trial design, for evaluation of rapidly evolving technologies. Tracker trials, which include randomized cohorts and which track changes and progress over time, provide unbiased comparisons at each stage in development. Evaluation of a new device-based treatment differs from that of a new drug or even a new operation. Variables that influence outcome include both operator experience and device design, so that both aspects need to be studied objectively. Issues of patient preference for less invasive intervention will further complicate the successful conduct of a trial comparing an interventional catheter treatment with surgery, even before outcomes become clear. Nevertheless, formal testing of the results of intervention in well-characterized cohorts of patients, comparison with alternative treatments, and influence on outcome will be critical for understanding the role of percutaneous pulmonary valve implantation.

Lifetime management strategies

Percutaneous pulmonary valve implantation has provided a unique opportunity to study the right ventricular responses to acute and chronic pressure and volume unloading without the confounding effects of surgery and cardiopulmonary bypass. Observations after implantation support the findings from surgical reports that show reduction of right ventricular dimensions and improvements in function and clinical well-being.

The availability of a simple, effective technique with low morbidity and excellent patient acceptability will undoubtedly result in a re-evaluation of the whole approach to lifetime management of right ventricular outflow tract reconstruction in patients with congenital heart disease. A policy of earlier intervention is likely to be adopted, as evidence accumulates that current strategies may produce disappointing benefits on the right ventricle. During the period within which we have performed both percutaneous pulmonary valve implantation and surgery, the total number of procedures undertaken has risen considerably, reflecting this shift in approach. A prospective randomized trial comparing intervention with conservative management for asymptomatic young individuals with pulmonary regurgitation would be invaluable to support 'evidence-based' medical practice.

A hybrid approach involving surgery and interventional catheterization is likely to be indicated for many patients. This, in some patients, will involve a change in the surgical strategy both during the primary repair and during reoperation to enable the emerging technologies of transcatheter valve implantation to be an option during later follow-up. For example, the homograft implanted in the initial repair should be of a size that could last up to adulthood and be suitable for percutaneous valve implantation when the homograft deteriorates. It may be advantageous to consider the future elastic properties of the right ventricular outflow tract, with avoidance of non-circumferential augmentation with distensible materials such as autologous pericardium. Surgical repair should not only result in early hemodynamic benefits but should also provide a platform for future catheter interventions.

Conclusion

Management of severe right ventricular outflow regurgitation in the postoperative patient has been limited to surgical reintervention. Percutaneous pulmonary valve implantation is the first human experience of transcatheter treatment for valvar regurgitation. Current experience is encouraging, and has provided a challenge to cardiologists and surgeons to rethink the lifetime management of many congenital cardiac defects. The importance of surgical involvement in the planning and implementation of a new interventional catheter program cannot be overemphasized. It is likely that new valves will be developed and that the indications and opportunities for percutaneous valve implantation will expand considerably in the near future. Systematic evaluation of results of different treatment options will be essential.

Major advances are being made in tissue engineering of heart valves, which will have an impact on both surgical and interventional catheter approaches to valve implantation. A multidisciplinary approach in research and development will shorten the time to clinical application. The exciting success of percutaneous pulmonary valve implantation will be a stimulus to extend transcatheter treatment to other dysfunctional cardiac valves, including the aortic valve. A number of approaches have already been attempted. Carefully conducted basic and clinical programs will ensure that these evolving technologies benefit a wide spectrum of patients with heart valve disease.

References

1. Boudjemline Y, Bonhoeffer P. Percutaneous valve insertion: a new approach? J Thorac Cardiovasc Surg 2003; 125: 741–2.
2. Rashkind WJ, Gibson J Jr. Interventional cardiac catheterization in congenital heart disease. Int J Cardiol 1985; 7: 1–11.
3. Bonhoeffer P, Boudjemline Y, Saliba Z, et al. Percutaneous replacement of pulmonary valve in a right-ventricle to pulmonary-artery prosthetic

conduit with valve dysfunction. Lancet 2000; 356: 1403–5.

4. Dore A, Glancy DL, Stone S, et al. Cardiac surgery for grown-up congenital heart patients: survey of 307 consecutive operations from 1991 to 1994. Am J Cardiol 1997; 80: 906–13.

5. Daliento L. Total correction of tetralogy of Fallot: late clinical follow-up. Ital Heart J 2002; 3: 24–7.

6. Gatzoulis MA, Balaji S, Webber SA, et al. Risk factors for arrhythmia and sudden cardiac death late after repair of tetralogy of Fallot: a multicentre study. Lancet 2000; 356: 975–81.

7. James FW, Kaplan S, Schwartz DC, et al. Response to exercise in patients after total surgical correction of tetralogy of Fallot. Circulation 1976; 54: 671–9.

8. Carvalho JS, Shinebourne EA, Busst C, et al. Exercise capacity after complete repair of tetralogy of Fallot: deleterious effects of residual pulmonary regurgitation. Br Heart J 1992; 67: 470–3.

9. Conte S, Jashari R, Eyskens B, et al. Homograft valve insertion for pulmonary regurgitation late after valveless repair of right ventricular outflow tract obstruction. Eur J Cardiothorac Surg 1999; 15: 143–9.

10. Tweddell JS, Pelech AN, Frommelt PC, et al. Factors affecting longevity of homograft valves used in right ventricular outflow tract reconstruction for congenital heart disease. Circulation 2000; 102(19 Suppl 3): III130–III135.

11. Therrien J, Siu SC, Harris L, et al. Impact of pulmonary valve replacement on arrhythmia propensity late after repair of tetralogy of Fallot. Circulation 2001; 103: 2489–94.

12. Bonhoeffer P, Boudjemline Y, Qureshi SA, et al. Percutaneous insertion of the pulmonary valve. J Am Coll Cardiol 2002; 39: 1664–9.

13. Boudjemline Y, Schievano S, Bonnet C, et al. Off-pump replacement of the pulmonary valve in large right ventricular outflow tracts: a hybrid approach. J Thorac Cardiovasc Surg 2005; 129: 831–7.

14. d'Udekem dY, Pasquet A, Van Caenegem O, et al. Reoperation for severe right ventricular dilatation after tetralogy of Fallot repair: pulmonary infundibuloplasty should be added to homograft implantation. J Heart Valve Dis 2004; 13: 307–12.

15. Coats L, Tsang V, Khambadkone S, et al. The potential impact of percutaneous pulmonary valve stent implantation on right ventricular outflow tract re-intervention. Eur J Cardiothorac Surg 2005; 27: 536–43.

7

Established techniques for repair/replacement of the pulmonary valve

Emile A Bacha

Introduction

It can be argued that the pulmonary valve has been considered as one of the least important valves of the heart. The most recent Executive Summary of the American College of Cardiology/American Heart Association Task Force on Practice Guidelines related to the management of patients with valvular heart disease has only a very short chapter (1/39 of the total pages) dealing with pulmonary stenosis and regurgitation.[1] Acquired pulmonary valve disease is almost unheard of (risk of infective endocarditis 0.94 per 10 000 patient-years[1]), and congenital pulmonary heart disease is mostly confined to pulmonary stenosis. The vast majority of patients with pulmonary stenosis are managed with balloon pulmonary valvotomy, which has enjoyed very good long-term success.[2,3] However, pulmonary regurgitation is a frequent sequelae of balloon pulmonary valvotomy. In addition, with increasing numbers of repaired tetralogy of Fallot patients surviving into adulthood, pulmonary regurgitation (PR) is becoming a fairly common diagnosis in adults with congenital heart disease.[4] Some of the long-term sequelae of PR are well known, and include right ventricle (RV) dilation, RV dysfunction, and arrhythmias.[4,5] A negative impact on left ventricle (LV) systolic function has also been demonstrated.[6] Other potential long-term effects of PR, such as the potential for sudden death from arrhythmias, decreased quality of life, and shortened life expectancy, are currently being investigated and may play a larger role in the indications for pulmonary valve repair or replacement. Pulmonary valve replacement in the setting of PR after repaired tetralogy of Fallot has been shown to improve ventricular function and functional class, stabilize QRS duration, and reduce atrial and ventricular arrhythmias.[7-9] The optimal timing of pulmonary valve replacement late after repair of tetralogy of Fallot remains controversial. If performed too late, in patients with impaired RV function, it may not be as beneficial.[10] However, despite many advances in the field of non-invasive diagnostics such as magnetic resonance imaging and tissue Doppler echocardiography, a good marker of preclinical RV dysfunction remains elusive.

Established techniques of pulmonary valve repair

The pulmonary valve again distinguishes itself from other cardiac valves in that pulmonary valve repair is a rarity. The valve can be repaired, the technique generally involving an incision taken through the pulmonary annulus and the anterior pulmonary cusp. The anterior pulmonary cusp is then reconstructed and augmented with a quadrangular patch. The transannular patch is then sutured as usual, anchoring the reconstructed anterior pulmonary cusp to the transannular patch. This technique has been used in selected patients during primary repair of tetralogy of Fallot and in patients with Noonan syndrome.[11,12]

Established techniques of pulmonary valve replacement

General information

Pulmonary valve replacement is a very safe procedure that carries minimal morbidity and mortality.[13,14] Most large series report a hospital mortality rate of less than 1–2%. The main risks arise from the potential difficulties with redo sternotomies, especially in cases where the RV outflow tract (RVOT) is located anterior and close to the posterior table of the sternum. Other potential risks involve accompanying defects that may need to be addressed. Tricuspid valvuloplasties, pulmonary artery plasties, or closure of residual ventricular septal defects are commonly performed at the time of pulmonary valve replacement. Anti-arrhythmic procedures such as the maze procedure of ablation can be added when indicated. In the absence of hemodynamically significant residual defects, postoperative care is usually routine.

Surgical technique

Redo sternotomy is performed as is routine. It is imperative that the status of the peripheral vasculature be known beforehand as the risk of serious hemorrhage from laceration of a vascular structure is always present. Most patients presenting for pulmonary valve replacement are older patients and therefore the groin vessels are usually suitable for emergency peripheral cannulation. However, some patients will have had multiple catheterizations and might have stenotic or occluded groin vessels. In younger children with small inguinal vessels, the neck vessels have been used for emergency cannulation, with good success.[15] The cannulation for and conduct of cardiopulmonary bypass is generally routine. Mild hypothermia may be employed. At the operating surgeon's discretion, the procedure can be performed with or without cardioplegic arrest. The main risk of cardioplegic arrest is the effect of ischemia on a compromised right ventricle. On the other hand, the main advantage of cardioplegic arrest is to provide a perfectly still operative bloodless field. Not using cardioplegic arrest, i.e. per-

forming a pulmonary valve replacement on cardiopulmonary bypass but with a beating heart, carries a risk of systemic air embolism. This technique should be used with great caution if intracardiac shunts are present. Air can then be aspirated from the opened right side of the heart to the left side. Another disadvantage of beating-heart surgery is the less than perfect exposure, although with judicious use of suckers, this is usually not a problem. Therefore, both techniques have definite advantages and drawbacks. Both, however, are perfectly safe provided appropriate preventive measures are taken, such as installing an aortic vent during beating-heart surgery. The RVOT (or the previous conduit) is opened longitudinally, and after making sure there are no proximal or distal stenoses, the prosthesis is inserted (Figure 7.1). It is usual to try to place an oversized prosthesis, especially in younger patients. An antifibrinolytic drug infusion (e.g. aprotinin or aminocaproic acid) is usually given during the procedure. Antibiotic prophylaxis is routine, as in any other valve surgery.

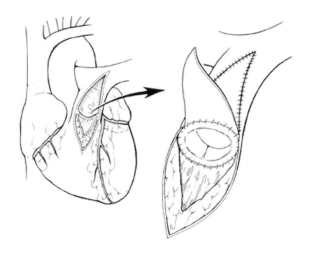

Figure 7.1

Technique of pulmonary valve insertion. A longitudinal incision is made in the main pulmonary artery (with extension into the right ventricular outflow tract (RVOT) if needed). After sizing the pulmonary annulus, a prosthetic valve is inserted by using continuous or interrupted sutures at the level of the annulus. After the pulmonary valve prosthesis is tied in place, a patch is used to augment the anterior portion of the RVOT and main pulmonary artery. The anterior edge of the pulmonary valve prosthesis is sutured to the patch.

Choice of prosthesis

Many choices of prosthesis exist when it comes to pulmonary valve replacement. Mechanical valves are essentially contraindicated because of the need for anticoagulation, the high risk of thrombosis despite adequate anticoagulation (likely due to the lower flow velocities on the right side of the heart), and last but not least the availability of other better prostheses.[16]

Pulmonary valve prostheses are placed orthotopically (i.e. in the bed of the previous pulmonary valve) in the vast majority of cases. Because an oversized valve is usually placed in an effort to increase longevity of the prosthesis, the 'native' RVOT or main pulmonary artery is usually not wide enough, and an anterior patch is usually required to complete RVOT closure (Figure 7.1).

The main categories to choose from are:

- prosthetic tissue valves (bioprosthetic valves) (Figure 7.2)
- biological conduits and homografts (Figure 7.3)
- monocusps.[17,18]

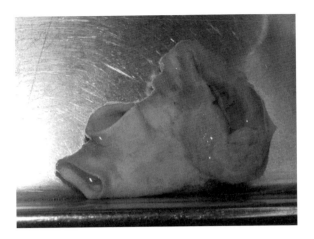

Figure 7.3

A pulmonary homograft as it comes out of the package. Both branch pulmonary artery ostia and the proximal right ventricular outflow tract muscle are visible. It has not yet been trimmed.

Prosthetic tissue valves (bioprosthetic valves)

There are many prosthetic tissue valves available on the market. They were all developed for aortic valve replacement. Prosthetic tissue valves can be divided into stented (i.e. the valve is mounted on a rigid stent that has typically three struts that correspond to each commissure; the stent also provides a sewing ring) or non-stented valves. Stented valves are usually easier to insert, since they require only a single suture line between the 'pulmonary annulus' and the sewing ring. A running suture technique or interrupted sutures can be used. The rigid struts are also sometimes useful in keeping the sternum from compressing the RVOT and the valve. Non-stented ('stentless valves') valves have been used less frequently (Figure 7.4). Insertion is more complex, since they require a proximal and a distal suture line. Their superiority over stented valves has not been demonstrated.[19,20] The most frequently used stentless valves are the Freestyle aortic root bioprosthesis (Medtronic, Inc., Minneapolis, MN) and the Toronto SPV (St Jude Medical, St Paul, MN), both of which are aortic

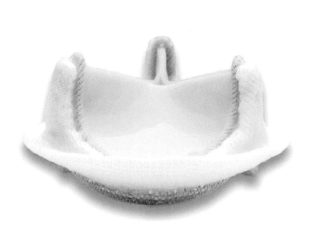

Figure 7.2

A typical bioprosthesis, built with bovine pericardium: the Carpentier–Edwards PERIMOUNT Magna Bioprosthesis. (Courtesy of Edwards Lifesciences, Inc., CA.)

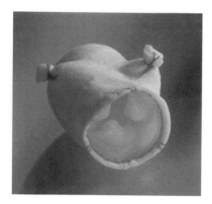

Figure 7.4

A stentless valve, the Freestyle aortic root bioprosthesis. (Courtesy of Medtronic, Inc., Minneapolis, MN.)

porcine valves. No one bioprosthetic tissue valve has been conclusively demonstrated to be superior to the others in terms of longevity. In fact, data reported in similar populations suggest equivalent actuarial and actual freedom from structural valve deterioration at 15 years for pericardial and porcine bioprostheses placed in either the mitral or the aortic position.[21] Some studies have shown superior outcomes of bioprosthetic tissue valves when compared with homografts, but those differences usually disappear when one adjusts for age, since most younger patients undergo homograft insertion and not bioprosthetic valve insertion due to size issues.[13] Younger patients usually calcify their prostheses more rapidly than older patients.[22] Most published series show a very low operative mortality rate, of the order of 1%.[10,13,14,23,24] The freedom from reoperation on the pulmonary valve after PVR is quite high, with a large recent series showing 100% freedom from reoperation at 8 years.[13]

Homografts and biological conduits

Biological conduits and homografts between the RV and pulmonary artery (PA) are frequently used in congenital heart surgery. Homografts are often chosen over bioprosthetic valves because they are available in small sizes. The smallest available size for bioprosthetic valves is usually 19 mm,

whereas homografts as small as 6–7 mm can be found. Hence, smaller and younger patients are more likely to require a homograft. This often skews long-term results towards better freedom from reoperation for bioprosthetic valves. However, if one adjusts for age, those differences usually disappear.[13] The homograft is usually inserted orthotopically using a proximal and a distal suture line. Either it can be placed in the native (usually enlarged) RVOT or it can be sutured as a de novo connection after having detached the native RV–PA connection. Another advantage of homografts is their greater flexibility with respect to distal PA reconstruction. They are very malleable, and one can use the distal conduit portion to reconstruct stenotic PAs. Many studies have looked at determinants of durability of RV–PA conduits and homografts.[22,25–28] The only factors that have been conclusively shown to affect longevity by multivariate analysis are younger age at insertion and smaller homograft size. Further analysis shows that this apparent age influence is mostly due to the small size of the valve at the time of insertion. Some recent biochemical modifications in the way in which homografts are preserved are promising in terms of increasing longevity. The SynerGraft homograft valve, for example, is a new acellular non-glutaraldehyde-fixed tissue heart valve that carries the possibility of autologous recellularization.[29]

Recently, other biological conduits have been made available. Most are not yet approved by the US Food and Drug Administration (FDA), but have been used extensively in Europe. The Contegra (Medtronic Inc., Minneapolis, MN) is a biological valved conduit consisting of a zero-pressure glutaraldehyde-preserved heterologous bovine jugular vein with a trileaflet venous valve with natural sinuses.[30] It has provided encouraging data after experimental studies in animals and in some clinical series. The Shelhigh No-React porcine pulmonic valve conduit is another bovine alternative.[31] Some reports have emerged of a high incidence of distal conduit stenosis due to intimal peel formation in the small-size category (diameter ≤14 mm).[32,33]

Monocusps

The third alternative to either prosthetic valves or RV–PA conduits in pulmonary valve replacement is monocusp valves. These are constructed during surgery by the operating surgeon. The material used is generally polytetrafluoroethylene (PTFE) (Goretex, Gore Inc., Flagstaff, AZ), but pieces of homograft, native pericardium, or bovine pericardium have also been used. By suturing a PTFE patch to the anterior transannular patch material and the anterior RVOT incision edge, the surgeon essentially creates a 'trap door' that allows blood to pass through in one direction only.[17,18] Proponents of monocusps point to the effectiveness at reducing PR in the short and possibly mid term, the ease of implantation, and the very low cost, especially compared with high-priced homografts and prosthetic valves. Opponents argue that the use of monocusps increases cardiopulmonary bypass and ischemic times, and has a fairly high risk of developing pulmonary stenosis in the long term.

In conclusion, pulmonary valve replacement is a very safe and increasingly employed procedure. A wide variety of biological conduits, homografts, and bioprosthetic tissue valves are available. Homografts are most often used in younger and smaller patients, while bioprosthetic valves are often used in older patients.

References

1. Bonow RO, Carabello B, de Leon AC, et al. Guidelines for the management of patients with valvular heart disease (Executive Summary). Circulation 1998; 98: 1949–84.

2. McCrindle BW. Independent predictors of long-term results after balloon pulmonary valvuloplasty. Circulation 1994; 89: 1751–9.

3. Peterson C, Schilthuis JJ, Dodge-Khatami A, et al. Comparative long-term results of surgery versus balloon valvuloplasty for pulmonary valve stenosis in infants and children. Ann Thorac Surg 2003; 76: 1078–82.

4. Therrien J, Marx GR, Gatzoulis MA. Late problems in tetralogy of Fallot – recognition, management and prevention. Cardiol Clin 2002; 3: 395–40.

5. Gatzoulis MA, Balaji S, Webber SA, et al. Risk factors for arrhythmias and sudden death in repaired tetralogy of Fallot; a multi-centre study. Lancet 2000; 356: 975–81.

6. Frigiola A, Redington AN, Cullen S, Vogel M. Pulmonary regurgitation is an important determinant of right ventricular contractile dysfunction in patients with surgically repaired tetralogy of Fallot. Circulation 2004; 110: II153–II157.

7. Eyskens B, Reybrouk T, Bogaert J, et al. Homograft insertion for pulmonary regurgitation after repair of tetralogy of Fallot improves cardiopulmonary exercise performance. Am J Cardiol 2000; 85: 221–5.

8. Therrien J, Siu SC, Harris L, et al. Impact of pulmonary valve replacement on arrhythmia propensity late after repair of tetralogy of Fallot. Circulation 2001; 103: 2489.

9. Oechslin EN, Harrison DA, Harris L, et al. Reoperation in adults with repair of tetralogy of Fallot: indications and outcomes. J Thorac Cardiovasc Surg 1999; 118: 245–51.

10. Therrien J, Siu SC, McLaughlin PR, et al. Pulmonary valve replacement in adults late after repair of tetralogy of Fallot: Are we operating too late? J Am Coll Cardiol 2000; 36: 1670–5.

11. Sung SC, Kim S, Woo JS, Lee YS. Pulmonic valve annular enlargement with valve repair in tetralogy of Fallot. Ann Thorac Surg. 2003; 75: 303–5.

12. Deleon SY, Dorotan J, Abdallah H, et al. Annular and leaflet augmentation in Noonan's syndrome with dysplastic pulmonary valve. Pediatr Cardiol 2003; 24: 574–5.

13. Kanter KR, Budde JM, Parks J, et al. One hundred pulmonary valve replacements in children after relief of right ventricular outflow tract obstruction. Ann Thorac Surg 2002; 73: 1801–7

14. Warner KG, O'Brien PK, Rhodes J, et al. Expanding the indications for pulmonary valve replacement after repair of tetralogy of Fallot. Ann Thorac Surg 2003; 76: 1066–71.

15. Delius RE, Buckley C, Walters HL 3rd. Cervical cannulation for resternotomy in pediatric patients. J Thorac Cardiovasc Surg 2003; 126: 2095–6.

16. Miyamura H, Kanazawa H, Hayashi J, Eguchi S. Thrombosed St. Jude Medical valve prosthesis in the right side of the heart in patients with tetralogy of Fallot. J Thorac Cardiovasc Surg 1987; 94: 148–50.

17. Turrentine MW, McCarthy RP, Vijay P, et al. PTFE monocusp valve reconstruction of the right ventricular outflow tract. Ann Thorac Surg 2002; 73: 871–80.

18. Gundry SR. Pericardial and synthetic monocusp valves: indication and results. Pediatr Cardiac Surg Annual Semin Thorac Cardiovasc Surg 1999; 2: 77–82.

19. Kanter KR, Fyfe DA, Mahle WT, et al. Results with the freestyle porcine aortic root for right ventricular outflow tract reconstruction in children. Ann Thorac Surg 2003; 76: 1889–95.

20. Chard RB, Kang N, Andrews DR, Nunn GR. Use of the Medtronic freestyle valve as a right ventricular to pulmonary artery conduit. Ann Thorac Surg 2001; 71: 361–4.

21. Bach DS. Choice of prosthetic heart valves: update

for the next generation. Am Coll Cardiol 2003; 42: 1717–19.

22. Forbess JM, Shah AS, St Louis JD, et al. Cryopreserved homografts in the pulmonary position: determinants of durability. Ann Thorac Surg 2001; 71: 54–9.

23. Yemets IM, Williams WG, Webb GD, et al. Pulmonary valve replacement late after repair of tetralogy of Fallot. Ann Thorac Surg 1997; 64: 526–30.

24. Discigil B, Dearani JA, Puga FJ, et al. Late pulmonary valve replacement after repair of tetralogy of Fallot. J Thorac Cardiovasc Surg 2001; 121: 344–51.

25. Stark J. The use of valved conduits in pediatric cardiac surgery. Pediatr Cardiol 1998; 19: 282–8.

26. Tweddell JS, Pelech AN, Frommelt PC, et al. Factors affecting longevity of homograft valves used in right ventricular outflow reconstruction for congenital heart disease. Circulation 2000; 102: III130–III135

27. Bando K, Danielson GK, Schaff HV, et al. Outcome of pulmonary and aortic homografts for right ventricular outflow tract reconstruction. J Thorac Cardiovasc Surg 1995; 109: 509–17.

28. Caldarone CA, McCrindle BW, Van Arsdell GS, et al. Independent factors associated with longevity of prosthetic pulmonary valves and valved conduits. J Thorac Cardiovasc Surg 2000; 120: 1022–31.

29. Bechtel JF, Muller-Steinhardt M, Schmidtke C, et al. Evaluation of the decellularized pulmonary valve homograft (SynerGraft). J Heart Valve Dis 2003; 12: 734–9.

30. Corno AF, Qanadli SD, Sekarski N, et al. Bovine valved xenograft in pulmonary position: medium-term follow-up with excellent hemodynamics and freedom from calcification. Ann Thorac Surg 2004; 78: 1382–8.

31. Marianeschi SM, Iacona GM, Seddio F, et al. Shelhigh No-React porcine pulmonic valve conduit: a new alternative to the homograft. Ann Thorac Surg 2001; 71: 619–23.

32. Pearl JM, Cooper DS, Bove KE, Manning PB. Early failure of the Shelhigh pulmonary valve conduit in infants. Ann Thorac Surg 2002; 74: 542–8.

33. Ishizaka T, Ohye RG, Goldberg CS, et al. Premature failure of small-sized Shelhigh No-React porcine pulmonic valve conduit model NR-4000. Eur J Cardiothorac Surg 2003; 23: 715–18.

8

Small intestinal submucosa – a new generation of valve replacement

Carlos E Ruiz, Ulf H Beier

Introduction

The past 20 years have brought remarkable improvements in valvular heart disease, including advances in prosthetic valve development and minimal invasive surgery techniques.[1] To date surgical valve replacement remains the cornerstone therapy for end-stage valvular disease and substantially improves its natural history.[2] There are two types of valve prostheses: mechanical and biological. The mechanical valves have an excellent performance record; however, they are associated with substantial risks of thromboembolism and hemolysis, and therefore need permanent anticoagulation.[3–6] The primary advantage of bioprostheses over mechanical prostheses is the reduction of thromboembolic complications, as opposed to their major disadvantages – mechanical deterioration, degeneration, and calcification.[3–6] Currently, their indication is restricted to patients with either life expectancies shorter than the time interval to repetitive surgery, when the risks of anticoagulation outweigh the benefits of durability, or whenever anticoagulation is not feasible, including females of childbearing age, who should not undergo anticoagulation during pregnancy.[7,8]

Considering advantages as well as disadvantages of currently used prosthetic valves, ongoing improvements in graft endurance, rejection, calcification, thromboembolism, and hemodynamic properties are essential to optimize clinical outcome. Therefore, small intestinal submucosa (SIS) has been introduced into valve replacement as a potential biological valve. SIS bioengineered tissue substitutes have previously been applied in urologic and orthopedic interventions, and

encouraging results have led to their introduction in cardiology and vascular surgery.[9,10] With regard to valvular replacement, however, the data remain contradictory. Up to now, SIS has been applied in porcine, canine, and sheep models.[11–18] Some of the data indicate encouraging results with regard to prolonged graft endurance due to tissue remodeling, growth adaptation, and the possibility of percutaneous delivery. However, problems reported with current valve models based on SIS, such as thickening and degradation as well as degeneration and functional failure, imply the need for caution at present.[19] Further studies will be necessary in order to establish improved versions of the SIS valve before a human application can be considered. This chapter focuses on the properties of SIS tissue, the results of applied SIS valve replacement from animal studies, and future perspectives for this technology.

Small intestinal submucosa

Porcine SIS is an acellular matrix extracted from the jejunum. It can be used as xenograft material because it induces variable degrees of tissue-specific remodeling in the organ or tissue into which it is placed.[9–18,20–23] It is mostly composed of type I collagen, although it has some collagen type III and IV in addition to other extracellular matrix molecules such as fibronectin, hyaluronic acid, chondroitin sulfate A and B, heparin, heparan sulfate, and some growth factors such as basic fibroblast growth factor 2, transforming growth factor β, and vascular endothelial growth factor.

SIS offers two major perspectives in tissue replacement technology. First, its composition has a very low immunogenicity, as a result of several factors. It is acellular, and therefore does not produce antigens that might induce an adverse response from the host. In addition, its extracellular matrix macromolecules are closely related to their human equivalents, which makes them unlikely to evoke rejection. Furthermore, the components of the SIS material are reabsorbed and processed in a matter of weeks to a point where they become virtually untraceable, which eliminates the possibility of inducing an adverse reaction. SIS interacts with the surrounding cells, and in a few weeks, the remodeling process into the tissue it is supposed to replace is significantly advanced. Epithelial cells as well as fibroblasts soon invade the SIS and start rearranging the graft. The spreading host cells multiply, while the SIS collagen undergoes a digestive process, most likely induced by matrix metalloproteinases and other digestive enzymes. New extracellular matrix proteins are secreted by the host cells, and continuously remodel the biological entity of the graft. The unique properties of SIS offer a broad potential for its application as a multifunctional tissue replacement. Even more interesting than remodeling is the potential of SIS to adapt to the challenges of somatic growth. Therefore, the possibility of a valve based upon SIS arose, and was tested in porcine and canine animal models. Nevertheless, its use in humans remains theoretical, since definite studies have yet to prove the concept.

SIS valve in an experimental porcine model

After completion of numerous in vitro experiments, which also included long-endurance extracorporeal cycling studies, the in vivo testing of the SIS valve in an animal model has been initiated.[19] Taking account of the previous work by Matheny et al,[11] who substituted a valve leaflet with SIS material, this experiment was designed to assess long-term hemodynamic as well as histologic properties up to 1 year after placement. The following questions needed to be answered: Can a valve made out of SIS replace a pulmonary valve with regard to its hemodynamic function? Does adaptation to the host tissue occur, as had

been previously reported, and, furthermore, up to a point where the complete SIS material has been entirely remodeled? Does rejection occur? How does the SIS valve react to growth-mediated demands, i.e. can it adapt to an expanding vascular system? Finally, this animal study was also intended to assess the modalities of percutaneous delivery of the SIS valve.

In this experiment, 12 female farm pigs were stented at the native pulmonary valve to induce pulmonary insufficiency. Once right ventricular (RV) dilatation occurred, the SIS valve was implanted. After placement, the animals were euthanized at 1 day, 1 month, 3 months, 6 months, and 12 months post valve implant. The pigs were followed-up by transthoracic Doppler echocardiography (TTE) and postmortem macroscopic and histologic evaluation of the implanted valves.[19]

Construction of the SIS valve

The pulmonary valve prostheses were constructed of square stents with four barbs (Cook Inc., Bloomington, IN) and a hydrated sheet of SIS (Cook Biotech Lafayette, IN), as previously described by Pavcnik et al.[16] The square stents were made of stainless steel wire (0.01905 mm in diameter), based on a SIS valve model previously described in a canine model,[14,15] and are self-expanding devices, which have four corners bent into spring-like coils to reduce stress and metal fatigue. The wire ends are extended 1 mm over the stent frame forming barbs on opposing stent corners to provide anchors for the stent during placement. Two more anchoring barbs were added by attaching a wire to the contralateral side of the stent frame. Two triangular pieces of SIS were sutured with 7.0 Prolene monofilament (Ethicon, Somerville, NJ) to the stent frame to form the valve. The layer of SIS sutured to the metal frame had a flap about 2 mm wide extending beyond the frame.[14,15] All valves were 17 mm in diameter. After construction, the valves were lyophilized and gas-sterilized. The lyophilized SIS sheet was 100–120 μm thick. The valves were then folded and front-loaded into an 8 Fr Teflon sheath 80 cm long (Cook Inc., Bloomington, IN) and delivered coaxially[14,15] (Figure 8.1). Extracorporeal cycling studies of this valve construction were conducted by the manufacturer in advance this experiment.

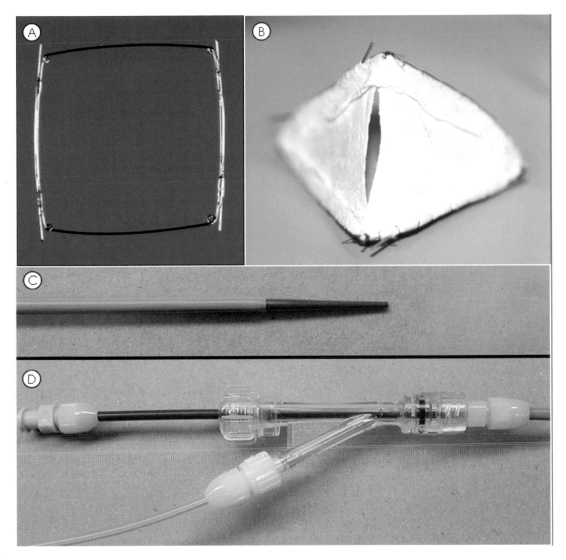

Figure 8.1

(A) Self-expanding square stent. (B) SIS material attached to the square stent; (C, D) Catheter delivery system, 8 Fr.

Preparation of animals with right ventricular failure

Twelve female farm pigs weighing 8–18 kg received sedation with intramuscular atropine 0.05 mg/kg and intravenous tiletamine (Telazol) 4.4 mg/kg and xylazine 2.2 mg/kg. The animals were endotracheally intubated and mechanically ventilated, and gas anesthesia was maintained at stage III, planes 1–2 with 2–3% isoflurane (Isothesia, Burns Veterinary Supply, Rockville Center, NY) in oxygen. The animals then underwent cardiac catheterization for stenting of the native pulmonary valve. Digital fluoroscopy images were obtained and stored with an OEC-9600 C-arm cardiac mobile system (GE Medical Systems, Waukesha, WI). The native pulmonary valve, the distal part of the right ventricular outflow tract (RVOT) and the proximal third of the main pulmonary artery (PA) were covered with two or three metallic stents (Cordis, Miami Lakes, FL). The stents were mounted on a 14.0 mm × 3.0 cm, 7.0 mm × 2.0 mm BIB balloon (NuMed, Hopkinton, NY) and deployed under simultaneous digital fluoroscopic and TTE guidance (Figure 8.2). Moderate to severe pulmonary regurgitation (PR) was documented by color flow Doppler in all animals. The animals were returned to their community cages for a 2- or 4-week period until significant RV dilatation was documented by TTE. One animal died of heart failure before the valve could be implanted.

Percutaneous valve implantation

The 11 surviving animals underwent percutaneous access of the right internal jugular vein under general anesthesia. Using a multipurpose catheter, the stented native pulmonary valve was crossed and an extra stiff Amplatz wire (AGA Medical Corp., Golden Valley, MD) was advanced to one of the distal PA branches. The multipurpose catheter was exchanged for the 8 Fr delivery system, which was advanced over the guidewire into the main PA just distal to the stented valve. The valve was deployed under fluoroscopic and TTE guidance (Figure 8.2). After deployment, the valve orifice was not crossed to prevent any dislodgement and the guidewire was pulled out. The intracardiac echo (ICE) probe (AcuNav, Acuson,

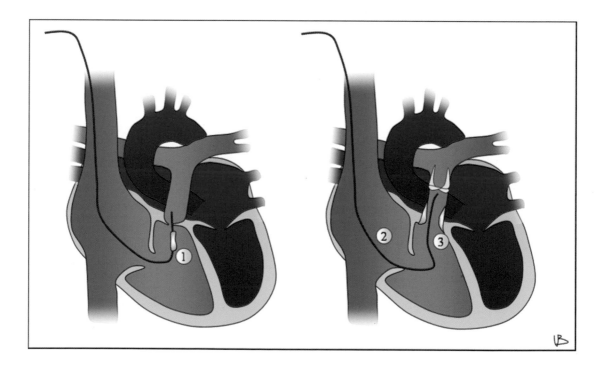

Figure 8.2

Preparation and placement of the SIS valve. Left: Preparation of the pig heart with a pulmonary valve stent (1), resulting in pulmonary insufficiency. Right: Advancement of a low-profile percutaneous delivery system (2) distal to the stented pulmonary valve (3) and placement of the SIS valve.

Mountain View, CA) was advanced to the mid superior vena cava to best visualize the newly implanted valve. The pigs received 100 U/kg of heparin at the beginning of the procedure, and it was not reversed at the end.

Serial follow-up

All 11 animals were placed on 325 mg/day oral aspirin, but no anticoagulants were used. The pigs underwent weekly TTE under sedation for the first 4 weeks following valve implantation. Echocardiograms were obtained using an Acuson Sequoia (Acuson, Mountain View, CA) and a 5 MHz transducer. The images were stored digitally as well as recorded on videotape. After the first 4 weeks post implant, serial TTEs were obtained every 2 weeks until euthanasia. The animals were sacrificed in the following order: one animal at 24 hours, one animal at 1 month, and three animals each at the 3-month, 6-month, and 1-year endpoints. Euthanasia was performed under general anesthesia using sodium pentobarbital 100 mg/kg. Prior to euthanasia, all animals received 50 000 U of heparin intravenously to prevent any postmortem clot formation, and underwent diagnostic cardiac catheterization, angiography, and ICE.

Histology and flow evaluation

Immediately postmortem, the distal RVOT to the PA bifurcation was carefully dissected and removed. The vessel was rinsed in saline and placed in a container with 0.9% sterile iced saline with gentamicin. The container was then placed on ice and sent to the histology laboratory. Prior to fixation and histologic processing, video footage of valve function was acquired. Unfixed valves were placed in tubing of appropriate size to hold the valve in place. Blood flow was simulated with an electric pump circulating 0.9% saline solution through the tubing containing the valve. An endoscope was placed close enough to the valve to capture video images of its function. Afterwards, the valves were placed in 10% neutral buffered formalin and allowed to fix for 24–48 hours. After fixation, the vessels were dehydrated and embedded

in polymethyl methacrylate plastic. After polymerization, the samples were cut on a plane perpendicular to the orifice of the valve. Longitudinal thick sections (approximately 50 μm) were cut with a rotary saw microtome and stained with hematoxylin and eosin (H&E). For immunohistochemical examination, sections of tissue were deparaffinized and rehydrated. Antigen retrieval was accomplished by an antigen retrieval solution (Dako Cytomation, Carpinteria, CA). Endogenous peroxidase was blocked for 15 minutes with 3% hydrogen peroxide. Non-specific immunoglobulin binding was blocked by incubation of slides for 10 minutes with a protein-blocking agent (Dako Cytomation, Carpinteria, CA) prior to application of the primary antibodies (all Dako Cytomation, Carpenteria, CA). Vimentin immunostain was used to document mesenchymal differentiation, desmin, and smooth muscle actin (SMA) for muscle cell differentiation, and von Willebrand factor (vWF) and CD31 for angioformative differentiation. A labelled streptavidin–biotin–peroxidase complex system (Dako Cytomation, Carpinteria, CA) was used to visualize all immune reactions. The immunoreaction was visualized with 3,3'-diaminobenzidine substrate (Dako Cytomation, Carpinteria, CA). Sections were counterstained with Mayer's hematoxylin. Positive immunohistochemical controls included lymph nodes and arteries from normal swine to which the appropriate antisera were added. For negative controls, the primary antibodies were replaced with homologous non-immune sera.[24] An independent, board-certified pathologist, experienced in the evaluation of chronically implanted vascular stents, performed qualitative histopathologic evaluation of the stented vessels. Slides were evaluated for remodeling of the valve material and to assess potential adverse effects with particular attention to the interface between the implant and the vessel wall, as well as to signs of graft rejection.

Adaptation of the SIS valve over 1 year

All 12 animals had their pulmonary valve stented successfully. One animal died of heart failure prior to valve implantation. The SIS valve was percutaneously implanted in 11 pigs (median

23.6 kg, range 17.5–34.4 kg). In 10 animals, the valves were implanted just distal to the distal stent, within the main pulmonary artery. In one animal expected to survive for 1 year, the valve was implanted at the origin of the right PA to minimize the mismatching effects of somatic growth between the valve and the vessel wall. There were no major clinical complications from any of the procedures nor were any observed during the follow-up period (i.e. valve thrombosis or infective endocarditis).

After 1 day the presence of moderate tricuspid regurgitation (TR) was observed post stent implantation in all animals, with an average

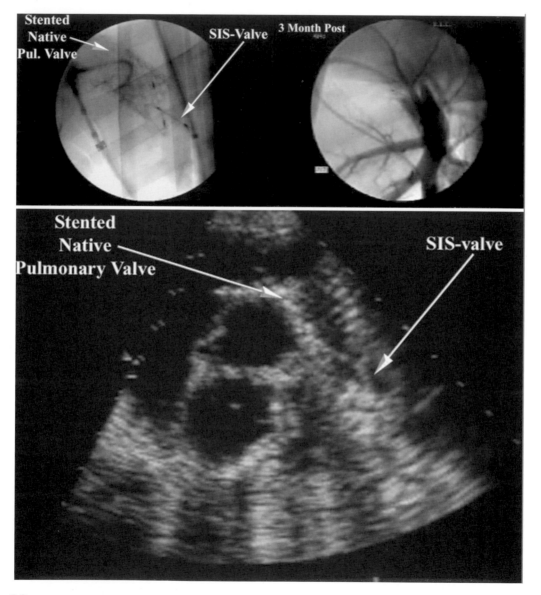

Figure 8.3

Three months post SIS valve placement: Upper panel: Angiography with and without contrast. Lower panel: Transthoracic echocardiography.

velocity of 2.45 m/s. After valve implantation, the TR improved to trace and the TR velocity decreased to 1.40 m/s. There was a moderate degree of perivalvular leak but there was no valvular regurgitation. Perivalvular leak was observed in all implants. The valve appeared well anchored to the pulmonary artery. The implant was attached to the vessel wall by the hooks; however, there was no tissue attachment between the leaflets and the arterial wall. Upon histologic evaluation, the valve leaflets were 17 mm in length and the diameter of the main pulmonary artery (MPA) was 13 mm, resulting in a valve/PA ratio of 1.3. There were no infiltrating host cells. The SIS collagen fibers were separated, resulting in marked edema of the leaflets by infiltration of serum, blood cells, minimal fibrin, and a few platelets. There were no signs of graft rejection.

After 1 month of placement, traces of TR were still present, and the TR average velocity was 1.08 m/s. There was a trivial central jet of pulmonary insufficiency on color flow Doppler and the perivalvular leak was still present in 3 of the 10 animals, although significantly decreased. Video recording of the prosthetic valve within the PA in a pump simulator revealed very pliable leaflets with complete coaptation. The base of the leaflets was firmly adhered to the vessel wall. The valve/PA ratio was 1.02. The leaflets were infiltrated with host fibroblasts and capillaries, but the SIS was still visible. A thin neointima covered large portions of the leaflet. Endothelium partially covered most of the leaflet – some areas only sporadically. There were few lymphocytes and plasma cells, which were not consistent with graft rejection in number and appearance.

Three months after placement, there was no change in the amount of TR and the mean velocity was 1.36 m/s. There was still a trivial central jet PR on color flow Doppler, which had not changed from the 1-month follow-up. There were no perivalvular leaks in any of the 9 animals at 3 months (Figure 8.3). The valve/PA ratios were 0.88. The valve was well anchored to the pulmonary artery. The prosthetic valve was well incorporated and firmly adhered to the vessel wall. There was a minimal progression of leaflet stiffening noted on in vitro video recording, with an apparent increase in leaflet thickness but with complete coaptation (Figure 8.4). The valves were firmly adhered to the vessel wall and the leaflets were

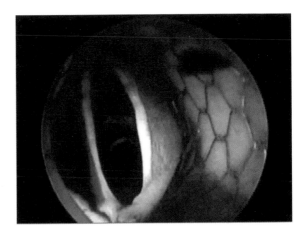

Figure 8.4

Endoscopic view of the SIS valve in situ immediately after euthanization.

slightly shorter (mean 15.6 mm). The base of the leaflets had a thin coating of neointima (usually 20 μm thick), which extended to the remainder of the leaflet as a neointimal coating one or two cells thick. In the middle, leaflets were approximately 200 μm thick and contained mostly dense collagen fibers, with a few capillaries and a few infiltrating host cells. Endothelium was present, but occasionally sporadic. There were no signs of graft rejection (Figures 8.5 and 8.6).

Half a year after implantation of the SIS valve, the TR was essentially unchanged, with a mean velocity of 1.49 m/s. There was no change in the amount of PR in any of the animals and there were no perivalvular leaks. The valve/PA ratios were 0.78. All the valves appeared well anchored to the PA. There was a slight further increase in stiffening and thickness of the leaflets, but they still had complete coaptation. The leaflets were slightly shorter (mean 14.4 mm) and thicker at the base and in the middle of the leaflet. Neointima was usually 50–150 μm thick at the base and tapered towards the tip of the leaflet. In the middle, leaflets were usually 200–400 μm thick (one was up to 1200 μm thick) and fully infiltrated with spindle-shaped host cells, capillaries, arterioles, covered with neointima 10–20 μm thick, and endothelium. There were no signs of graft rejection (Figures 8.5 and 8.6).

Finally 1 year after implantation of the SIS valve, there was an increase in the amount of TR secondary to dilatation of the RV, which

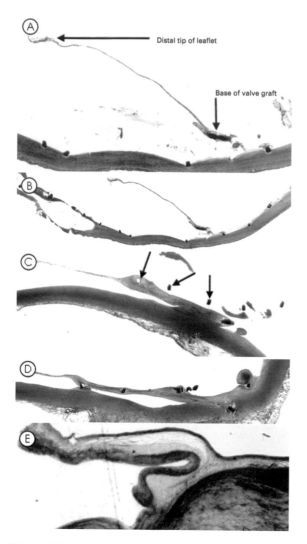

Figure 8.5

Progressive thickening of the SIS valve post placement (H&E staining, ×50 magnification): (A) 1 month post placement; (B) 3 months post placement; (C) 6 months post placement; (D) 1 year post placement; (E) native valve.

progressed from the 10- and 11-month follow-up in the two animals that had had the valve implanted in the MPA. By the 12th month, both

animals had wide open PR and in both animals the valve stent was noted to be broken and separated on one side from the PA wall. The animal that had had the valve implanted in the right PA had trivial PR through the valve and there was no gradient across the valve. All three animals had significant pericardial and pleural effusion. At autopsy, the two animals with the implanted valve in the MPA had dilated RV and right atrium (RA) with large pericardial and pleural effusion. The valve/PA ratio was 0.48. In one animal, a fragment of the stent was noted protruding through the MPA wall. The prosthetic valves implanted in the MPA were both fractured and separated on one side from the PA wall. The valve leaflets were torn on one side and there was a significant mismatch between the valve stent frame diameter (17 mm) and the size of the MPA (34.8 mm) at the time of euthanasia. The animal that had the valve implanted at the origin of the right PA had no fractures of the stent, and the valve was well incorporated within the artery with no tears noted. The valve leaflets ranged from 200 to 1200 μm thick and measured 9 mm. In the middle, leaflets were fully infiltrated with fibroblasts, capillaries, arterioles, and a few scattered lymphocytes, and were covered with neointima 10–20 μm thick and endothelium. A few thick dense collagen fibers were present in the core of the leaflet. Immunohistochemically, the core of the leaflet was phenotypically fibroblastic cells intermixed with dense collagen and capillaries. A layer of spindle-shaped cells that were phenotypically similar to smooth muscle cells surrounded the core. Inflammation was mostly absent. By comparison, native pulmonary leaflets were approximately 5 mm long and ranged from 1 mm thick at the base to approximately 100–300 μm over most of its length. The valve was composed of dense collagenous connective tissue and elastic fibers forming bands under the endothelium on both surfaces. The central surface of the valve, which was continuous with the endocardium, had slightly thicker connective tissue (approximately 100 μm thick) than the peripheral side (<50 μm thick) (Figures 8.5–8.8).

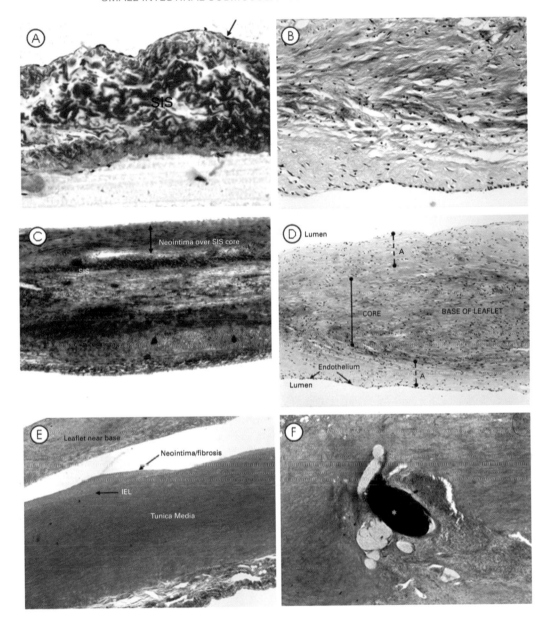

Figure 8.6

H&E staining of the SIS valve samples showing progressive remodeling: (A) ×200 magnification 1 month post placement, showing endothelium and occasional fibroblasts; (B) ×200 magnification 3 months post placement, showing remodeling of the valve core with fibroblasts; (C) ×100 magnification 6 months post placement and (D) ×100 magnification 1 year post placement, showing ongoing remodeling demonstrating the presence of smooth muscle cells and fibroblasts, as well as the gradual disappearance of the original SIS material. (E, F) Adverse reactions: (E) H&E staining, ×100 magnification showing intimal fibrosis; (F) H&E staining, ×500 magnification demonstrating fibrosis and calcification around the square stent.

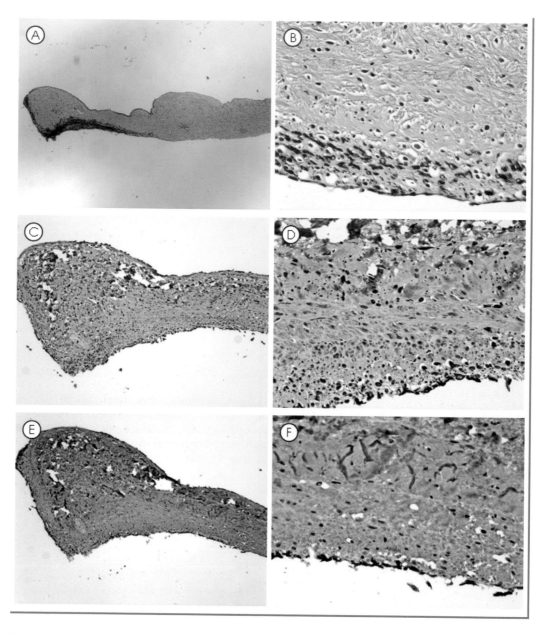

Figure 8.7

Immunohistochemistry, 1 year post placement: (A, B) ×50 and ×200 magnification smooth muscle antibody; (C, D) ×100 and ×200 magnification vimentin antibody; (E, F) ×100 and ×200 magnification von Willebrand antibody.

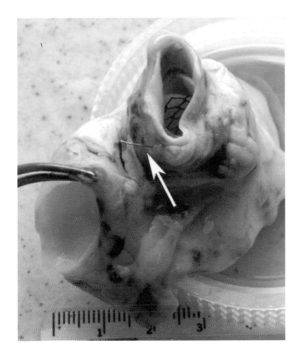

Figure 8.8

At 1 year post implant in the main pulmonary artery, there were fractures of the valve stent in one animal. A fragment of the stent from the SIS valve perforated the wall of the pulmonary artery.

Implications for current valve replacement strategies

The results of the recent work on the SIS valve based upon a metal string support the tissue remodeling and low immunogenicity as beneficial for graft endurance and adaptation; however, it also revealed weaknesses with regard to tissue thickening and paravalular leakage. The implications of the data presented are discussed below.

Valvular graft endurance

Valve replacement using bioprosthetic valves has been performed for more than 30 years; however, the graft endurance of biological tissue valves after placement is still a significant problem, with only little improvement in recent decades.[25,26] The

mechanisms by which biological valves degrade are multifactorial, with involvement of immunologic rejection, mechanical wear, calcification, and enzymatic digestion with subsequent loss of the original histologic integrity.[27–29] Recent work on SIS valves suggests that they provide substantial improvements in many aspects associated with early tissue remodeling as well as lack of significant immunologic rejection, which is frequently assessed by histology, suggesting prolonged graft survival.[30,31] This observation is likely to be explained by the lack of antigens and the histologic remodeling of the SIS material, leading to the expression of host antigens.

The mechanisms of bioprosthetic valve degeneration are an area of great interest. Simionescu et al[28] investigated the influence of bioprosthetic valve preparation during manufacture and whether this can influence durability in a swine model. They found that glutaraldehyde preservation of bioprosthetic valves failed to prevent the breakdown of glycosaminoglycans and elastin-associated microfibrils. The latter have important mechanical functions in addition to protecting elastin from calcification.[32–34] Recently, several attempts have been made to prevent glutaraldehyde-treated valves from calcifying. Vasudev et al[35] found calcification to be slowed by iron and magnesium supplements. In contrast, the SIS valve does not need pretreatment with glutaraldehyde, thus avoiding early calcification. Furthermore, the induction of early remodeling of the SIS leads to de novo synthesis of extracellular matrix macromolecules, including elastin-associated microfibrils. A comparable approach avoiding glutaraldehyde preparation has been attempted by O'Brien et al,[36] who introduced an artificially decellularized porcine valve (the SynerGraft valve). However, its application to humans did not meet the expectations arising from the preclinical trials. Bechtel et al[37] reported a reduced immunologic response after SynerGraft pulmonary homograft implantation; however, this did not translate into any clinical advantage. The experience from the SynerGraft valve implied that decellularization was effective in decreasing rejection and avoiding calcification, without any improvement in endurance. The ability of the SIS material to become remodeled might be the key point in creating a valve replacement more closely resembling native valves and contributing to prolonged graft survival.

Adaptation to somatic growth

Somatic growth of juvenile cardiac outflow tract vessels is a significant challenge to the adaptation and durability of a prosthetic valve in the pediatric population. All current prosthetic valves lack the ability to adapt to somatic growth, and are therefore far from ideal for patients with an anticipated relevant growth of the heart vessels.[38] In children, pulmonary autografts are the treatment of choice for aortic valve replacement, mainly because of their preferable adaptation to somatic growth.[38,39] The ability of the SIS valve to remodel suggests that it might be able to adapt to somatic growth once it has been implanted. However, there are a number of limitations of the currently investigated SIS valve types. The SIS valves currently used include a square metal stent, which cannot expand beyond its physical limits. Therefore, current SIS valves need to be placed at those points in the vascular system where the vessel diameter does not exceed the size of the metal square stent frame. However, there are investigations underway that might further improve the SIS valves and make them more adaptable to somatic growth.

SIS valve in low-profile percutaneous placement

Currently, surgical procedures still make up the vast majority of valve replacements.[40,41] There are certain subtypes of valvular disease, such as ischemic and rheumatic mitral insufficiency, for which repair has been shown to be superior to replacement.[42] The problem of surgery in these instances is that the outcome of surgical valve replacement, regarding intraoperative risks and the long-term results with the implanted valve, force clinicians to balance risks versus benefits, and so the high rate of complications tends to delay surgical valve replacement for as long as possible. A major consideration of surgery for valve replacement is the need for cardiopulmonary bypass, which leads to a number of secondary complications including ischemic brain injuries and damage to other organs.[1,43] At the time of surgical replacement, there are often irreversible changes to heart function. These place a further burden on the heart after the procedure. This may change in the future, if new valves with fewer side-effects and minimally invasive replacement procedures emerge, enabling an early indication for valve replacement.

Percutaneous catheter-based systems for the treatment of valvular heart disease have been studied in animal models for several years, including valve replacement as well as repair procedures.[18,44–48] The major advantage of this approach is that it does not require surgery. Nevertheless, surgical procedures still make up the vast majority of valve replacements.[40] In 2002, Bonhoeffer et al,[43] using a bovine jugular vein valve mounted on a stent, performed the first in-human percutaneous implantations of artificial valves in children with RV-to-PA prosthetic conduits. In addition, Cribier et al[49] described one case report of a successful percutaneous valve replacement in a 57-year-old man. Subsequent experiments in eight patients with aortic stenosis substantiated this valve replacement technique, and showed an improvement of left ventricular global and regional systolic function evidenced by tissue Doppler imaging.[50] The percutaneous placement of valve grafts is a particularly interesting alternative for patients with medical conditions contraindicating an invasive surgical procedure.[51,52]

Current implantation procedures are based on large delivery systems. Bonhoeffer et al[43] used 22 Fr catheters for pulmonary valve placement and Cribier and colleagues[49,50] used 22 and 24 Fr for aortic valve placement. In previous experiments with SIS valves, 8 and 9 Fr catheter delivery systems were used. These results suggest that the percutaneous placement procedure could be made even less invasive using low-profile delivery systems, and might therefore substantiate the potential of this upcoming technology.

SIS valves: future perspective

Current data from preclinical in vivo SIS testing are ambiguous. On the one hand, there is strong support for the ability of SIS valves to remodel and to adopt the histologic properties of the original valve. However, the data also suggest ongoing thickening of the valve leaflets, which might indicate a potential source of problems in exposures lasting longer than 1 year. Furthermore, the design of current SIS valves needs to be improved. Even though initial hemodynamic properties were promising, ongoing vessel expansion finally overcame the ability to compensate for somatic growth and led to paravalvular leakage. There are several ways to approach this problem. The metal ring, which, with its current composition, cannot expand beyond its physical limits, could be removed and a valve constructed from SIS tissue and other soluble materials, or the metal ring could be replaced by a structure that allows expansion after placement.

Conclusion

The current state of investigation of SIS valves is at an advanced preclinical in vivo stage, with the need for crucial improvements in design in order to respond to the main concerns regarding current construction, before clinical trials can be undertaken. Future SIS valves need to be able to compensate for growth adaptation, and they require further proof of long-term endurance, especially with regard to leaflet thickening. The potential of SIS-based valve replacement remains, since current data support their advantages of tissue remodeling and the lack of host rejection reactions contributing to degeneration. Furthermore, excellent low-profile percutaneous placement results encourage ongoing investigations to reach a final version of this valve. Therefore, further animal studies will be necessary, which will cover an improved valve, larger sample numbers, and prolonged testing intervals. Finally, if these experiments are successful, a controlled clinical trial could conclude the development of this promising new approach to valvular heart disease.

References

1. Carabello BA, Crawford FA. Valvular heart disease. N Engl J Med 1997; 337: 32–41.
2. Braunwald E. Valvular heart disease. In: Braunwald E (ed). Heart Disease, 4th edn. Philadelphia: WB Saunders, 1992: 1007–77.
3. Vongpatanasin W, Hillis LD, Lange RA. Prosthetic heart valves. N Engl J Med 1996; 335: 407–16.
4. Hammermeister KE, Sethi GK, Henderson WG, et al. Outcomes 15 years after replacement with a mechanical versus bioprosthetic valve: final report from the Veterans Affairs randomized trial. J Am Coll Cardiol 2000; 36: 1152–8.
5. Rahimtoola SH. Choice of prosthetic heart valve for adult patients. J Am Coll Cardiol 2003; 41: 893–904.
6. Bloomfied P, Wheatley DJ, Prescott RJ, et al. Twelve-year comparison of a Björk–Shiley mechanical heart-valve with porcine bioprosthesis. N Engl J Med 1991; 324: 573–9.
7. Reimold SC, Rutherford JD. Valvular heart disease in pregnancy. N Engl J Med 2003; 349: 52–9.
8. Hung L, Rahimtoola SH. Prosthetic heart valves and pregnancy. Circulation 2003; 107: 1240–6.
9. Aiken SW, Badylak SF, Toombs JP. Small intestinal submucosa as an intra-articular ligamentous graft material: a pilot study in dogs. Vet Comp Orthoped Trauma 1994; 7: 124–8.
10. Knapp PM, Lingeman JE, Siegel YI, et al. Biocompatibility of small intestinal submucosa in urinary tract as augmentation cystoplasty graft and injectible suspension. J Endourol 1994; 8: 125–30.
11. Matheny RG, Hutchinson ML, Dryden PE, et al. Porcine small intestinal submucosa as a pulmonary valve leaflet substitute. J Heart Valve Dis 2000; 9: 769–75.
12. Badylak SF, Lantz GC, Coffey A, Geddes LA. Small intestinal submucosa as a large diameter vascular graft in the dog. J Surg Res 1989; 47: 74–80.
13. Badylak SF, Voytik SL, Kokini K. The use of xenogeneic small intestinal submucosa as a biomaterial for Achilles tendon repair in a dog model. J Biomed Mater Res 1995; 29: 977–85.
14. Lantz GC, Badylak SF, Coffey A, et al. Small intestinal submucosa as a small-diameter arterial graft in the dog. J Invest Surg 1990; 3: 217–27.
15. Lantz GC, Badylak SF, Coffey AC, et al. Small intestinal submucosa as a superior vena cava graft in the dog. J Surg Res 1992; 53: 175–81.
16. Pavcnik D, Uchida BT, Timmermans HA, et al. Percutaneous bioprosthetic venous valve: a long-term study in sheep. J Vasc Surg 2002; 35: 598–602.
17. Brountzos E, Pavcnik D, Timmermans HA, et al. Remodeling of suspended small intestinal submucosa venous valve: an experimental study in sheep to assess the host cells' origin. J Vasc Interv Radiol 2003; 14: 349–56.
18. Pavcnik D, Machan L, Uchida B, et al. Percutaneous prosthetic venous valves: current state and possible applications. Tech Vasc Interv Radiol 2003; 6: 137–42.
19. Ruiz C, Iemura M, Medie S, et al. Transcatheter placement of a low-profile biodegradable pulmonary valve made of small intestinal submucosa: a long-term study in a swine model. J Thorac Cardiovasc Surg 2005; 130: 477–84..
20. Badylak SF. Small intestinal submucosa (SIS): A biomaterial conducive to smart tissue remodeling. In: Bell E (ed). Tissue Engineering: Current

Perspectives. Cambridge, MA: Birkhaüser, 1993: 179–89.

21. Cobb MA, Badylak SF, Janas W, et al. Histology after dural grafting with small intestinal submucosa. Surg Neurol 1996; 46; 389–93.

22. Prevel CD, Eppley BL, Summerlin DJ, et al. Small intestinal submucosa: utilization as a wound dressing in full-thickness rodent wounds. Ann Plast Surg 1995; 35: 381–5.

23. Prevel CD, Eppley BL, Sumerlin DJ, et al. Small intestinal submucosa (SIS): utilization for repair of rodent abdominal wall defects. Ann Plast Surg 1995; 35: 374–80.

24. Patrick DJ, Kiupel M, Gerber V, et al. Malignant granulosa–theca cell tumor in a 2-year-old miniature horse. J Vet Diagn Invest 2003; 15: 60–3.

25. Barratt-Boyes BG, Roche AH, Subramanyan R, et al. Long-term follow-up of patients with antibiotic-sterilized aortic homograft valve inserted freehand in the aortic position. Circulation 1987; 75: 768–77.

26. Lund O, Chandrasekaran V, Grocott-Mason R, et al. Primary aortic valve replacement with allografts over twenty-five years: valve-related and procedure-related determinants of outcome. J Thorac Cardiovasc Surg 1999; 117: 77–91.

27. Green MK, Walsh MD, Dare A, et al. Histological and immunohistochemical responses after aortic valve allografts in the rat. Ann Thorac Surg 1998; 66: 216–20.

28. Simionescu DT, Lovekamp JJ, Vyavahare NR. Degeneration of bioprosthetic heart valve cusp and wall tissues is initiated during tissue preparation: an ultrastructural study. J Heart Valve Dis 2003; 12: 226–34.

29. Simionescu DT, Lovekamp JJ, Vyavahare NR. Glycosaminoglycan-degrading enzymes in porcine aortic heart valves: implications for bioprosthetic heart valve degeneration. J Heart Valve Dis 2003; 12: 217–25.

30. Chen Y, Demir Y, Valujskikh A, et al. Antigen location contributes to the pathological features of a transplanted heart graft. Am J Pathol 2004; 164: 1407–15.

31. Weiser AC, Franco I, Herz DB, et al. Single layered small intestinal submucosa in the repair of severe chordee and complicated hypospadias. J Urol 2003; 170: 1593–5.

32. Lillie MA, David GJ, Gosline JM. Mechanical role of elastin-associated microfibrils in pig aortic elastic tissue. Connect Tissue Res 1998; 37: 121–41.

33. Pereira L, Lee SY, Gayraud B, et al. Pathogenetic sequence for aneurysm revealed in mice underexpressing fibrillin-1. Proc Natl Acad Sci USA 1999; 96: 3819–23.

34. Wallin R, Wajih N, Greenwood GT, et al. Arterial

calcification: a review of mechanisms, animal models, and the prospects for therapy. Med Res Rev 2001; 21: 274–301.

35. Vasudev SC, Chandy T, Umasankar MM, Sharma CP. Inhibition of bioprosthesis calcification due to synergistic effect of Fe/Mg ions to polyethylene glycol grafted bovine pericardium. J Biomater Appl 2001; 16: 93–107.

36. O'Brien MF, Goldstein S, Walsh S, et al. The Syner-Graft valve: a new acellular (nonglutaraldehyde-fixed) tissue heart valve for autologous recellularization first experimental studies before clinical implantation. Semin Thorac Cardiovasc Surg 1999; 11: 194–200.

37. Bechtel JF, Muller-Steinhardt M, Schmidtke C, et al. Evaluation of the decellularized pulmonary valve homograft (SynerGraft). J Heart Valve Dis 2003; 12: 734–9.

38. Elkins RC, Knott-Craig CJ, Ward KE, et al. Pulmonary autograft in children: realized potential growth. Ann Thorac Surg 1994; 57: 1387–94.

39. Solymar L, Südow G, Holmgren D. Increase in size of the pulmonary autograft after the Ross operation in children: growth or dilation. J Thorac Cardiovasc Surg 2000; 119: 4–9.

40. Schwarz F, Baumann P, Manthey J, et al. The effect of aortic valve replacement on survival. Circulation 1982; 66: 1105–10.

41. Morris JJ, Schaff HV, Mullany CJ, et al. Gender differences in left ventricular functional response to aortic valve replacement. Circulation 1994; 90: 183–9.

42. Tribouilloy CM, Enriquez-Sarano M, Schaff HV, et al. Impact of preoperative symptoms on survival after surgical correction of organic mitral regurgitation: rationale for optimizing surgical indications. Circulation 1999; 99: 400–5.

43. Bonhoeffer P, Boudjemline Y, Qureshi SA, et al. Percutaneous insertion of the pulmonary valve. J Am Coll Cardiol 2002; 39: 1664–9.

44. Davies H. Catheter mounted valve for temporary relief of aortic insufficiency. Lancet 1965; 1: 250.

45. Andersen HR, Knudsen LL, Hasemkam JM. Transluminal implantation of artificial heart valves: description of a new expandable aortic valve and initial results with implantation by catheter technique in closed chest pigs. Eur Heart J 1992; 13: 704–8.

46. Kaye D, Byrne M, Alferness C, Power J. Feasibility and short-term efficacy of percutaneous mitral annular reduction for the therapy of heart failure-induced mitral regurgitation. Circulation 2003; 108: 1795–7.

47. Fann J, St Goa FG, Komtebedde J, et al. Beating heart catheter-based edge-to-edge mitral valve

procedure in a porcine model: efficacy and healing response. Circulation 2004; 110: 988–93.

48. Boudjemline Y, Bonnet D, Sidi D, Bonhoeffer P. Percutaneous implantation of a biological valve in the aorta to treat aortic valve insufficiency – a sheep study. Med Sci Monit 2002; 8: 113–16.

49. Cribier A, Eltchaninoff H, Bash A, et al. Percutaneous transcatheter implantation of an aortic valve prosthesis for calcific aortic stenosis: first human case description. Circulation 2002; 106: 3006–8.

50. Bauer F, Eltchaninoff H, Tron C, et al. Acute improvement in global and regional left ventricular systolic function after percutaneous heart valve implantation in patients with symptomatic aortic stenosis. Circulation 2004; 110: 1473–6.

51. Cribier A, Eltchaninoff H, Tron C, et al. Early experience with percutaneous transcatheter implantation of heart valve prosthesis for the treatment of end-stage inoperable patients with calcific aortic stenosis. Am J Coll Cardiol 2004; 43: 698–703.

52. Eltchaninoff H, Tron C, Cribier A. Percutaneous implantation of aortic valve prosthesis in patients with calcific aortic stenosis: technical aspects. Ann Interv Cardiol 2003; 16: 515–21.

9

Available transcatheter pulmonary valves: Perventricular technique with the Shelhigh valve

Zahid Amin

Introduction

The era of pediatric cardiac surgery began when Walton Lillehi performed the first successful procedure for closure of ventricular septal defect using the patient's mother as cross-circulation. Despite significant advances in cardiopulmonary bypass (CPB) techniques, there are unknown risks associated with CPB that led physicians to devise new ways to avoid it. Minimally invasive surgery and percutaneous techniques have progressed significantly; more and more hybrid procedures are being employed to optimize patient care. The full range of side-effects of CPB in the pediatric population remains unknown, and their severity may be related to the length of CPB as well as the patient's age. It can be speculated that in children who are in a developmental stage, the effects may be worse than in an adult.[1]

The pioneering work of percutaneous pulmonary[2,3] and aortic valve[4] placement is well known. There are, however, some limitations of the pulmonary valve procedures in the pediatric population. These procedures require a large sheath size and may be difficult or not feasible in patients with smaller body surface area. In addition, some patients have a very dilated pulmonary outflow tract and would require valves that are larger than those being investigated.[5]

Perventricular closure of ventricular septal defects was introduced by us in 1997 and published in 1998.[6,7] It is now an accepted hybrid procedure for closure of difficult ventricular septal defects in small patients where percutaneous closure is not feasible or increases the chance of complications.[8]

Pulmonary valve placement is recommended in patients with severe pulmonary insufficiency due to native or bioprosthetic valve dysfunction. These patients' diagnoses include truncus arteriosus, Ross operation, pulmonary atresia with or without ventricular septal defects, and others.[5] The detrimental effects of pulmonary insufficiency on right ventricular outflow are being recognized with increasing frequency.[9] Depending upon the diagnosis and the type of repair, the morphology of the right ventricular outflow tract (RVOT) differs from one patient to another. Most of the patients who are candidates for valve placement may have significantly dilated RVOT and they may require valves larger than 20 mm.

In order to have a valve available for large outflow tracts, we decided to evaluate the applicability of the Shelhigh pulmonary valve in a self-expanding tracheobronchial stent (Cook-Z stent).

Methods

All animals received humane care in compliance with the 'Guide for the Care and Use of Laboratory Animals'.[10]

The stent

A Cook-Z stent (Gianturco–Rosch tracheo-bronchial design; Cook, Bloomington, IN) was used for the study (Figure 9.1). This is a self-expanding stent available in single-body and multibody configurations to increase malleability. Available sizes include 15, 20, 25, and 30 mm. Its outer surface has hooks pointing in opposite directions to prevent antegrade or retrograde slipping of the stent. The stent is crimpable after expansion and has excellent hoop strength. It was modified so that each body was 2.5 cm in length, with two bodies measuring 5.0 cm in total length. The diameter of the stent chosen for this study was 20 mm.

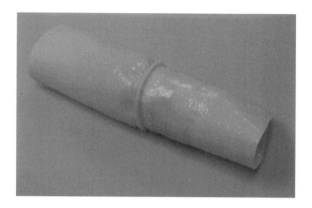

Figure 9.2

The Shelhigh pulmonary valve tube.

The Shelhigh valve conduit

The Shelhigh valve porcine pulmonary valve conduit is approved by the US Food and Drug Administration (FDA) (Figure 9.2). It has been used in the pulmonary position in the pediatric population with equivocal results.[11,12] The valve is

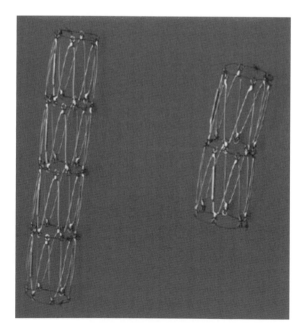

Figure 9.1

The Cook-Z stent: two-body (right) and multibody (left).

coated with No-React™ material, which appears to decrease calcification of the valve after implantation. It is available in an array of sizes ranging up to 26 mm diameter. The valve and part of the pulmonary tube were trimmed and sutured inside the Cook-Z stent (Figure 9.3). The inner surface of the stent was covered with a sleeve of bovine pericardium. After the valve was sewn into the stent, the stent was crimped into the delivery gun and loaded (Figure 9.3). The tip of the delivery gun was tapered to ease its introduction through the right ventricular free wall. The diameter of the delivery gun was 24 Fr.

The study was conducted in a sheep model weighing 35–45 kg. The perventricular technique remains the same as has been described in our previous studies.[7–9]

All procedures were performed under general anesthesia. The animal was placed on its back and the chest was shaved. The animal was prepped and draped in sterile fashion. The chest was opened via median sternotomy; in one sheep, a right thoracotomy was performed. The pericardium was opened longitudinally and cradled with stay sutures. A purse-string suture was placed on the right ventricle. Epicardial echocardiography was performed during the procedure. The diameter of the pulmonary valve was measured by 2D echocardiography. The diameter of the pulmonary valve was also measured directly with the help of calipers. Based upon the diameter, an appropriately sized stented valve was loaded into the delivery gun. A purse-string suture was placed on the free wall of the right ventricle;

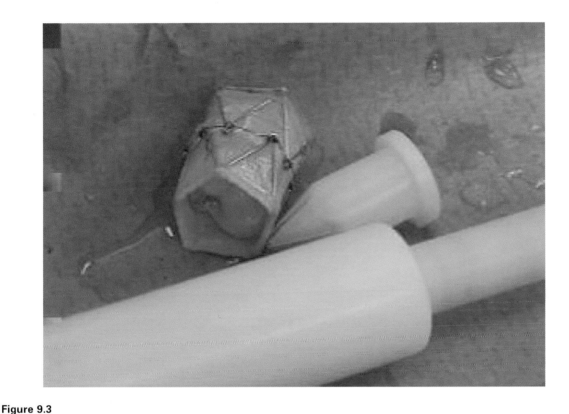

Figure 9.3

Cook-Z stent with pericardial sleeve and stent sutured (top left). The delivery gun and the introducer are also shown.

this suture was reinforced with Shelhigh bovine pericardial strips. The right ventricle was punctured with a sharp knife. The tip of the delivery gun was advanced through the right ventricular free wall and the pulmonary valve was crossed. By pulling the outer tube that carried the pulmonary valve, in the RVOT, we deployed the stented valve. Care was taken to completely cover the pulmonary valve with the stented valve so that the native valve would not be effective. Epicardial echocardiography was performed to ensure proper positioning of the stented valve. The chest was closed in the routine fashion and the animal extubated the same day.

The animals were followed for 7 months. At the conclusion of follow-up, the animal was brought to the cardiac catheterization laboratory. Femoral venous access was obtained and a wedge catheter was advanced through the femoral venous sheath to the right atrium, right ventricle, and pulmonary artery, to obtain hemodynamics.

Angiograms were performed with a Berman angiographic catheter. Transthoracic echocardiography was also performed during the catheterization to obtain maximal information, although the picture quality was not good because of poor acoustic windows.

The animals were euthanized at the conclusion of cardiac catheterization. The chest was opened and the heart was separated from adhesion and removed. Gross and microscopic examinations were performed of the valve and stent.

Results

The procedure was successful in all sheep. The first sheep was euthanized after the procedure to obtain acute results. The hooks of the stent were embedded into the pulmonary artery, and the stent appeared stable. The integrity of the valve was checked with saline and found to be normal.

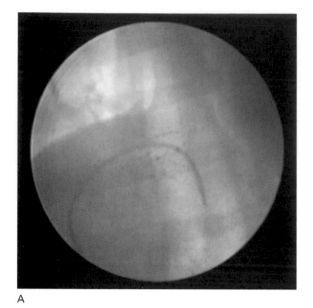

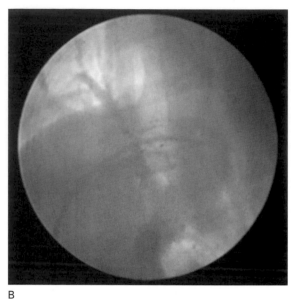

A

B

Figure 9.4

(A, B) Contrast injection in the branch pulmonary arteries. Cine angiograms showing the stented valve in place. No pulmonary insufficiency is present.

Cardiac catheterization data in the animals that were euthanized after 7 months revealed no gradient across the stented valve. Angiograms revealed a wide-open RVOT with well-functioning pulmonary conduit (Figure 9.4A). The integrity of the valve was maintained. In one sheep, mild pulmonary insufficiency was noted. The branch pulmonary arteries were wide open (Figure 9.4B).

After explanting the heart, the right ventricle was opened and the RVOT was exposed. Gross examination revealed that the stent was covered with neo-endocardium that was continuous with the surrounding endocardium (Figures 9.5 and 9.6). The native valve was completely covered with the stent, rendering it non-functional. There was no evidence of external injury because of the hooks on the outer surface of the Cook-Z stent.

The microscopic examination revealed that the new fibrovascular tissue surrounded the wires of the stent. This tissue was continuous from the surface of the pulmonary valve. Low magnification of the slides revealed normal response of the body to stent valve tissue (Figure 9.7). Higher magnification adjacent to the valve leaflet revealed endothelial cell-like lining (Figures 9.8 and 9.9).

Conclusions

The perventricular approach for stented valve placement was successfully applied in this experiment. This is ongoing work and more sheep will undergo such experiments in the future. A similar approach has been described by Zhou et al.[12] There are several distinct advantages to the perventricular approach. It is feasible in smaller patients as there are no vascular issues involved with this approach. Although sternotomy is required, CPB is avoided. This feature will help decrease morbidity and mortality. The hospital stay is shortened. The potential complications of CPB for vital organs are avoided and the procedure time is shorter. If for any reason the placement of the stented valve is not possible, a stentless Shelhigh or other pulmonary valve can be placed by placing the patient on CPB; hence the success rate will be extremely high. In addition, all potential complications of the cardiac

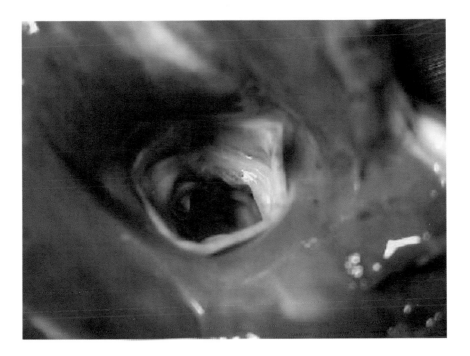

Figure 9.5

The stent after opening the pulmonary artery. Nice endothelialization is seen that is continuous with the surrounding pulmonary artery tissue.

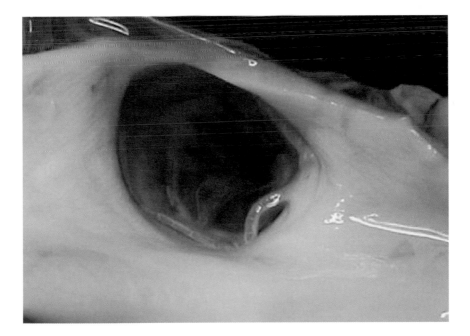

Figure 9.6

The right ventricular aspect of the stented valve. The stent appears to be endothelialized completely. The valve is wide open.

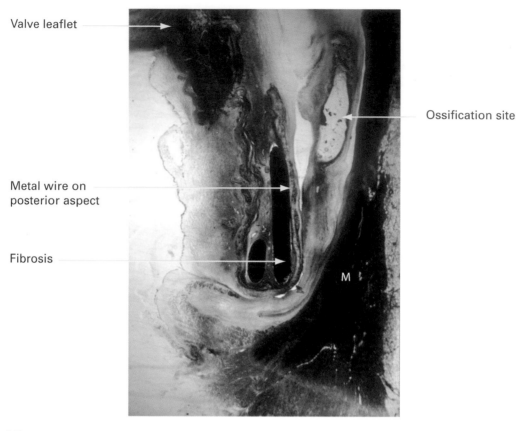

Valve leaflet

Ossification site

Metal wire on
posterior aspect

Fibrosis

M

Figure 9.7

Microscopic examination of the laser-cut portion of the valve. A normal response of the body to metal and the valve is seen. M, muscle tissue.

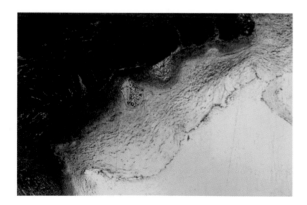

Figure 9.8

Microscopic examination (higher magnification) of the valve leaflet. The multifilament suture (bottom right) can be seen, and covering this multifilament and native tissue are endothelial cells.

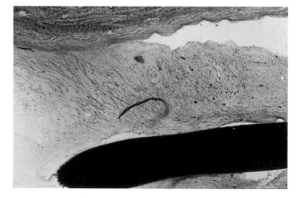

Figure 9.9

Higher magnification of the valve leaflet shows endothelial-like cells. The dark shadow at the bottom is a magnified stent wire.

catheterization laboratory – technical, stented-valve-related, access-related, and fluoroscopy-related – can be avoided.

The Shelhigh valve is already approved by the FDA and the results in the pediatric population are promising. The No-React treatment will prevent the valve from early calcification,[12] which will improve the durability of the valve, ultimately benefiting the patient.

The Cook-Z stent is not approved by the FDA for intravascular use, although experimental animal data are suggestive of good results (personal communication). It is a self-expandable stent with excellent hoop strength. The hooks prevent migration of the stent, once it has been released, towards the pulmonary artery or the RVOT. The disadvantage of the stent is that it is not retrievable once deployed. The hooks on the stent appear to cause no injury to the outflow tract or the pulmonary artery. Although no deleterious effects of the stent were seen in this experiment, long-term investigation is imperative before human trials can be conducted.

Histologic studies have shown that the stented valve endothelializes well. The growth of endothelial-like cells over the valve leaflet is heartening and may increase the longevity of the valve leaflets.

Future direction with this technique will include decreasing the delivery sheath size to 20 Fr or less, so that a percutaneous technique can be employed. If the procedure is performed using a percutaneous technique, a delivery system that will maintain the integrity of the valve will need to be available. The stented valve should be able to follow the acute turns in the RVOT well, since it is a multibody stent and can fold easily.

Acknowledgments

This study was supported by Shelhigh Company and would not have been possible without the expert opinion and guidance of Dr Shlomo Gabbay. The experiments were carried out at the Robert W Johnson Hospital, NJ under the guidance of Dr Schulz, Chief of Cardiothoracic Surgery. His expert opinion and suggestions are appreciated very much.

I very much appreciate Mr Jay Leonard and Ms Sarah Guillian of Cook Corporation, who were instrumental in modifying the stent and who supplied the stent free of charge for this study. Thanks are due to Mr Brian Bates for his unconditional support of this project.

Finally, I am indebted to Janson Emmanual, who did histologic work on the explanted valves.

References

1. Kwern FH, Hickey PR. The effects of cardiopulmonary bypass on the brain. In: Jonas RA (ed). Cardiopulmonary Bypass in Neonates and Infants and Young Children. Boston: Blackwell Science, 1994: 263–78.

2. Bonhoeffer P, Boudjemline Y, Saliba Z, et al. Transcatheter implantation of a bovine valve in a pulmonary position. Circulation 2000; 102: 813.

3. Bonhoeffer P, Boudjemline Y, Qureshi S, et al. Percutaneous insertion of the pulmonary valve. J Am Coll Cardiol 2002; 39: 1664–9.

4. Cribier A, Eltchaninoff H, Tron C, et al. Early experience with percutaneous transcatheter implantation of heart valve prosthesis for the treatment of end-stage inoperable patients with calcific aortic stenosis. J Am Coll Cardiol 2004; 43: 698–703.

5. Khambadkone S, Bonhoeffer P. Nonsurgical pulmonary valve replacement: Why, when and how? Catheter Cardiovasc Interv 2004; 62: 401–8.

6. Amin Z, Berry JM, Foker J, et al. Intraoperative closure of muscular ventricular septal defect in a canine model and application of the technique in a baby. J Thorac Cardiovasc Surg 1998; 115: 1374–6

7. Amin Z, Gu X, Berry JM, et al. Perventricular closure of ventricular septal defects without cardiopulmonary bypass. Ann Thorac Surg 1999; 68: 149–54.

8. Bacha EA, Cao QL, Starr JP, et al. Perventricular device closure of muscular ventricular septal defects on the beating heart: technique and results. J Thorac Cardiovasc Surg 2003; 126: 1718–23.

9. Davlouros PA, Kilner PJ, Hornung TS, et al. Right ventricular function in adults with repaired tetralogy of Fallot assessed with cardiovascular magnetic resonance imaging: detrimental role of right ventricular outflow aneurysms or akinesia and adverse right-to-left ventricular interaction. J Am Coll Cardiol 2002; 40: 2044–52.

10. Guide for the Care and Use of Laboratory Animals. NIH Publication 86–23, revised 1985.

11. Marianeschi SM, Iacona GM, Seddio F, et al. Shelhigh No-React porcine pulmonic valve conduit: A new alternative to the homograft. Ann Thorac Surg 2001; 71: 619–23.

12. Zhou JQ, Corno AF, Huber CH, et al. Self-expandable valved stent of large size: off-bypass implantation in pulmonary position. Eur J Cardiothorac Surg 2003; 24: 212–16.

10

Available transcatheter pulmonary valves: Bonhoeffer valve

Sachin Khambadkone, Younes Boudjemline, Philipp Bonhoeffer

Introduction

Percutaneous implantation of valves is a fast-evolving field in the practice of interventional cardiology.[1–3] Interventions on the pulmonary outflow tract are quite commonly performed after repair of congenital heart disease. The impact of pulmonary valvular dysfunction on right ventricular (RV) function and the understanding of its progression from a compensated reversible stage to a decompensated irreversible stage has led to earlier intervention.[4,5] The importance of a technique with lower morbidity and mortality, good patient acceptance, and efficacy that is comparable with surgery cannot be underestimated.

In this chapter, we describe the Bonhoeffer valve and early results from our clinical experience with this valve.

The device

Most devices involving percutaneous implantation of valves rely on stents to hold the valve and aid its implantation. Stents have been used in the RV outflow tract (RVOT) to relieve conduit obstruction that does not respond to balloon dilatation.[6,7] Despite being successful in relieving obstruction, it leaves no intact valvular mechanism, and regurgitation becomes a problem. Implantation of a valved stent has techniques similar to stent implantation in the outflow tract.

Many herbivorous animals have a venous valve in their jugular veins that prevents stasis of blood during feeding. The bovine jugular venous valves can have perfectly formed bicuspid or tricuspid arrangements (Figure 10.1). After harvesting,

they can be used with preservation of the valvular mechanism. Surgical implantation of the venous valve conduit has been successfully performed in the RVOT.[8,9]

The biologic valve is harvested from the jugular vein of fresh bovine cadavers, trimmed, and tanned to reduce the thickness of the wall to permit it to be sutured inside the stent. The valve is sutured inside the pre-expanded stent (Numed, Hopkinton, NY) (Figure 10.2). The stent is made of platinum–iridium wire welded together with gold. The valve itself can undergo multiple compression and re-expansion inside the stent. The valved stent assembly is crimped on a custom-made delivery system, which is based on a front-loading mechanism. The tip of the delivery system is 21 Fr with an inner diameter of 18 Fr

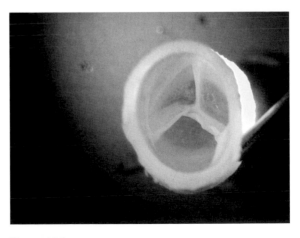

Figure 10.1

Bovine jugular venous valve with three leaflets.

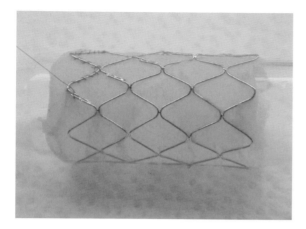

Figure 10.2

Valve sutured inside the stent.

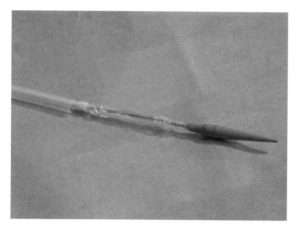

Figure 10.3

Delivery system for the Bonhoeffer valve.

(Figure 10.3). After crimping the valved stent on the balloon-in-balloon (BIB) system, it is covered by the sheath during its entry through the skin and uncovered only before deployment at the implantation site. The distal part of the sheath is not radio-opaque and a marker at the proximal end of the sheath indicates that the stent is uncovered before deployment. Once the valve is uncovered, the outer sheath can be used for angiography by injection through the side-port at the proximal end. The balloons are inflated in succession, the inner balloon first, which helps further in positioning the stent, followed by the outer one, which deploys the device. After deployment of the stent, the delivery system is removed very carefully to prevent any part of it being caught in the valve.

Animal studies

Eleven lambs 2 months old and weighing 16–18 kg underwent catheterization for transcatheter pulmonary valve replacement.[10] All lambs were treated according to the European Regulations for Animal Experimentation. Anesthesia was induced with 10 mg/kg of thiopental sodium and maintained with halothane in mechanically ventilated lambs. The right internal jugular vein was prepared for catheterization. Heparin (100 IU/kg) and penicillin were administered prophylactically. After the procedure, the jugular vein was preserved to allow for repeat catheterizations. Through the internal jugular approach, a guidewire was positioned in the pulmonary artery. The valved stent was then hand-crimped onto the inflatable portion of an 18, 20, or 22 mm balloon catheter. The size of the balloon was dependent on the size of the pulmonary artery measured by angiography. To limit the risk of dislodgment or slipping of the balloon, the assembly was front-loaded in a 16 Fr Mullins long sheath. After the loading onto the previously positioned guidewire, the whole system was advanced and implanted percutaneously. The position of the valved stent was easily tracked fluoroscopically because of the highly radio-opaque material of the stent. The valved stent was then balloon-expanded and deployed in the native pulmonary valve of the lamb to impinge upon the function of this native valve and to fix the device on the pulmonary wall. The balloon was subsequently deflated, and the catheter was removed, leaving the replacement valve assembly in the desired position. Hemodynamic and angiographic evaluation was performed before and after valve implantation.

The valves were retrieved after 2 months and were studied macroscopically, tested in vitro, and then studied histologically.

Seven of the eleven animals had successful implantation of the valved stent with technical failures in four, due to acute angulation between the tricuspid and pulmonary valves. In the successful implants, there were no significant complications during the procedure and early follow-up. No early or late stent migration was noted. Six of the seven valved stents were competent angiographically; one was mildly stenotic with a gradient of 15 mmHg between the right ventricle and the pulmonary artery. Four of the five valves implanted in satisfactory position on macroscopic examination showed competence with no calcification. The remaining one had macroscopic evidence of calcification with some degeneration of cusps, which could be attributed to suboptimal sterilization in the early experience. The two stents implanted in unsatisfactory position (adjacent to the native pulmonary valve) were not functional, mainly due to growth of tissue into the valves. In vitro, the valve leaflets could be seen after removal of the fibrous tissue as thin and pliable. The microscopic examination showed fibrin deposition at the margins of the stent. There was an endothelial cell-like layer in the luminal portion of the stent; however, the leaflets seemed free of this layer. The valve, which was stenotic, showed evidence of calcification, inflammatory infiltration, and neovascularization, which was probably contributed to by suboptimal sterilization protocol.

The animal experiments suggested that percutaneous implantation of valves was feasible when mounted inside the stents, with results comparable to those after surgical implantation.

The patient in clinical practice

The patient cohort likely to form the major bulk of the clinical population who would require transcatheter pulmonary valve implantation are those with previous operations on the RVOT as a part of their primary repair of congenital heart disease. Tetralogy of Fallot complex is the most common diagnosis leading to surgical pulmonary valve replacement.[11–13]

Patients were considered for percutaneous pulmonary valve implantation if they had previously undergone surgery on the RVOT during repair of congenital heart disease and had symptoms or RVOT dysfunction of a sufficient degree to warrant further surgical intervention based on conventional practices for surgical indications.[12–15] This included RV hypertension ($\geqslant$2/3 of systemic

blood pressure) with outflow tract obstruction, significant pulmonary insufficiency, RV dilatation, or RV failure.

All patients had a detailed clinical examination, ECG, chest radiograph, and echocardiography including color Doppler and continuous- and pulsed-wave Doppler studies to assess RV function, outflow obstruction, and pulmonary regurgitation. Magnetic resonance imaging was used to assess the morphology of the RVOT, to assess RV volumes and function, and to quantify pulmonary regurgitation.

Procedure

All procedures are performed under general anesthesia. Standard right heart catheterization with invasive systemic arterial pressure monitoring is undertaken for hemodynamic assessment. Angiography is performed in frontal, lateral, and oblique orthogonal projections to determine the anatomy of the RVOT, the implantation site, and the branch pulmonary arteries in order to confirm feasibility, select the appropriate site of deployment, and aid the choice of delivery system. It is quite important to assess any additional areas of stenosis, which, if not relieved, may affect the result of the valve implantation. The length of stenosis at the implantation site should also be adequately covered by the valved stent for an optimal result.

A Judkins right coronary catheter or a balloon-tipped catheter is used to cross the tricuspid valve to enter the right ventricle. The catheter is then positioned into the distal branch pulmonary artery until it is wedged. A 0.035-inch hydrophilic wire may be used to achieve a good stable position of the catheter. A stiff exchange wire is then used to achieve a good stable position to track the delivery system. The wire may need a pre-fashioned curve to facilitate a stable position. A Multitrack angiographic catheter is then used to measure pressure in the RV and the pulmonary artery and perform angiography to outline the RVOT and assess pulmonary regurgitation. The area of calcification and stenosis in the homografts usually provide a good landmark to choose an implantation point.

The valve is prepared by washing off the glutaraldehyde preservative with three 5-minute washes in saline. The delivery system is flushed and prepared. The BIB system is de-aired and the outer sheath is flushed and de-aired. The stent is then crimped down to a smaller diameter, and then crimped down further directly onto the outer balloon of the BIB system. The most important thing is to orientate the valve stent appropriately in the direction of flow. The sutures on the valve stent have different colors matching with the colors on the delivery system. The distal end of the valve is sutured with a blue suture, which matches with the blue tapered tip of the delivery system. The outer sheath is then used to cover the valve stent, ensuring that the whole of the latter is covered and remains stable on the balloon. Before introduction of the delivery system, the vein is dilated with an 18–22 Fr dilator to facilitate easy entry. The delivery system is then tracked under fluoroscopy to an appropriate position based on the angiographic reference images. Once the valve stent is in an appropriate position, it is uncovered by pulling back the outer sheath; this can sometimes facilitate advancement of the system. Angiography can be performed through the side-arm of the outer sheath and fine adjustment can be made to the position of the valve. The inner and outer balloons are then inflated sequentially to deploy the valve stent. The delivery system is then carefully withdrawn, keeping the guidewire position intact. Hemodynamics and angiography are then performed to assess the results. In the presence of a residual gradient, a high-pressure balloon has been used successfully with inflation up to 8–10 atm without any disruption of the valvular mechanism and good relief of the residual stenosis.

Results

Between January 2000 and September 2004, we implanted valves percutaneously in 58 patients. The median age was 16 years (range 9–43 years) and the median weight 56 kg (range 25–110 kg). Thirty-six (61%) patients had variants of tetralogy of Fallot, the majority (18) with pulmonary atresia, three with absent pulmonary valve syndrome, and the rest with severe pulmonary stenosis (Table 10.1). The majority of patients had a homograft conduit after surgery on the RVOT (46 of 59, 79%). Only three patients had had a 'native' RVOT that had been augmented with a pericardial or homograft patch.

Table 10.1   Patient characteristics

Age	Median 16 years (range 9–43 years)
Weight	Median 56 kg (range 25–110 kg)
Diagnosis:	
Tetralogy of Fallot variants	36
Transposition of the great arteries, ventricular septal defect, or pulmonary stenosis	9
Ross operation	6
Truncus arteriosus	4
Others	4

After valve implantation, the RV systolic pressure (64.4±17.2 mmHg to 50.4±14 mmHg; p <0.005) and outflow gradient (33±24.6 mmHg to 19.5±15.3 mmHg, p <0.005)(Figure 10.4) fell significantly without any significant change in the systemic arterial pressure (103.4±18.4 mmHg to 109.6±16.1 mmHg, p = 0.64). There was a significant increase in the pulmonary artery diastolic pressure (9.9±3.7 mmHg to 13.5±5.3 mmHg; p <0.005). There was a decrease in the RV end-diastolic pressure (RVEDP) (11.5±3.7 mmHg or 10.5±4.2 mmHg; p = 0.005). Angiography showed

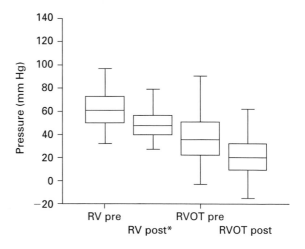

Figure 10.4

Hemodynamic improvement after percutaneous pulmonary valve implantation. Reduction in right ventricular pressure and outflow gradient (*p <0.005).

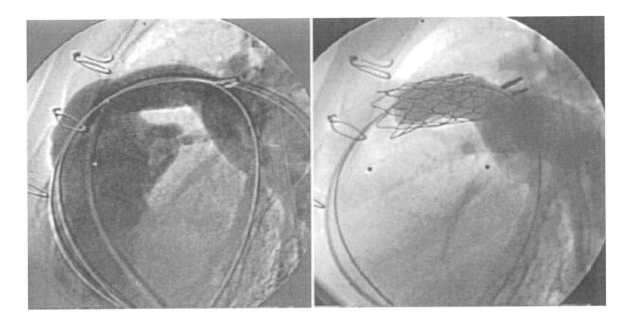

Figure 10.5

Lateral angiogram showing complete relief of pulmonary regurgitation after percutaneous pulmonary valve implantation.

a significant improvement in regurgitation, with none having more than trivial to mild regurgitation after the procedure (Figure 10.5).

In the predominant stenosis group (peak-to-peak gradient of ⩾30 mmHg measured during cardiac catheterization), there was a significant drop in the RV systolic pressure (71±15.3 mmHg to 52.3±14.5 mmHg; *p* <0.005) and gradient across the RVOT (44.6±24.3 to 24.4±15.2 mmHg; *p* <0.005) after valve implantation. Furthermore, there was a significant drop in RVEDP (11.7±3.4 mmHg to 10±3.9 mmHg; *p* <0.05).

In the predominant regurgitation group (peak-to-peak gradient <30 mmHg during cardiac catheterization), however, there were no changes in these parameters immediately after valve implantation (RV systolic pressure 49.4±10.5 mmHg to 47.2±14.1 mmHg (*p* = 0.45); RVOT gradient 14.5±9.3 mmHg to 11.8±12.1 mmHg (*p* = 0.26); RVEDP 10.7±2.8 mmHg to 11.4±4.6 mmHg (*p* = 0.43). There was, however, a significant increase in the pulmonary artery diastolic pressure (10.1±3.6 mmHg to 15.4±7.6 mmHg; *p* <0.005). New York Heart Association (NYHA) functional class, assessed during the latest follow-up, improved after valve implantation, with 57% in class I after implantation, compared with only 8.6% before the procedure (*p* <0.001).

Complications

There have been no procedural or late deaths after percutaneous pulmonary valve implantation.

Two patients had stent instability. In one, it was during the procedure, and the patient had surgical explantation with placement of a surgical homograft. The other patient developed displacement of the stent into the right ventricle 4 hours after the procedure and needed emergency surgery. There was one life-threatening bleed into the mediastinum due to homograft rupture, which was treated successfully by transfusion and surgical repair of the bleeding site.

There were seven minor complications: one minor dissection of a homograft (treated conservatively), two detachments of the distal tip of the delivery system, and four local bleeds, which were controlled without transfusion.

Follow-up

The mean follow-up was 9.8±1.4 months and was 100% complete for mortality and freedom from explantation.

Echocardiography performed 24 hours after valve implantation revealed a significant reduction in the tricuspid regurgitation velocity (4.0±0.6 m/s to 3.6±0.7 m/s; p <0.005) and RVOT gradient (63.4±23.4 mmHg to 40.5±18.2 mmHg, p <0.001). There was a significant reduction in the grade of pulmonary regurgitation, with all patients having grade ≥2 regurgitation before, and none with more than grade 2 after the procedure (p <0.001).

Device-related adverse events

During follow-up, there were device-related problems in 14 patients.

Device-related adverse events with clinical impact resulted from stent fracture in seven patients, a median 9 months after percutaneous pulmonary valve implantation. During meticulous follow-up, clinical problems were observed in two patients. In one, an increase in RVOT gradient developed and the patient was successfully treated with a second valve implantation. In the other, there was stent embolization 9 months after the procedure. Elective surgical explantation was performed and a homograft conduit was implanted.

The most common impact of a device-related event was stenosis. In seven patients, in-stent stenosis was observed due to a 'hammock effect' in which the valve separated from the stent in between the sutured ends of the venous segment (Figure 10.6). Prior to recognition of this phenomenon, the device was explanted surgically, but once the design of the valve had been changed, a second valve was implanted within the first in three patients, with successful relief of stenosis. Those valves with the new design where the venous wall was sutured along its length did not show a hammock effect.

In the remaining patients who required explantation, a major indication was residual stenosis, and two mechanisms of obstruction were observed. In two patients, there was external compression of the conduit despite the presence of the stent, and in the other two, the device

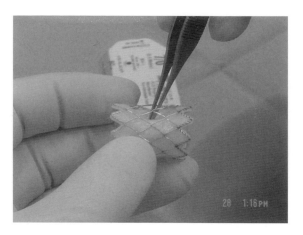

Figure 10.6

'Hammock effect'. Mechanism of re-stenosis due to separation of the venous wall from the stent.

could not be fully deployed at implantation (one of these was associated with intravascular hemolysis).

One patient developed endocarditis after a dental procedure without prophylaxis and required explantation of the valve for failure of medical therapy.

The explanted valves, whenever available for gross examination, showed competent leaflets on in vitro testing, except for the one with endocarditis.

Serial echocardiography showed that the early decrease in RVOT gradient was sustained at latest follow-up (mean 9.8 months) (63.4±23.4 mmHg to 48.8±24.2 mmHg, p <0.01). The improvement in regurgitation was also sustained, with only one patient having moderate regurgitation due to endocarditis of the valve.

All of the re-interventions thus far have been for stenosis, with no intervention required for regurgitation.

Late follow-up

The freedom from explantation for valve failure was 89% (95% confidence interval 80–97%) at 6 months, 83.3% (69.5–97.2%) at 12 months, 79.7% (67.2–92.2%) at 24 months, and 69.8% (48.4–91.1%) at 36 months (Figure 10.7).

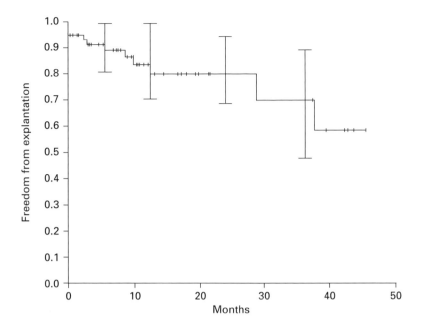

Figure 10.7

Kaplan Meier graph for freedom from explantation.

Surgical homograft valve insertion was successful in all patients after explantation of the device. However, in two patients, early homograft stenosis occurred. In one of these patients, the stenosis was successfully treated with valve implantation; the other is awaiting this procedure.

All procedures were performed through femoral (56 patients) or internal jugular (2 patients) access. The median procedure time was 102 minutes (interquartile range 67–124 patients) and the median fluoroscopy time was 21 minutes (range 11–36 minutes). Five additional procedures were performed at the time of valve implantation: stenting of distal pulmonary arteries (2), ventricular septal defect closure (1), atrial septal defect closure (1), and occlusion of a paraprosthetic leak through a mechanical aortic valve (1).

All patients with successful valve implantation were ambulatory within 24 hours of the procedure.

Future directions

The Bonhoeffer percutaneous pulmonary valve has been used successfully in patients with RVOT dimensions up to 22 mm. There is a large cohort of patients with dilated aneurysmal RVOT where the current device cannot be implanted due to a discrepancy of dimensions. Most of these outflows have transannular patch repair with homograft tissue, autologous pericardium, or prosthetic materials. The dynamic changes in dimensions due to distensible tissue in the RVOT make assessment of the size of the implantation point difficult. Use of 3D imaging helps to understand the difficulty of obtaining the maximum and minimum dimensions in 2D imaging modalities. Construction of 3D models of the RVOT with data derived from 3D reconstruction of magnetic resonance images has expanded our understanding of variations in the RVOT. However, assessment of dynamic changes in the RVOT during the cardiac cycle and differential stresses and strains on separate parts of the RVOT is still elusive.

We have shown in animal models that this device can be implanted in the large RVOT with the use of RVOT reducers.[16] The valve was loaded into a specially designed nitinol stent, which was shaped like a conduit with a central restriction to 18 mm diameter, and the assembly stabilized in the large RVOT. The entire length of this device was 5.5 cm. Downsizing of the RVOT was possible from 30 mm to 18 mm, with good stability of the device. We are in the process of developing a similar application for use in the patient cohorts with dilated and aneurysmal RVOT.

Stent fractures have been seen as a part of device failure in our series. A better understanding of metal behavior in the dynamic RVOT and the use of different materials may help in overcoming this problem.

Finally, the long-term behavior of this biologic valve still remains to be seen. Calcification, leaflet degeneration, and fibrosis are known problems in biologic valves used in surgical series. Although the longevity of biologic valves (especially homografts) has been judged in several surgical series, the bovine jugular venous valve implanted surgically has shown encouraging results in the early and medium term.[9] There is no reason to believe that the percutaneous valve will not behave in the same manner. Indeed, the problems related to dilatation of the venous wall in some cases may be prevented by the support of the stent.[17] The major advantage is the ability to implant a second valve within the first one, with successful relief of stenosis or regurgitation, a technique which has been performed with good results in our series.

References

1. Boudjemline Y, Bonnet D, Sidi D, Bonhoeffer P. Percutaneous implantation of a biological valve in the aorta to treat aortic valve insufficiency – a sheep study. Med Sci Monit 2002; 8: BR113–BR116.
2. Boudjemline Y, Bonhoeffer P. Steps toward percutaneous aortic valve replacement. Circulation 2002; 105: 775–8.
3. Pavcnik D, Wright KC, Wallace S. Development and initial experimental evaluation of a prosthetic aortic valve for transcatheter placement. Work in progress. Radiology 1992; 183: 151–4.
4. Therrien J, Siu SC, McLaughlin PR, et al. Pulmonary valve replacement in adults late after repair of tetralogy of Fallot: Are we operating too late? J Am Coll Cardiol 2000; 36: 1670–5.
5. Therrien J, Siu SC, Harris L, et al. Impact of pulmonary valve replacement on arrhythmia propensity late after repair of tetralogy of Fallot. Circulation 2001; 103: 2489–94.
6. Almagor Y, Prevosti LG, Bartorelli AL, et al. Balloon expandable stent implantation in stenotic right heart valved conduits. J Am Coll Cardiol 1990; 16: 1310–14.
7. Pedra CA, Justino H, Nykanen DG, et al. Percutaneous stent implantation to stenotic bioprosthetic valves in the pulmonary position. J Thorac Cardiovasc Surg 2002; 124: 82–7.
8. Breymann T, Thies WR, Boethig D, et al. Bovine valved venous xenografts for RVOT reconstruction: results after 71 implantations. Eur J Cardiothorac Surg 2002; 21: 703–10.
9. Corno AF, Qanadli SD, Sekarski N, et al. Bovine valved xenograft in pulmonary position: medium-term follow-up with excellent hemodynamics and freedom from calcification. Ann Thorac Surg 2004; 78: 1382–8.
10. Bonhoeffer P, Boudjemline Y, Saliba Z, et al. Transcatheter implantation of a bovine valve in pulmonary position: a lamb study. Circulation 2000; 102: 813–16.
11. Kanter KR, Budde JM, Parks WJ, et al. One hundred pulmonary valve replacements in children after relief of right ventricular outflow tract obstruction. Ann Thorac Surg 2002; 73: 1801–6.
12. Discigil B, Dearani JA, Puga FJ, et al. Late pulmonary valve replacement after repair of tetralogy of Fallot. J Thorac Cardiovasc Surg 2001; 121: 344–51.
13. Bove EL, Kavey RE, Byrum CJ, et al. Improved right ventricular function following late pulmonary valve replacement for residual pulmonary insufficiency or stenosis. J Thorac Cardiovasc Surg 1985; 90: 50–5.
14. Warner KG, O'Brien PK, Rhodes J, et al. Expanding the indications for pulmonary valve replacement after repair of tetralogy of Fallot. Ann Thorac Surg 2003; 76: 1066–71.
15. Vliegen HW, van Straten A, de Roos A, et al. Magnetic resonance imaging to assess the hemodynamic effects of pulmonary valve replacement in adults late after repair of tetralogy of Fallot. Circulation 2002; 106: 1703–7.
16. Boudjemline Y, Agnoletti G, Bonnet D, et al. Percutaneous pulmonary valve replacement in a large right ventricular outflow tract: an experimental study. J Am Coll Cardiol 2004; 43: 1082–7.
17. Boudjemline Y, Bonnet D, Agnoletti G, Vouhe P. Aneurysm of the right ventricular outflow following bovine valved venous conduit insertion. Eur J Cardiothorac Surg 2003; 23: 122–4.

11

Extending the present indications for percutaneous pulmonary valve replacement to small patients and large ventricular outflow tracts

Younes Boudjemline, Philipp Bonhoeffer

Introduction

Pulmonary valve replacement through a trans-catheter technique is presently limited to the small group of patients who have a right ventricular outflow tract (RVOT) <22 mm in diameter and a weight of at least 20–25 kg.[1–3] Expansion of the indications for the technique to both small infants and large RVOTs will allow the present indications to be extended to the whole spectrum of patients in need of pulmonary valve replacement.

Off-pump pulmonary valve replacement in patients with RVOT >22 mm

Background

As reported elsewhere in this book, efforts have been made to implant percutaneously a device that reduces the size of the main pulmonary artery (PA). Two approaches have been investigated: a one-step procedure in which the device already contained a valve and a two-step procedure in which the device allowed for subsequent valve insertion.[4] Unfortunately, the anatomy of RVOT in patients operated for tetralogy of Fallot in infancy varies greatly in length, size, and geometry, making the use of a symmetrical device as we designed it unlikely in all patients.

During the last year, we have been imaging and building models of the RVOT from patients with aneurysmal RVOT in need of pulmonary valve replacement. Virtual implantation of the so-called 'infundibulum reducer' in those models was adequate in less than 50%, making this device clearly not universal. Incomplete expansion leading to both lengthening of the device and improper sealing was the typical drawback observed. For this reason, in parallel to the development of a modified 'infundibulum reducer', we have investigated an alternative approach to encompass these difficulties. We adopted a hybrid approach involving both surgeons and cardiac interventionists, with the first step being a surgical pulmonary artery banding to a diameter that allows further pulmonary valve replacement.

Device preparation for downsizing the diameter of the pulmonary trunk

Two rings made of a 0.27 mm self-expandable alloy wire (AMF, Reuilly, France) encapsulated in a plastic tube were prepared (Figure 11.1). The rings had a diameter of 18 mm and could be straightened in order to be placed around the pulmonary artery. The purpose of these rings was to reduce the diameter of the pulmonary artery as

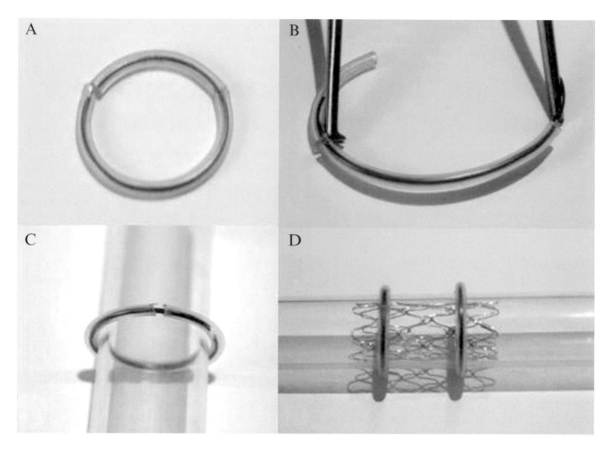

Figure 11.1

In vitro views of the various phases of the procedure. (A) The ring used for the pulmonary artery (PA) banding is made of nitinol and has a spontaneous diameter of 18 mm. (B) The ring is opened and straightened before its passage around the main PA represented by the glass tube. (C) View showing the aspect of the ring around a glass tube. (D) View showing the aspect of a stent placed inside the glass tube after placement of two rings.

well as to provide support to the valved stent and to assist in its precise placement under fluoroscopic guidance. The rings were placed as a first step in eight ewes. Following complete right heart catheterization, all animals had a surgical reduction of the PA diameter through a thoracotomy, using the rings without cardiopulmonary bypass. The rings were subsequently straightened and inserted proximally around the main PA. The second ring was placed 1.5–2 cm more distally than the first. The rings were secured to the PA with a discontinuous suture. After banding was performed, right heart catheterization was repeated and compared with basal data. For valve placement, valved stents (Numed/Medtronic Inc.)

were used without any modification. The delivery system (Numed Inc., Hopkinton, USA) was also identical. In four animals, the valve was delivered percutaneously through the left jugular vein. The valved stent was advanced, uncovered, and deployed in the pulmonary trunk between the two inserted rings. In the remaining four animals, the valved stent was inserted through a transventricular incision using the surgical access performed for PA banding. For that purpose, a purse-string suture was performed about 3 cm below the native pulmonary valve. The right ventricle (RV) was punctured in the middle of the purse-string with a needle, and a wire was inserted in the lumen of the needle, advanced in the PA, and exchanged for a 0.035-inch extra-stiff guidewire, on which the loaded delivery system was advanced. The valved stent was finally inserted as previously described. After retrieval of the delivery system and wire, bleeding was controlled by tightening the purse-string. Right heart catheterization was performed and the animals were sacrificed after evaluation.

Animal experience: study results

The mean size of the pulmonary trunk decreased from 30±1.6 mm to 17.6±0.5 mm after insertion of the rings around the pulmonary artery. The RV systolic pressure increased from 25±3 mmHg to 36±6 mmHg. All valved stents were successfully implanted using a 22 mm balloon catheter. The mean diameter of the main PA increased significantly after valve insertion to 21.1±0.8 mm as compared with the post-banding procedure. The mean systolic transprosthetic gradient decreased from 14±9.7 mmHg to 6.4±2.1 mmHg after valve insertion. The mean ratio between the RV and aortic pressures was <35% (27.8%±3.6%) in all animals. There was no early migration of any valved stents. On angiographic evaluation, the implants were in the desired position between the two rings (Figure 11.2), the valves were

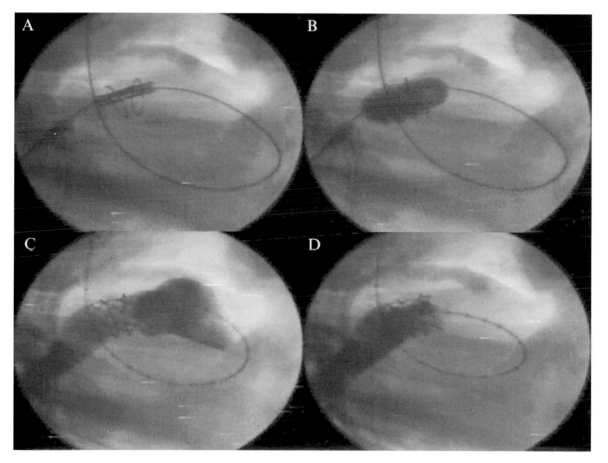

Figure 11.2

Angiograms showing implantation of the valved stent through a percutaneous approach. (A) The valved stent has been advanced from the jugular vein in the main pulmonary artery. (B) The balloons are inflated in order to expand the stent. (C) Proximal angiogram showing the sealing of the device. (D) Distal angiogram demonstrating the competence of the implanted valve.

competent, and there was no paravalvular leak around the devices.

Animal experience: study limitations and unanswered questions

First, only animals with no previous heart surgery were evaluated. Patients with tetrology of Fallot are often operated on several times, making the chest opening and dissection more difficult each time. The creation of the banding could, at least in theory, be difficult in such situations because of the history of previous interventions.

Second, as advocated by surgeons, the investigated approaches do not retrieve the aneurysmal and akinetic portion of the RVOT. If demonstrated, this could limit the improvement of the RV function of the patients and would favor on-pump surgical procedures with resection of the aneurysmal part. This should, however, be balanced by the repercussions of cardiopulmonary bypass for ventricular function. Moreover, the superiority of pulmonary valve replacement with RVOT remodeling over standard pulmonary valve replacement has not been clearly shown.[5] Randomized controlled studies will be necessary to address this question, in which various techniques including off-pump hybrid approaches and on-pump pulmonary valve replacement with and without RVOT remodeling should be compared prospectively.

Third, because no chronic data are available at present, the long-term performance of this approach remains unknown and more experimental studies are needed before human application, to address in particular the risks of secondary erosion and migration of the rings and valved stents. In further chronic studies, various techniques could be used to reduced or cancel the risk of migration. Limiting the dissection posteriorly of the pulmonary artery to two small spaces rather than one large space is one way to limit the tendency of the bands to migrate. Suturing the rings to the pulmonary artery wall might also reduce this risk. Similarly, to avoid embolization of the valved stent, the latter can be secured by suturing the stent to the bands. Flaring the end part of the stent using a larger balloon might additionally help to reduce this risk.

In conclusion, we have overcome the present limitation of percutaneous valve insertion in large RVOTs by a collaborative approach involving both surgeons and interventionists. This approach allows for off-pump pulmonary valve insertion either percutaneously or through a small ventriculotomy, extending the present indications for minimally invasive pulmonary valve replacement to patients with large RVOTs.

Pulmonary valve replacement in patients weighing <20–25 kg

Background

Prosthetic valved or valveless conduits have been used surgically to re-establish continuity between the RV and the pulmonary artery as a part of the complete repair of some congenital heart defects involving the RVOT.[6] Over the past 40 years, various types of conduits have been developed according to the type of valve incorporated and the structure supporting this valve. Despite major advances in terms of durability, the life span of these conduits is still limited because of valvular calcific degeneration, accumulation of intimal peel within conduits, and/or inability to grow with patients.[7] Therefore, patients are committed to multiple reoperations to replace outgrowth or degenerated conduits. Transcatheter techniques (i.e balloon dilatation, bared stent placement, or valved stent insertion) have been proposed to delay the need for reoperation.[8] However, these techniques have limited efficacy in children with small conduits, mainly because of the inability to expand the balloon over the nominal size of the conduit. Based on our experience of valve insertion through a transcatheter technique, we investigated the possibility to implant a stented conduit surgically in order to fashion a dilatable conduit. It can be inserted in small children and dilated percutaneously to follow the growth until the weight of 25 kg, at which time a valved stent can be implanted.

Preparation of the dilatable conduit

A 'non-prepared' 18 mm Contegra conduit was sutured inside a CP stent. The stent was slightly different from the one used for percutaneous valve replacement. It had only three rows and a total length of 14 mm when inflated to 18 mm.

Insertion of the dilatable valved conduit

Five sheep have been included so far in the study. Surgery was performed under general anesthesia via a left thoracotomy. The grafts were implanted in the main pulmonary artery with a beating heart and without myocardial protection. Access to cardiopulmonary bypass was gained via the femoral artery and the right atrium with a cannula introduced from the right jugular vein. Under full car-

diopulmonary bypass flow, the main pulmonary artery was cross-clamped below its bifurcation, and opened transversally 1 cm above the pulmonary annulus. The native valve was excised by resecting each leaflet. The annulus was preserved. The conduits were fashioned in length according to each animal's anatomy. The prepared conduits, dilated to 16 mm diameter, were inserted in place of the excised main pulmonary artery (Figure 11.3). After weaning off bypass, hemodynamic and angiographic data were obtained to assess valvular function and gradient across the conduit. For long-term observation, sheep were transferred to a farm and assessed monthly or sooner if any symptoms occurred by echocardiography. At 2 months or

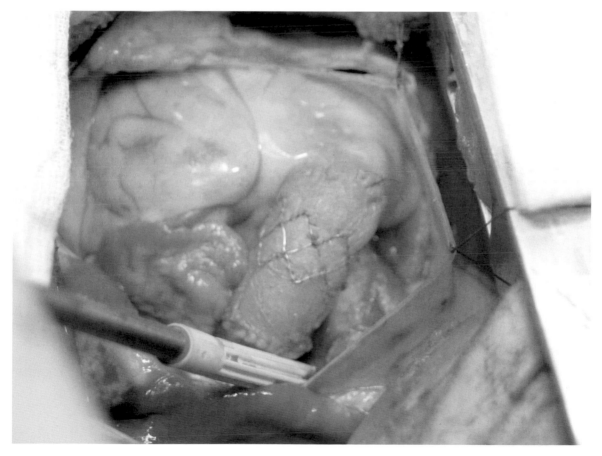

Figure 11.3

The dilatable valved conduit has been surgically placed between the pulmonary annulus and the pulmonary artery bifurcation. Note the length of the stent covering the valved conduit.

when echocardiographic data were inappropriate or showed a significant increase in transvalvular gradient, cardiac catheterization was performed with the aim of dilating the surgically inserted conduit with an 18, 20, or a 22 mm balloon catheter (Tyshak II, Numed Inc., NY). Prior and after dilatation, hemodynamic and angiographic data were acquired to assess the function of the implanted valve, the efficacy of dilatation, and the occurrence of vascular rupture. If dilatation led to severe pulmonary regurgitation, a 22 mm valved stent was implanted through a transcatheter technique into the previously placed dilatable conduit with a device and technique described previously. Following this insertion, the animals were sacrificed.

Animal experience: study results

The dilatable valved conduit was implanted surgically in all included animals. Acute hemodynamic assessment showed a perfectly functioning valve. The postoperative course was complicated in two out of five animals. Two needed slow weaning off cardiopulmonary bypass and postoperative inotropic support and one recovered. Despite low transprosthetic gradient, a balloon dilatation using a larger balloon was attempted in two animals in an attempt to reduce the afterload of the failing RV. In one, a rupture of the suture occurred, leading to fatal thoracic bleeding. The remaining three animals had a simple postoperative course and were followed according to the

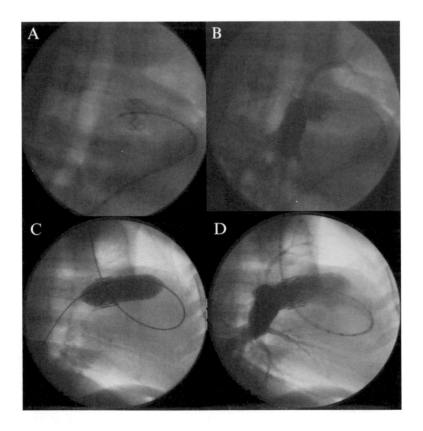

Figure 11.4

(A, B) Angiograms performed just after dilatable conduit insertion, showing good valvular function. (C) Balloon dilatation with a 22 mm balloon catheter 2 months after conduit insertion. (D) Angiogram showing moderate to severe pulmonary regurgitation.

protocol. Monthly echocardiography showed a moderate increase in the transprosthetic gradient (from 10 mmHg to 40 mmHg), in parallel with an increase in the animal's weight (from 25 kg to 44 kg). Valve competency decreased from grade 0–1 to grade 2–3. Balloon dilatation was performed electively after a mean period of 2 months (Figure 11.4). Systolic RV pressure dropped from 55 mmHg to 26 mmHg after the dilatation. The diameter increased from 15.6 mm to 20 mm. Transcatheter valve implantation has been attempted with success in two animals so far (Figure 11.5). Two animals are waiting for further valvulation. No early migration occurred. Diastolic pressure increased from 8 mmHg to 14 mmHg, reflecting the excellent valvular function.

Animal experience: study limitations and unanswered questions

Due to the unavailability of a small circuit for extracorporeal circulation, we were unable to include small animals with a high growth capability. This leads to an inability to create a rapid and significant gradient over the conduit, despite long follow-up. We have, however, demonstrated the possibility of dilating the conduit from 16 mm to 22 mm in a small number of animals. Moreover, we were able to dilate this conduit ex vivo to 30 mm without any rupture of the pulmonary artery. There is therefore no reason why this conduit could not be dilated from 12 to 22 mm or more. These results are very encouraging,

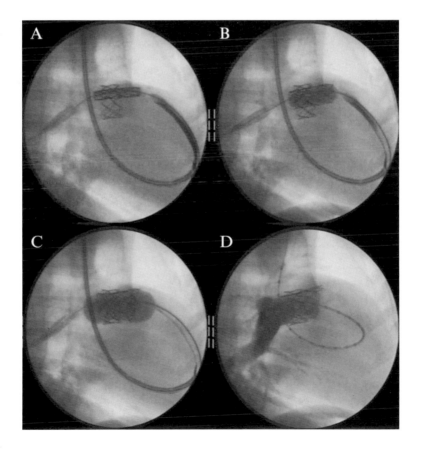

Figure 11.5

(A–D) Angiograms showing percutaneous valve placement inside a failing dilatable conduit.

but are still preliminary, since more animals are expected to be included in the experimental study. Similarly, questions regarding the possibility of compression of adjacent structures (in particular, the coronary arteries) remain unanswered, in particular with regard to small patients, and need further investigation before human introduction. Because, with time, the conduit can be imbedded in fibrotic tissue, its dilatability could be impaired or reduced. We have not encountered this drawback. However, it is more likely to occur after a long time period – longer than our period of follow-up. If we want to answer this question, longer follow-ups are required. Alternatively, we might consider dilating those conduits electively every 6–12 months before any appearance of conduit stenosis.

Conclusion

The life span of RV–PA conduits is limited due to valvular degeneration or conduit outgrowth. We have reported the development and application of a valved conduit allowing for repeated dilatations to follow growth and to a diameter that permits non-surgical implantation of a pulmonary valve. If demonstrated in a larger number of animals, this new application might extend the indications for transcatheter valve replacement and may have an important role to play in the management of right-sided congenital heart diseases.

Acknowledgments

The authors thank the veterinary surgeons of the Animal Laboratory and Numed Inc. for its technical support. The study was made possible through the support of a Program Grant from the British Heart Foundation (Grant BHF#1BUZ).

References

1. Bonhoeffer P, Boudjemline Y, Saliba Z, et al. Transcatheter implantation of a bovine valve in pulmonary position: a lamb study. Circulation 2000; 102: 813–16.
2. Bonhoeffer P, Boudjemline Y, Saliba Z, et al. Percutaneous replacement of pulmonary valve in a right-ventricle to pulmonary-artery prosthetic conduit with valve dysfunction. Lancet 2000; 356: 1403–5.
3. Bonhoeffer P, Boudjemline Y, Qureshi SA, et al. Percutaneous insertion of the pulmonary valve. J Am Coll Cardiol 2002; 39: 1664–9.
4. Boudjemline Y, Agnoletti G, Bonnet D, et al. Percutaneous pulmonary valve replacement in a large right ventricular outflow tract: an experimental study. J Am Coll Cardiol 2004; 43: 1082–7.
5. Therrien J, Siu SC, McLaughlin PR, et al. Pulmonary valve replacement in adults late after repair of tetralogy of Fallot: Are we operating too late? J Am Coll Cardiol 2000; 36: 1670–5.
6. Razzouk AJ, Williams WG, Cleveland DC, et al. Surgical connections from ventricle to pulmonary artery: comparison of four types of valved implants. Circulation 1992; 86(Suppl II): II-154–II-158.
7. Champsaur G, Robin J, Curtil A, et al. Long-term clinical and hemodynamic evaluation of porcine valved conduits implanted from the right ventricle to the pulmonary artery. J Thorac Cardiovasc Surg 1998; 116: 793–804.
8. Powell AJ, Lock JE, Keane JF, Perry SB. Prolongation of right ventricular to pulmonary artery conduit life span by percutaneous stent implantation: intermediate-term results. Circulation 1995; 92: 3282–8.

Section 2

The aortic valve

12

Aortic stenosis: Pathophysiologic, clinical, and echocardiographic manifestations

R Parker Ward, Roberto M Lang

Introduction

Aortic stenosis is a disease in which left ventricular (LV) outflow obstruction results in progressive LV hypertrophy, typical symptoms, and (if left untreated) death. The presentation, clinical course, and treatment of aortic stenosis are dependent on the cause and severity of the outflow obstruction. Echocardiography represents the primary non-invasive imaging modality for the diagnosis of aortic stenosis. In this chapter, we will review the clinical manifestations, pathophysiology, and echocardiographic features of aortic stenosis.

Differential diagnosis

Aortic stenosis can be caused by subvalvular, valvular, or supravalvular obstruction to LV outflow. While the majority of aortic stenoses occur with an abnormality of the aortic valve, obstruction above and below the valve may have a similar clinical presentation and confound the diagnosis.

Supravalvular aortic stenosis

Supravalvular aortic stenosis is the least common form and is due to a congenital narrowing of the ascending aorta, usually beginning just above the sinuses of Valsalva. This defect generally occurs in association with other congenital malforma-

tions such as elfin facies, peripheral pulmonic stenosis, and hypercalcemia. The diagnosis of supravalvular aortic stenosis can usually be made using Doppler echocardiography and should be entertained in a young person with an LV outflow murmur.

Subvalvular aortic stenosis

Discrete subvalvular stenosis accounts for 8–10% of all congenital aortic stenosis and is more common in males.[1] This abnormality usually occurs as a fibromuscular membrane or a tunnel-like narrowing of the LV outflow tract (LVOT). Subvalvular stenosis is frequently associated with aortic regurgitation, resulting from chronic trauma to the aortic valve leaflets caused by the turbulent high-velocity systolic jet. The diagnosis should be suspected on echocardiography in patients with unexplained increased velocities across the LVOT in the presence of normal aortic valve leaflet excursion, or with evidence for early aortic valve closure. While the subvalvular membrane itself can occasionally be visualized with transthoracic echocardiography, transesophageal echocardiography is often helpful in confirming the diagnosis. The treatment of discrete subvalvular aortic stenosis requires surgical resection of the membrane, and the timing depends on the degree of obstruction and severity of aortic regurgitation. Although controversial, surgical resection may be considered, even in the absence of critical obstruction, to prevent progressive aortic regurgitation, which ultimately would require aortic valve replacement.[2,3]

Valvular aortic stenosis

The majority of aortic stenoses occur due to an abnormality of the aortic valve leaflets. The causes of valvular aortic stenosis can be divided into congenital, rheumatic, and degenerative. Congenital aortic stenosis accounts for the majority of cases of valvular aortic stenosis in young adults, while degenerative aortic stenosis is most common in the elderly and accounts for the majority of cases in adults overall.[4] Historically, rheumatic aortic stenosis was prevalent, but now it is increasingly rare.

Congenital aortic stenosis

Congenital abnormalities of the aortic valve may be unicuspid, bicuspid, or tricuspid. A bicuspid aortic valve is the most common congenital cardiac malformation (occurring in 1–2% of the general population) and is more common in males.[1] While bicuspid aortic valves may present with significant functional stenosis in childhood, more commonly the resulting turbulent flow leads to progressive fibrosis and calcification of the valve leaflets, with the clinical presentation of aortic stenosis in adulthood. The two leaflets are typically of unequal size, commonly with the larger leaflet having a raphe, which can give the appearance of a tricuspid valve (Figures 12.1 and 12.2). Bicuspid valves may also present with aortic regurgitation or infective endocarditis, or may be associated with other congenital anomalies such as coarctation of the aorta. Bicuspid aortic valves may be associated with aortic root enlargement and represent a risk factor for aortic dissection.

Unicuspid valves produce severe obstruction in infancy and thus are rarely encountered in adults. Congenital tricuspid aortic stenosis involves mild abnormalities of the aortic valve leaflets, including partial commissural fusion and unequal cusp size.

Rheumatic aortic stenosis

Rheumatic aortic abnormalities may include commissural fusion, thickening, and calcification of the leaflet tips and systolic doming of the leaflets, although the findings are frequently nonspecific. As the mitral valve is preferentially affected in rheumatic heart disease, definitive diagnosis of rheumatic aortic stenosis frequently requires associated mitral valve involvement.

Degenerative aortic stenosis

Degenerative (or senile calcific) aortic stenosis develops after years of mechanical stress on an otherwise-normal aortic valve. It occurs due to progressive calcium deposition at the leaflet bases, which limits leaflet excursion (Figure 12.2). Degenerative aortic stenosis is the most common etiology of aortic stenosis in patients referred for aortic valve replacement.[5] Risk factors for degenerative aortic stenosis are similar to those for coronary artery disease, including hypertension and hypercholesterolemia, and coexisting atherosclerotic heart disease is common.[6]

Pathophysiology

The obstruction of LV outflow in patients with aortic stenosis typically develops gradually over many years. For congenital causes, the aortic valve orifice area shows little change, but as the child grows, the degree of obstruction increases. In degenerative aortic stenosis, the valve mobility and orifice area typically decrease over time. Progressive obstruction leads to increasing LV pressure overload and reactive concentric LV hypertrophy. This compensatory mechanism allows the LV to maintain normal size and normal cardiac output for many years without symptoms, despite a significant pressure gradient across the aortic valve. Gradually, as LV afterload continues to increase, the first symptoms frequently develop as a consequence of increasing LV diastolic pressures due to diastolic dysfunction and/or myocardial ischemia. When the LV

Diastole   Systole

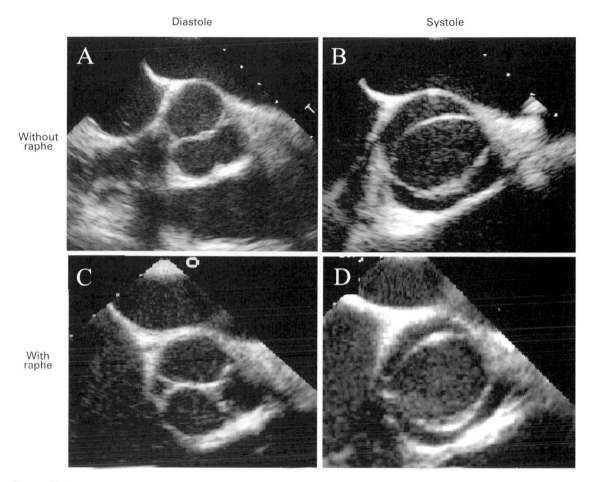

Figure 12.1

Transesophageal short-axis view in systole and diastole of bicuspid aortic valves without (A, B), and with (C, D) a raphe.

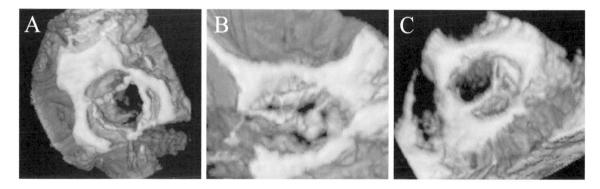

Figure 12.2

Three-dimensional echocardiography short-axis view of a normal trileaflet aortic valve (A), a trileaflet valve with degenerative aortic stenosis (B), and a bicuspid aortic valve with a raphe (C).

can no longer compensate for the increasing obstruction, LV dilation and progressive LV dysfunction occur.

Clinical presentation

Aortic stenosis is typically associated with a long latent period in which patients remain asymptomatic. Diagnosis during this stage is usually made after evaluation of a heart murmur noted on physical examination. The classic presenting symptoms in aortic stenosis are angina, syncope, and dyspnea due to congestive heart failure. Angina frequently occurs even in the absence of significant epicardial coronary artery disease, as a result of myocardial oxygen supply demand mismatch due to diminished coronary flow to the hypertrophied LV. Syncope in aortic stenosis may be due to mechanical obstruction to LV outflow, ventricular arrhythmias, or an abnormal vasodepressor reflex in the setting of a high LV diastolic pressure. With the onset of LV dysfunction, symptoms of dyspnea and volume overload are common.

Physical examination of a patient with severe aortic stenosis classically reveals a loud late peaking systolic ejection murmur, often heard with equal intensity at the apex and base, slow and late carotid upstrokes, and a diminished loudness of A_2. As aortic stenosis becomes more severe, the systolic murmur typically moves later in systole as it takes the LV longer to generate the systolic pressure to initiate systolic ejection (Figure 12.3). The A_2 may become increasingly inaudible due to the prolonged aortic ejection murmur and to progressive restriction of leaflet excursion. Ultimately, as critical aortic obstruction develops or with the development of significant LV dysfunction, the intensity of the systolic murmur may decrease due to diminished transaortic flow.

The natural history of untreated aortic stenosis is closely tied to symptoms (Figure 12.4). During the asymptomatic latent period, morbidity and mortality, even with severe aortic stenosis, are low, although a small risk of sudden cardiac death (approximately 1% per year) has been noted.[7] Once symptoms develop, prognosis is poor.[1,8] Average survivals in patients with aortic stenosis with angina, syncope, and heart failure have been reported to be 5, 3 and <2 years, respectively.[1,8]

Treatment of aortic stenosis is discussed in detail elsewhere in this book, but in symptomatic adults, aortic valve replacement can restore an excellent long-term prognosis.[8]

Echocardiography for the assessment of aortic stenosis

Two-dimensional and Doppler echocardiography is the primary imaging modality for the diagnosis of aortic stenosis. In addition to the identification of the level of LV outflow obstruction (supravalvular, valvular, or subvalvular), echocardiography frequently allows determination of etiology (i.e. congenital, rheumatic, or degenerative), multiple ways to categorize the severity of the LV obstruc-

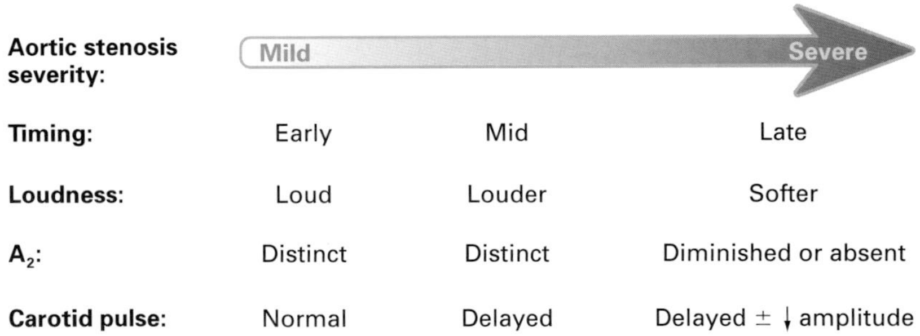

Aortic stenosis severity:	Mild → Severe		
Timing:	Early	Mid	Late
Loudness:	Loud	Louder	Softer
A_2:	Distinct	Distinct	Diminished or absent
Carotid pulse:	Normal	Delayed	Delayed ± ↓ amplitude

Figure 12.3

Physical examination findings in patients with mild, moderate, and severe aortic stenosis.

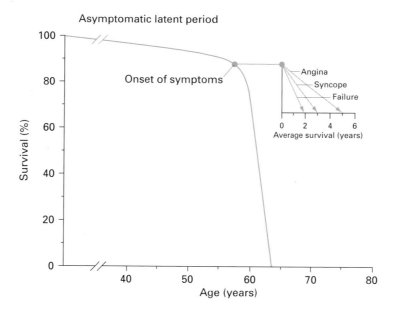

Figure 12.4

Natural history of aortic stenosis. (Adapted from Ross J, Braunwald A. Circulation 1968; 37(Suppl V): 61[8] with permission from Lippincott Williams & Wilkins.)

tion, and visualization of other associated cardiac findings vital to clinical decision making for the patient with aortic stenosis (i.e. LV dysfunction and coexistent valve disease).

Assessment of severity

Aortic pressure gradient

The pressure gradient across the aortic valve is arguably the most clinically important parameter for assessing the severity of aortic stenosis. The pressure gradient represents the load that the LV must overcome to maintain stroke volume. The pressure gradient is determined not only by the aortic valve orifice area but also by other factors such as LV performance. Doppler-derived pressure gradients are calculated using the modified Bernoulli equation

$$\Delta P = 4(V_1^2 - V_2^2)$$

where ΔP is the pressure gradient, V_1 is the velocity proximal to the stenosis (generally in the LVOT), and V_2 is the velocity at the aortic valve (where the flow velocity is greatest). This equation is commonly simplified further to

$$\Delta P = 4V_2^2$$

This simplification is acceptable provided that there is no significant acceleration of flow prior to the aortic valve. Examples of situations where it is important to use the full V_1, V_2 equation include patients with coexistent aortic regurgitation or dynamic LVOT obstruction (i.e. hypertrophic cardiomyopathy), in which the velocity across the LVOT (V_1) will also be elevated.

Aortic pressure gradients determined with Doppler echocardiography are maximum instantaneous pressure gradients (defined as the maximum pressure gradient across the aortic valve at any one point in time) and mean pressure gradients. Mean pressure gradients are derived by tracing the Doppler profile and are calculated automatically using standard echocardiographic analysis programs. Carefully obtained Doppler mean pressure gradients correlate well with mean pressure gradients derived by cardiac catheterization.[9] Catheter-derived maximal instantaneous pressure gradients also correlate with Doppler-derived maximum pressure gradients; however, peak-to-peak gradients commonly reported at cardiac catheterization do not. Peak LV and peak aortic pressures do not occur simultaneously (Figure 12.5); thus, there is no directly comparable Doppler-derived measurement. For consistency, transaortic gradients should be clearly identified as 'mean systolic', 'maximum instantaneous', or 'peak-to-peak' gradients.

Aortic valve area by continuity equation

The continuity equation is the primary means of calculating aortic valve area with echocardiography. This calculation relies on the principle that blood flow through the LVOT must be equal to blood flow through the aortic valve (Figure 12.6). Blood flow (Q) through any orifice is equal to the product of the cross-sectional area (CSA) and the time–velocity integral (TVI) at that specific location:

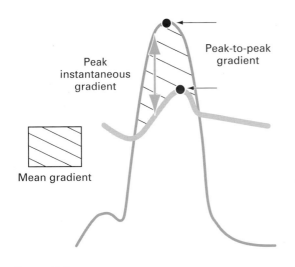

Figure 12.5

Simultaneous LV and ascending aortic pressure waveforms in a patient with aortic stenosis demonstrating the difference between the peak instantaneous gradient and the peak-to-peak gradient. The mean aortic pressure gradient is the mean of the peak instantaneous pressure gradients within the cross-hatched area.

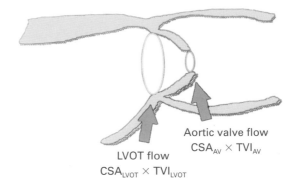

Figure 12.6

Practical application of the continuity equation: The CSA of the LVOT can be determined from a measurement of the LVOT diameter (D) using the equation: $CSA_{LVOT} = \pi (D/2)^2$. The TVI of the LVOT and aortic valve can be determined by tracing the appropriate Doppler profile using standard echocardiographic analysis programs. The aortic valve area (CSA_{AV}) can then be determined.

$$Q = CSA \times TVI$$

The TVI is generally obtained with Doppler echocardiography by tracing the Doppler profile and is automatically calculated using standard echocardiographic analysis programs. The CSA of the LVOT is calculated by measuring the LVOT diameter (D), which is best obtained from the parasternal long-axis view:

$$CSA_{LVOT} = \pi (D/2)^2$$

Consequently, the blood flow through the LVOT can be derived:

$$Q_{LVOT} = \pi (D/2)^2 \times TVI_{LVOT}$$

Because the blood flow through the LVOT must equal the blood flow through the aortic valve, the cross-sectional area of the aortic valve (CSA_{AV}) can be determined from the following continuity equation (Figure 12.7):

$$CSA_{AV} = \frac{CSA_{LVOT} \times TVI_{LVOT}}{TVI_{AV}}$$

This equation can be simplified by substituting the peak LVOT and aortic valve velocities with

$$CSA_{LVOT} \times TVI_{LVOT} = CSA_{AV} \times TVI_{AV}$$

$$CSA_{AV} = \rule{6cm}{0.4pt}$$

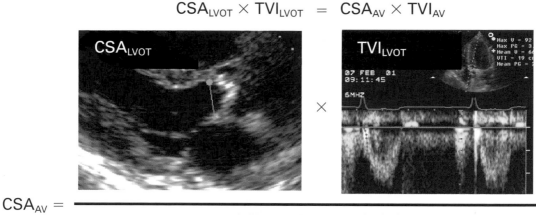

Figure 12.7

Basic principal of the continuity equations: blood flow through the LVOT ($CSA_{LVOT} \times TVI_{LVOT}$) must equal blood flow through the aortic valve ($CSA_{AV} \times TVI_{AV}$) AV, aortic value; CSA, cross sectional area; LVOT, left ventricular outflow tract; TVI, time velocity integral.

acceptable results. Additional attempts to simplify this equation generally sacrifice accuracy. As the LVOT diameter directly varies with patient body size, it is important to measure LVOT diameter directly for accurate aortic valve area calculations. However, LVOT diameters are generally stable in the same patient over time, so differences on serial studies are more likely to be due to measurement error than a real change. Thus, similar LVOT diameters should be used for calculation of CSA_{AV} in serial studies in order to obtain a true assessment of disease progression.

An additional consideration when assessing the severity of aortic stenosis with aortic valve area is patient size. Aortic valve area will vary with patient size, such that a valve area of 1.0 cm^2 in a large patient might represent significant obstruction of LV outflow, while the same valve

area in a very small patient may not. A common way to correct for patient body size is to 'index' the valve area for body surface area (BSA): CSA_{AV}/BSA (Table 12.1). This calculation is particularly important to perform in large or small patients, or in

Table 12.1	Measures of aortic stenosis severity		
Aortic stenosis severity	Aortic valve area (cm^2)	Aortic valve index (cm^2/m^2)	Mean aortic gradient (mmHg)
Mild	>1.5	>0.9	<25
Moderate	1.0–1.5	0.6–0.9	25–50
Severe	<1.0	<0.6	>50
Critical	<0.8	<0.4	>75

patients in whom the valve area and transaortic pressure gradients are discordant.

Aortic valve area by planimetry

Aortic valve area can also be directly measured by tracing the aortic valve orifice in a short-axis view. Accurate planimetry tracing generally requires transesophageal echocardiography (Figure 12.8), which allows for higher-resolution visualization of the aortic valve leaflets due to the closer proximity to the valve and the lack of attenuating structures (chest wall, bone, and lungs). Transesophageal planimetry of the aortic valve correlates well with measurement of aortic valve area by the continuity equation and should be considered in patients with technically suboptimal transthoracic images or when there are conflicting conclusions of aortic stenosis severity from other diagnostic modalities.[10,11]

Other measures of aortic stenosis severity

The ratio of LVOT velocity to aortic valve velocity can also be used to assess aortic stenosis severity. The advantage of a velocity ratio is that patient body size is not considered; thus, it allows direct comparison of stenosis severity across a broad population. A velocity ratio of 0.5 indicates that the aortic valve area is half the normal size, while a velocity ratio of 0.3 or less is generally present in patients with severe aortic stenosis. The velocity ratio is most useful for assessing progression of aortic stenosis in an individual patient, or as a quick screen to identify patients in whom a full evaluation with continuity equation will be required (i.e. a patient with increased velocities across the aortic valve due to moderate aortic insufficiency but without obvious two-dimensional evidence of aortic stenosis).

Aortic valve resistance has been suggested as a less flow-dependent measurement of aortic

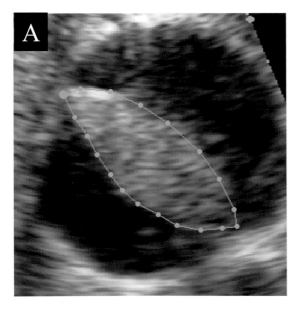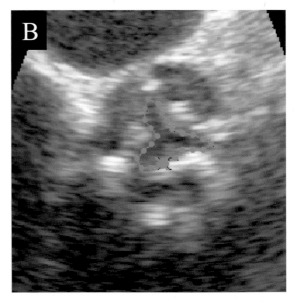

Figure 12.8

Transeophageal short-axis view of a bicuspid aortic valve (A) and a trileaflet aortic valve with degenerative aortic stenosis (B), demonstrating the use of planimetry for determination of aortic valve area.

stenosis severity, but recent studies suggest that it adds little to aortic valve area and has not gained widespread clinical acceptance.[13,14]

Progression of aortic stenosis

Clinical decisions regarding treatment and follow-up of patients with aortic stenosis frequently depend on the expected rate of progression of the disease. Aortic valve area decreases on average at a rate of 0.12 cm²/year, with an average increase in mean gradient of 7 mmHg/year; however, the rate of progression for the individual can be highly variable.[13] Over the last decade, echocardiographic findings such as a peak aortic jet velocity >4.0 m/s, an increase in peak aortic jet velocity of >0.3 m/s per year, and evidence of moderate or severe aortic valve calcification have been shown to predict symptom onset and need for aortic valve replacement in patients with aortic stenosis (Figure 12.9).[14,15]

Pitfalls in the echocardiographic diagnosis of aortic stenosis

Quantitative assessment of aortic valve stenosis severity with echocardiography correlates well with invasive assessment of aortic stenosis using the Gorlin formula.[16–18] However, each of these modalities has some technical limitations that can lead to measurement variability. It is important to be aware of the limitations and potential sources of error, particularly when results do not fit the clinical picture or are discordant with other diagnostic modalities. We will discuss some of the potential pitfalls of echocardiography here.

Technical considerations

LVOT diameter   This should be measured in the parasternal long-axis view in mid-systole. Because the LVOT diameter is squared [$CSA_{LVOT} = \pi (D/2)^2$] for determination of the LVOT area, small differences in LVOT diameter can cause

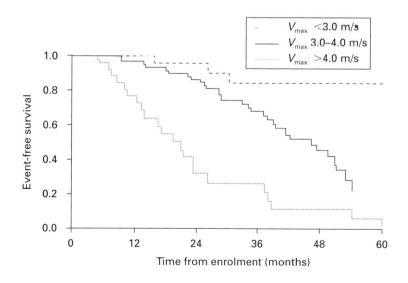

Figure 12.9

Event-free survival without valve replacement in patients with asymptomatic aortic stenosis. A maximal aortic velocity (V_{max}) >4.0 m/s predicts a poor event-free survival. (Adapted from Otto et al. Circulation 1997; 95: 2262–70[16] with permission from Lippincott Williams & Wilkins.)

significant differences in aortic valve area. In order to minimize this limitation, multiple LVOT measurements should be obtained in all patients and similar LVOT diameters should be used for serial studies in individual patients.

Aortic valve velocities   As with all Doppler-derived velocities and pressure gradients, the ultrasound beam and the jet of blood flow must be parallel for accurate measurement. If there is any deviation from this, the velocity and pressure gradient will be underestimated. Aortic velocities should be obtained from multiple transducer positions to obtain the highest possible velocities. The apical and suprasternal views commonly yield the best alignment with the highest velocities. Only complete Doppler signals with crisp edges over the entire systolic ejection period should be used for tracing.

LVOT velocities   LVOT velocities may be obtained with either continuous-wave or pulsed-wave Doppler echocardiography, and they should be similar when both can be adequately obtained. However, continuous-wave LVOT profiles are frequently inadequate for measurement, so caution should be used when only continuous-wave Doppler analysis is available. The pulsed-wave LVOT velocity determination should be performed at the same point as the LVOT diameter measurement, although this can be difficult to ensure in practice. Care should be taken to note if the pulsed-wave LVOT Doppler profile is obtained too close to the aortic valve where flow acceleration occurs prior to the stenotic orifice, as this will lead to underestimation of aortic valve area. Routine acquisition and measurement of multiple LVOT samples can help avoid these potential sources of error.

Patient factors

Rhythm other than sinus   When the patient has an irregular rhythm, the stroke volume for each beat changes. Thus, multiple samples of the LVOT and aortic valve velocities (about 10) need to be acquired and averaged to get true assessments of transaortic pressure gradients and aortic valve areas. On a continuous-wave Doppler profile, the ratio of the LVOT velocity to the aortic valve velocity for each beat should be similar, although multiple measurements should still be obtained, because differences in aortic valve opening may occur with beat-by-beat differences in transaortic flow.

Coexistent mitral regurgitation   Mitral regurgitation is commonly present in patients with aortic stenosis and can complicate the assessment of aortic stenosis. In patients with significant mitral regurgitation, transaortic gradients may be relatively low despite significant aortic stenosis and preserved LV function due to diminished transaortic forward flow. Additionally, even a small amount of mitral regurgitation can occasionally lead to misdiagnosis of aortic stenosis. Because the aortic ejection jet in apical views can be parallel and in close proximity to an eccentric mitral regurgitant jet, a high-velocity mitral regurgitant jet can sometimes be included in the continuous-wave Doppler sample across the aortic valve. This leads to the erroneous appearance of a markedly increased transaortic velocity (5–6 m/s) despite a normally appearing aortic valve. Care should be taken to take note of the mitral regurgitation and the characteristics of the mitral regurgitant jet, and to correlate the two-dimensional appearance of the aortic valve with the Doppler analysis for aortic stenosis.

Low-gradient aortic stenosis   A dilemma in the clinical management of aortic stenosis is the patient with severe aortic stenosis by aortic valve area (<1.0 cm^2) but a relatively low transaortic gradient (mean gradient <30 mmHg). This occurs most commonly in patients with significant LV dysfunction, but may arise from two different etiologies: (1) true severe aortic stenosis with a resulting weak LV that cannot generate a high gradient, or (2) pseudosevere aortic stenosis in which there is limited transaortic flow due to unrelated LV dysfunction that cannot fully open a calcified aortic valve with relatively mild aortic stenosis. These two situations would require markedly different treatments, with aortic valve replacement generally indicted for the former and treatment aimed at the LV dysfunction for the latter. Dobutamine echocardiography can frequently be used to differentiate between 'pseudo aortic stenosis' and true aortic stenosis in these patients (Figure 12.10).[19]

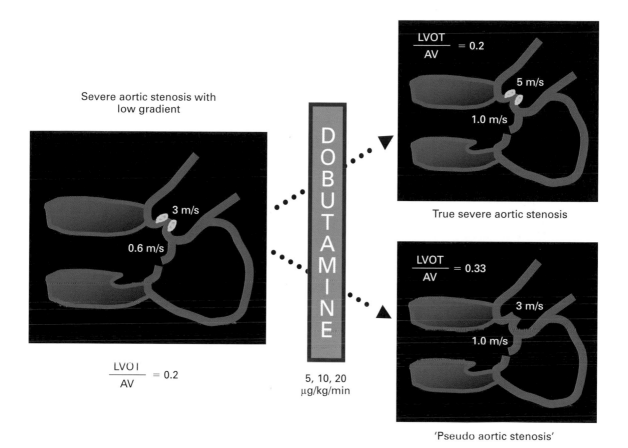

Figure 12.10

Use of dobutamine to evaluate low-gradient aortic stenosis. In a patient with a low LVOT/aortic valve (AV) velocity ratio (0.2) suggestive of severe aortic stenosis, but only a modestly elevated peak AV velocity (3.0 m/s), the addition of dobutamine can help distinguish true severe aortic stenosis from 'pseudo aortic stenosis'. Dobutamine will increase, flow through the LVOT and aortic valve. In true severe aortic stenosis, the LVOT and AV velocities will both increase resulting in a similar LVOT/AV velocity ratio. In 'pseudo aortic stenosis', the increased flow with dobutamine will facilitate improved opening of the AV. The peak velocity through the larger AV orifice will have little change, and thus the LVOT/AV velocity ratio will increase, suggesting that the aortic stenosis is not severe, and therapies aimed at improving forward flow should predominate.

Conclusion

Aortic stenosis is a disease characterized by progressive LV outflow obstruction resulting in typical symptoms, classic physical examination findings, and (if left untreated) death. Echocardiography represents the primary non-invasive imaging modality for the diagnosis of aortic stenosis and plays a vital role in the diagnosis, follow-up, and management of these patients. A thorough understanding of the clinical manifestations, pathophysiology, and echocar- diographic features of aortic stenosis is vital for all cardiovascular physicians.

References

1. Braunwald E, Zipes DP, Libby P (eds). Heart Disease: A Textbook of Cardiovascular Medicine, 6th edn. Philadelphia: WB Saunders, 2001.
2. Brauner R, Laks H, Drinkwater DC, et al. Benefits of early surgical repair in fixed subaortic stenosis. J Am Coll Cardiol 1997; 30: 1835–42.
3. Parry AJ, Kovalchin JP, Suda K, et al. Resection of

subaortic stenosis; Can a more aggressive approach be justified? Eur J Cardiothorac Surg 1999; 15: 631–8.

4. Passik CS, Ackerman DM, Pluth JR, Edwards WD. Temporal changes in the causes of aortic stenosis: a surgical pathologic study of 646 cases. Mayo Clin Proc 1987; 62: 119–23.

5. Otto CM, Lind BK, Kitzman DW, et al. Association of aortic valve sclerosis with cardiovascular mortality and morbidity in the elderly. N Engl J Med 1999; 341: 142.

6. Stewart BF, Siscovick D, Lind BK, et al. Clinical factors associated with calcific aortic valve disease. J Am Coll Cardiol 1997; 29: 630–4.

7. Bonow RO, Carabello B, de Leon AC Jr, et al. Guidelines for the management of patients with valvular heart disease: executive summary. Circulation 1998; 98: 1949–84.

8. Ross J, Braunwald E. The influence of corrective operations on the natural history of aortic stenosis. Circulation 1968; 37(Suppl V): 61.

9. Currie PJ, Seward JB, Reeder GS, et al. Continuous-wave Doppler echocardiographic assessment of severity of calcific aortic stenosis: a simultaneous Doppler-catheter correlative study in 100 adult patients. Circulation 1985; 71: 1162–9.

10. Kim C, Berglund H, Nishioka T, et al. Correspondence of aortic valve area determination from transesophageal echocardiography, transthoracic echocardiography, and cardiac catheterization. Am Heart J 1996; 132: 1163–72.

11. Hoffman R, Flachskampf FA, Hanrath P. Planimetry of orifice area in aortic stenosis using multiplane transesophageal echocardiography. J Am Coll Cardiol 1996; 22: 529–34.

12. Blais C, Pibarot P, Dumesnil JG, et al. Comparison of valve resistance with effective orifice area regarding flow dependence. Am J Cardiol 2001; 88: 45–52.

13. Mascherbauer J, Schima H, Rosenhek R, et al. Value and limitations of aortic valve resistance with particular consideration of low flow–low gradient aortic stenosis: an in vitro study. Eur Heart J 2004; 25: 787–93.

14. Otto, CM, Burwarsh IG, Legget ME, et al. A prospective study of asymptomatic valvular aortic stenosis: clinical, echocardiographic and exercise predictors of outcome. Circulation 1997; 95: 2262–70.

15. Rosenhek R, Binder T, Porenta G, et al. Predictors of outcome in severe, asymptomatic aortic stenosis. N Engl J Med 2000; 343: 611–17.

16. Skjaerpe T, Hegrenaes L, Hatle L. Noninvasive estimation of valve area in patients with aortic stenosis by Doppler ultrasound and two-dimensional echocardiography. Circulation 1985; 72: 810–18.

17. Zoghbi WA, Farmer KL, Soto JG, et al. Accurate noninvasive quantification of stenotic aortic valve area by Doppler echocardiography. Circulation 1986; 73: 452–9.

18. Teirstein P, Yeager M, Yock PG, Popp RL. Doppler echocardiographic measurement of aortic valve area in aortic stenosis: a noninvasive application of the Gorlin formula. J Am Coll Cardiol 1986; 8: 1059–65.

19. DeFilippi CR, Willett DL, Brickner ME, et al. Usefulness of dobutamine echocardiography in distinguishing severe from nonsevere valvular aortic stenosis in patients with depressed left ventricular function and low transvalvular gradient. Am J Cardiol 1995; 75: 191–4.

13

Hemodynamic evaluation of aortic valve disease and indications for repair/replacement

Joseph D Kay, John D Carroll

Overview

Abnormalities of the aortic valve are generally categorized as involving incompetence of the valve, i.e. aortic regurgitation or insufficiency, versus obstruction of the valve, i.e. aortic stenosis. In some valves, both abnormalities may be present. In this chapter, the hemodynamic abnormalities of these two prototypic lesions will be described, emphasizing methods used in the cardiac catheterization laboratory. This is particularly relevant to the emerging era of percutaneous aortic valve replacement, which requires hemodynamic measurements before and after the intervention. Furthermore, the indications for intervention on the aortic valve, either incompetent or stenotic, will be described and put in the context of percutaneous aortic valve replacement.

The assessment of the patient with aortic valve disease begins with an assessment of the hemodynamic severity of the valvular abnormality. Additional factors involved in decision-making, including the decision for surgical or percutaneous intervention, are shown in Figure 13.1.

There is also a need to assess hemodynamics after intervention. Prosthetic valves are not perfect, and it is expected that some may be relatively obstructive while others may have some degree of incompetence from inherent design limitations, unusual patient anatomy, technical problems at the time of implantation and degeneration. Of particular concern is the issue of patient–prosthetic mismatch, which results when the prosthetic valve has a degree of obstruction,

e.g. a postimplantation transvalvular gradient, that may prevent symptomatic improvement, regression of left ventricular (LV) hypertrophy and dilatation, and improved prognosis.[1] Elderly females with small aortic roots have been the major at-risk group in the surgical valve replacement era, and percutaneous valve replacement may or may not show a patient–prosthetic mismatch problem. Pressure gradient measurement and assessment of regurgitation with aortography are therefore methods that need to be used immediately post implantation of percutaneous valves.

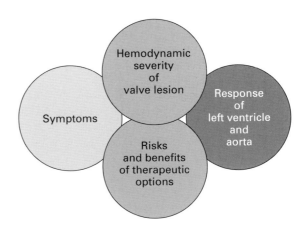

Figure 13.1

Hemodynamic assessment of aortic valve abnormalities is one of several key issues in patient management, including percutaneous valve replacement.

Aortic stenosis

Hemodynamics of aortic stenosis

Before presenting current methods of quantifying aortic stenosis using anatomic and hemodynamic measures, it is important to review the obstructive physiology of aortic stenosis. Obstruction can be described by its impact on blood flow and pressures. A large transvalvular gradient generally indicates severe obstruction, but may also be seen with moderate obstruction in the setting of high-flow states such as anemia, severe obesity, hyperthyroidism, and coexisting severe aortic regurgitation. Many patients may have lower than expected gradients with reduced transvalvular flow. Thus, it is important to understand flow and pressure alterations in aortic stenosis.

Aortic stenosis can be thought of as having multiple distinct hemodynamic zones with unique pressure and blood flow characteristics and relationship to the anatomic valve orifice (Figures 13.2 and 13.3 and Table 13.1). Using micro-

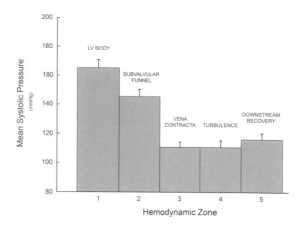

Figure 13.3

In a group of 35 patients with symptomatic aortic stenosis, the mean systolic pressure was measured in each of the five hemodynamic zones. Presented here are the averages and standard errors. Note the downstream pressure recovery of 5 mmHg.

manometer catheters with imbedded high-fidelity pressure and blood velocity sensors, these zones can be readily recorded. These types of recordings and the use of these expensive catheters are not routinely performed, but do provide a better description of obstructive physiology and understanding of how routine methods of measuring pressure and blood velocity still need to be performed and interpreted carefully.[2–4]

Any narrowing in the circulation causes local blood flow acceleration and potentially a transition to turbulence. We have previously described how the high-frequency oscillations recorded on high-fidelity transducers can give a measure of the intensity of turbulence and its variations with stroke volume.[5] The turbulent flow field caused by aortic stenosis and occupying the ascending aorta during systole disappears rapidly downstream. Turbulence causes energy loss associated with the stenosis, and produces the murmur.

The transvalvular pressure gradient is the hallmark of aortic valve obstruction. Using an upstream pressure waveform (i.e. LV) and a downstream pressure waveform (aortic or more commonly iliac–femoral), the gradient can be characterized. The need to adjust for the later arrival and often greater amplitude of the femoral artery pressure versus the ascending aortic waveform is well known. Typically, the pressure in the

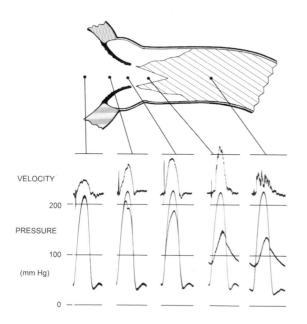

Figure 13.2

The hemodynamic zones below, at, and downstream of the stenotic orifice are shown using waveforms of high-fidelity pressure and blood velocity from transducers mounted on a catheter that was pulled back from the left ventricle to the aorta. See Table 13.1.

Table 13.1   Hemodynamic zones of aortic stenosis

Zone	Blood velocity	Pressure	Anatomic location
1	Laminar, normal velocity	LV waveform with maximal systolic pressure	LV beneath funnel of valve
2	Laminar, increasing velocity	LV waveform with decreasing systolic pressure	LV in funnel
3	Laminar, peak velocity	Aortic waveform	Orifice and vena contracta immediately above orifice
4	Turbulent	Aortic waveform with high-frequency oscillations and pressure loss especially in early to mid-systole	Ascending aorta within a few centimeters of valve orifice
5	Laminar, normal velocity	Aortic waveform with smooth but slow upstroke and having some pressure recovery relative to zone 4 aortic waveform	Downstream in aorta a variable distance in different patients

ascending aorta is recorded with the pressure from the femoral artery sheath to determine their absolute difference as well as the degree of delay in the femoral pressure waveform. In elderly adults with non-compliant systemic arterial systems, pulse wave velocity is elevated such that there is a small delay when compared with children or young adults. There also may be little systolic pressure differential between the central aorta and the iliac or femoral artery in older adults.

The arterial waveform undergoes shape and amplitude changes with distal propagation. In aortic stenosis, there are also changes in the pressure waveform with distal propagation due to changes in the blood flow characteristics, i.e. turbulent to laminar flow. As seen in Figure 13.4, the arterial pressure waveform undergoes major changes downstream for a stenotic aortic valve with a variable degree of pressure recovery. The location of pressure measurement could influence the calculation of a transvalvular gradient.[6]

Transvalvular pressure gradients are described as peak-to-peak or mean from catheter-based measurements, and instantaneous gradients are recorded with Doppler methods. Mean pressure gradients are the standard of hemodynamic assessment of the stenotic aortic valve, and an absolute mean pressure of less than 20 mmHg usually means that the degree of obstruction is not critical. On the other hand, the dependence of pressure gradient on flow leads to a mental

adjustment of the physiologic importance of a given pressure gradient when it is known that the patient's cardiac output is significantly reduced and/or LV systolic function is poor.

Hemodynamic testing with dobutamine or nitroprusside can be useful in assessing the degree of aortic stenosis in patients with a mean pressure gradient of less than 30 mmHg.[7,8] The

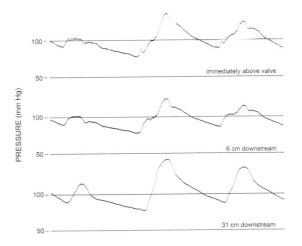

Figure 13.4

Simultaneously recorded high-fidelity pressure measurements at the valve and 6 and 31 cm downstream were taken from this patient with severe aortic stenosis. Note the change in the waveforms, including the later arrival of turbulent oscillations.

failure to increase the pressure gradient when flow increases implies that the stenosis is not severe. Nitroprusside may also be safely used to treat decompensated systolic heart failure despite severe aortic stenosis.[9]

Finally, the systolic ejection period must be assessed to finalize the assessment of the severity of aortic stenosis. Rapid heart rates reduce the systolic ejection period and atrial fibrillation makes it variable. Automated cardiac catheterization laboratory recording systems may be very inaccurate in the assessment of systolic ejection period. The onset of aortic valve opening, usually denoted by the initial aortic pressure waveform upstroke, and aortic valve closure, usually denoted at the dicrotic notch (if still visible), are the two time landmarks needed to measure the systolic ejection period. In compensated aortic stenosis, it is typical that ejection is prolonged, but with the onset of LV dysfunction it shortens.

Flow measurements in the cardiac catheterization laboratory are usually performed with either thermodilution or with calculation of arteriovenous oxygen differences, with an assumed oxygen consumption yielding an estimated Fick cardiac output. Thermodilution-determined cardiac outputs become less accurate with low cardiac outputs and in the face of tricuspid regurgitation.

Calculated indices of the severity of aortic stenosis

The clinical need for quantification of aortic stenosis severity has led to the development and testing of different indices, typically expressed as a single number. Using transvalvular gradient alone is problematic because of the common occurrence of moderate to high gradients in asymptomatic patients with a compensated LV on the one hand and the low flow states in the setting of LV dysfunction on the other hand. As displayed in Figure 13.1, the hemodynamic severity is put in the context of other issues before decisions are made on management. With this in mind, the calculated indices of aortic stenosis severity summarize the hemodynamic measurements either in the form of resistance units or by converting the hemodynamics into a calculated orifice size.

Aortic valve area

Despite valve area being part of the dogma of clinical cardiology, it is a calculated description fraught with some error and potential misrepresentation of aortic stenosis severity in a significant number of patients. The calculation of aortic valve area utilizes the Gorlin equation and requires an assessment of transvalvular flow, the mean pressure gradient, and the systolic ejection period and heart rate:

$$\text{aortic valve area (in cm}^2\text{)} = \frac{CO}{44.3 \times SEP \times HR \times \sqrt{(\text{mean gradient})}}$$

where CO is cardiac output (in ml/min), SEP is systolic ejection period (in s), and HR is heart rate (in beats/min); the mean gradient is in mmHg. The limitations of the Gorlin equation are numerous and well described by Ford et al.[10] One of the most common problems is the frequent overestimation of the severity of aortic stenosis when cardiac output is low from the excessive flow dependence of the equation or errors in transvalvular flow determination.

A calculated aortic valve area of less than 0.75 cm^2 remains a reasonable cut-off for clearly severe aortic stenosis and an area of up to 1.0 cm^2 represents a value that may represent obstruction capable of producing symptoms in some but not all patients. It is wise to always report the mean pressure gradient and the cardiac output rather than the valve area alone. Further nuances of valve area calculations have been reviewed.[11]

The derivation of calculated valve areas is appealing to the physician and helps explain the malady to patients. The oversimplified visualization of the orifice as a circular structure is apparent in most cases of adult aortic stenosis with irregular orifices.

Aortic valve resistance

This calculated variable also utilizes measured pressures and flow:

$$\text{aortic valve resistance (in dyn} \cdot \text{s/cm}^5\text{)} = \frac{\text{mean gradient}}{\text{flow}}$$

$$= \frac{1.33 \times \text{mean gradient} \times SEP \times HR}{CO}$$

A plot of calculated aortic valve area and resistance shows that a value of resistance below 250 $dyn \cdot s/cm^5$ corresponds to a valve that is not generally considered critical (i.e. >0.75 cm^2). As the true orifice becomes smaller, the valve resistance increases markedly out of proportion to further reductions in calculated orifice. This fits well with clinical evidence that symptoms and clinical deterioration progress rapidly once the valve narrows into this severe range.[12] Others have found that resistance calculations are also flow-dependent and therefore not the perfect index of aortic stenosis severity.[13]

The assessment of changes in aortic stenosis severity after balloon valvuloplasty has shown the residual obstruction commonly remaining with this simple balloon technique.[14] Similar post-implantation hemodynamic studies with percutaneous aortic valve replacement will need to be performed.

Direct visualization of aortic stenosis

Echocardiography, magnetic resonance imaging (MRI), and cardiac computed tomography (CT) are all capable of visualizing the stenotic aortic valve, although rarely is this anatomic assessment adequate for clinical purposes. In the era of percutaneous valve replacement in the cardiac catheterization laboratory, the recent refinement of intracardiac echocardiography (ICE) has provided the interventional cardiologist with the ability to visualize structures before, during, and after interventions. The current catheter contains a 10 MHz ultrasound transducer mounted on a 10 Fr catheter. Release of a lower-profile 8 Fr catheter is expected in 2005, which will allow safer use in smaller children. With the transducer in close proximity to the cardiac valves, increased spatial resolution of the aortic valve is possible, with images equivalent or superior to transesophageal echocardiography (Figure 13.5). Preliminary studies have shown that ICE assessment of aortic valve area correlates closely with invasive hemodynamic assessment using the Gorlin equation ($r = 0.78$) and more closely with pathologic in vitro direct measurement of aortic valve area ($r = 0.98$).[15,16]

With the development of 3D reconstructions from a variety of imaging modalities, it will be possible to quantify the tapering or non-tapering nature of the region immediately below the orifice. Valve shape, orifice roughness, and aortic root size all have an impact on the hemodynamics of aortic stenosis.[17]

The left ventricle in aortic stenosis

The hypertrophic response of the LV to the increased resistance of ejection through a narrowed aortic valve is an expected adaptive response that corresponds to the maintenance of a compensated clinical and hemodynamic state until fairly late in the disease process. It is quite remarkable that the LV can grow and easily generate systolic pressures that are two to three times greater than normal.

Eventually, the adaptation of the LV becomes inadequate. The response to the LV varies from patient to patient with aortic stenosis. Some of this variation is caused by additional disease, such as coronary artery disease.

Some patients present with marked systolic dysfunction and grossly elevated filling pressures indicative of a myopathic LV. Secondary mitral regurgitation is a common finding in these patients with dilated LV at end-diastole as well as end-systole. These individuals are more likely to be men and the degree of reversibility of the LV dysfunction is variable.[18] The lowered forward stroke volume causes the mean transvalvular gradient to be less than expected for the severity of aortic stenosis and may lead to provocative testing to increase transvalvular flow and reassessment of the valve gradient. Other measures, such as visualization of the valve by transthoracic, intracardiac, or transesophageal echocardiography, are needed to detect the severity of valve abnormality.

Some patients, particularly elderly women, present with symptomatic aortic stenosis with a small ventricle, a thick wall, a high-pressure gradient, and an elevated ejection fraction.[18] There may be significant elevation of LV filling pressures. These patients may be smaller, and concerns with patient–prosthetic mismatch have led to better prosthetic valve design. Despite this, some still need aortic valve outflow tract widening procedures. Others may have a subvalvular component

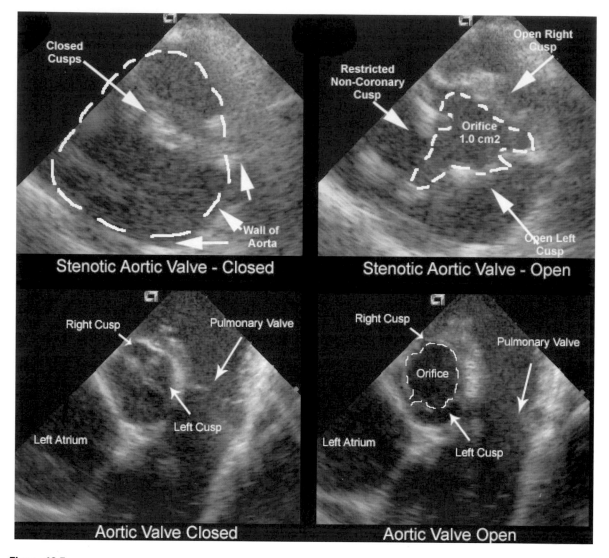

Figure 13.5

Intracardiac ultrasound of a stenotic aortic valve with slight magnification (top two images), and a normal aortic valve (bottom two images). The images during systole provide a new tool to assess aortic stenosis severity in a format similar to the parasternal short axis from transthoracic echocardiography, with the special resolution of a transesophageal echocardiogram, although not requiring the deep sedation needed for prolonged transesophageal imaging.

of obstruction that only becomes obvious when the valvular stenosis is relieved. Septal myomyectomy may be necessary.

The hemodynamics of aortic stenosis and associated changes in LV function have implications for percutaneous aortic valve replacement. The small chamber may also make percutaneous valve procedures challenging. Balloon positioning across the valve may be difficult, with hyperdynamic chamber function and runs of ventricular tachycardia with LV guidewires. After valve implantation, there is the potential for the emergence of a subvalvular gradient from the hypertrophic septum and the hyperdynamic chamber that would need to be recognized and corrective actions instituted such as beta-blocker therapy

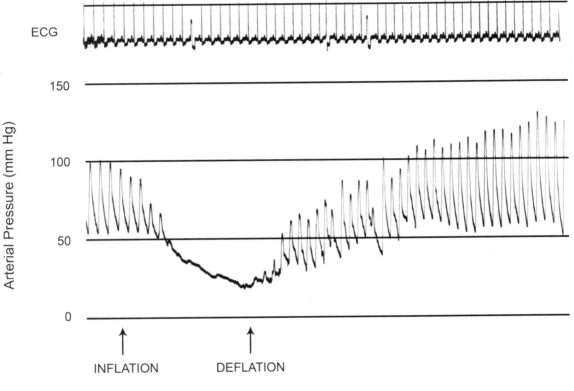

Figure 13.6

Balloon valvuloplasty of the aortic valve produces transient severe hypotension with a subsequent pressure rebound that is usually due to lessened obstruction and increased sympathetic tone.

and volume expansion. On the other hand, the severely myopathic LV may poorly tolerate the rapid pacing and transient occlusion of the aortic orifice during valve implantation (Figure 13.6).

Additional special hemodynamic subsets

Aortic stenosis and systolic hypertension

It is considered inconsistent to have elevated systolic arterial pressures and severe aortic stenosis. While this may be true for younger adults, it is common in aortic stenosis of the elderly to have systolic hypertension. The mechanism has not been well studied, but observations suggest that there is clearly a reflex vasoconstriction that occurs in the systemic vascular bed as aortic stenosis progresses. This may be, from a physiologic viewpoint, an adaptive means to maintain central aortic perfusion pressure while resting cardiac output starts to decline in severe to critical aortic stenosis. In addition, these elderly patients have very stiff or rigid large arteries, and the magnification of reflective waves and increased pulse pressure despite a lowered stroke volume both act to increase systolic pressure. As a result, the LV must eject not only against a stenotic aortic valve but also into an arterial system that has markedly reduced large artery compliance and increased peripheral vascular resistance.[7,9,19]

Aortic stenosis and pulmonary hypertension

Unlike mitral stenosis, the finding of pulmonary hypertension does not seem part of the pathophysiology of severe aortic stenosis. Patients with severe aortic stenosis undergoing aortic valve surgery may have important pulmonary hypertension. Surgical mortality is higher in those with pulmonary hypertension, but the hypertension appears to reverse after valve replacement, suggesting a linkage to the aortic stenosis – perhaps the commonly present LV diastolic dysfunction.[20]

Indications for aortic valve replacement/repair

As outlined in Figure 13.1, the management of patients with aortic stenosis is determined by multiple factors. Therapy should bring relief or substantial improvement of symptoms and a better prognosis at a reasonable risk to the patient. Percutaneous valve therapy will be evaluated in this general context of medical decision-making.

In children with hemodynamically severe aortic stenosis, with or without symptoms, the recommendation is surgical or balloon commissural incision/tearing. In this way, aortic valve replacement can be delayed, potentially for several decades.

In adults, the indications for aortic valve replacement have been symptoms or the development of LV systolic dysfunction in the setting of hemodynamically severe aortic stenosis. Balloon valvuloplasty is reserved as a bridging treatment to surgical valve replacement in severely decompensated patients. The use of balloon valvuloplasty as a palliative therapy when surgery is not reasonable due to comorbid conditions is routine in some centers but controversial in others.

The American College of Cardiology/American Heart Association (ACC/AHA) Guidelines for Management of Patients with Valvular Heart Disease, originally released in 1998,[21] are expected to be published in revised form in 2005.

Aortic regurgitation

Pathophysiology of aortic regurgitation

The volume load from aortic insufficiency stimulates compensatory changes in the LV to minimize increased diastolic wall stress. The LV dilates via the production of new sarcomeres, thus allowing for the eccentric hypertrophy.[22] Stroke volume increases with preservation of the cardiac output. Despite the preserved ejection fraction, the increased LV volume results in an increased systolic wall stress and afterload, stimulating additional concentric hypertrophy.[22,23] Although the LV can adapt to this combined excessive afterload and preload reserve for many years, eventually an afterload mismatch develops. A further increase in afterload leads initially to asymptomatic increased filling pressures, and eventually systolic dysfunction, followed by symptoms of exercise intolerance and congestive heart failure. As described earlier, the ventricular function may recover, with normalization of LV size and hypertrophy over 6 months to a year, provided that aortic valve replacement is performed promptly.

Hemodynamics of aortic regurgitation

Pressure waveforms and blood flow patterns are abnormal in aortic regurgitation. The arterial waveform in chronic aortic regurgitation shows an increased systolic pressure, a widened pulse pressure, and a decreased diastolic pressure. LV end-diastolic pressure may be normal or elevated, depending on LV adaptations and the chronicity of the regurgitation.

The major abnormality of blood flow is the substantial reversal of flow in diastole. Quantification of this abnormality is described below.

Changes in the ascending aorta

As with all valvular abnormalities, both the chambers upstream and downstream from the diseased valve are affected. In aortic insufficiency, therefore, the aorta as well as the LV is frequently found to dilate over time, occasionally requiring surgical resection at the time of valve replacement. This dilation in itself may lead to further annular dilation and an increase in the regurgitant fraction. Earlier studies have suggested that significant aortic dilation was not the norm, with only a 19% incidence.[24] More recent studies have refuted that number, with 30–50% having significant ascending aortic dilation.[25] Careful attention to the ascending aorta is therefore also required at serial follow-up, as well as prior to surgery, to reduce the risk of spontaneous aortic rupture and/or dissection, particularly in patients with a congenitally bicuspid aortic valve who have an increased risk for aortic complications.

Calculated indices of the severity of aortic regurgitation

Regurgitant volumes and fraction

Although echocardiography has replaced invasive catheterization assessment of aortic insufficiency severity in many centers, invasive-derived measurements of regurgitant fractions have shown to be useful predictors of regression of LV size after surgery. Calculation of regurgitant fraction may also be done with MRI. Calculation of the regurgitant fraction in the cardiac catheterization laboratory first requires validated quantitative angiography and the determination of forward cardiac output with Fick or thermodilution methods. Inaccuracies in any of these determinations will substantially change the calculated regurgitant volume and fraction.

Calculation of the LV volume from LV angiocardiography may be completed in either an anteroposterior or 30° RAO projection via the area–length method as described by Dodge and colleagues.[26,27] The short-axis diameter of each ventricular image is calculated from the equation $D = 4A/\pi L$, where D is the chamber diameter, A is the chamber area, and L is the length of the chamber. Volume (V) in systole and diastole is then calculated from the equation $V = (\pi/6)LD_aD_b$, where L is the longer measured length of two orthogonal projections and D_a and D_b are the calculated transverse diameters. With single-place angiography, the true volume is calculated from the regression equation $V_{true} = 0.928V_{measured} - 3.8$ ml. This has been simplified more recently with computer-automated software available with most cardiac imaging systems. The stroke volume is then SV = end-diastolic volume (EDV) − end-systolic volume (ESV). Cardiac output and index are then calculated as previously described

via either thermodilution or the Fick method. In the absence of aortic valve disease, stroke volumes calculated via angiocardiography and the Fick or thermodilution method (CO/HR) have a close correlation, with $r = 0.97$ and $r = 0.87$, respectively.[28,29] The regurgitant stroke volume (RSV) is simply the angiographic stroke volume minus the forward stroke volume. Regurgitant fraction (RF%) is then the regurgitant volume divided by the angiographic stroke volume. Severe aortic regurgitation typically has an RF% of 60% or more. Fioretti et al[30] demonstrated that patients with a preoperative RSV/LV end-diastolic volume greater than 0.28 had an 83% chance of normalization of postoperative LV dimension, compared with 50% persistent LV postoperative dilation in those with a ratio of less than 0.29.

Aortography

Because of its simplicity, the most common method of assessing the severity of aortic regurgitation invasively is a visually derived qualitative scale with grades from 1+ to 4+, based upon an angiographic injection of contrast into the ascending aorta, as described by Cohn et al.[31] Faint opacification of a small portion of the LV that clears with each systole is graded as 1+; 2+ requires LV opacification to a degree less than the aorta, but not clearing with each systole; 3+ is for LV opacification equal to that of the aorta after several beats; and 4+ is when the LV is completely opacified within 1 beat to an extent equal to or greater than the aorta. This method, however, has been shown to have only a modest correlation with the quantitative approach, with significant overlap in the absolute regurgitant fraction in each grade, and therefore only a modest correlation coefficient ($r = 0.56$).[28,29] The two methods are therefore not interchangeable and physicians should therefore choose one of the two in their laboratory for internal consistency.

Indications for aortic valve replacement

Delaying aortic valve replacement until the development of symptoms in patients with aortic regurgitation, unlike those with aortic stenosis, would lead to increased early and late surgical mortality in some patients. Early hemodynamic studies have identified an elevation of the LV end-diastolic pressure of 10 or greater as a risk for death with aortic valve replacement, and that increased ventricular filling pressures are seen prior to the development of symptoms.[32,33] More recent studies have shown that the best predictors in adults for remaining asymptomatic after aortic valve replacement are an end-systolic dimension less than 5.0 cm, an end-diastolic dimension less than 7.0 cm, the rate of change of the LV dimensions in the prior 6–12 months, and normal LV systolic function.[34–36] Aortic valve replacement promptly after the identification of LV dysfunction will frequently result in normalization of LV systolic function postoperatively.[37] Unlike patients with aortic stenosis, medical therapy has been shown to decrease LV size, and may potentially be useful in delaying the need for aortic valve replacement, but it is not a substitute for replacement when indications are met.[38–40]

References

1. Rahimtoola SH. Valve prosthesis–patient mismatch: an update. J Heart Valve Dis 1998; 7: 207–10.
2. Bird JJ, Murgo JP, Pasipoularides A. Fluid dynamics of aortic stenosis: subvalvular gradients without subvalvular obstruction. Circulation 1982; 66: 835–40.
3. Carroll JD, Feldman T, Chiu YC. Four distinct hemodynamic zones in valvular aortic stenosis. Circulation 1989; 80: II-648.
4. Laskey WK, Kussmaul WG. Subvalvular gradients in patients with valvular aortic stenosis. Circulation 2001; 104: 1019–25.
5. O'Toole MF, Carroll JD, Feldman T. Turbulence intensity in aortic stenosis: frequency characteristics and effects of alterations in left ventricular function. J Heart Valve Dis 1993: 2: 94–101.
6. Garcia D, Dumesnil JG, Durand LG, et al. Discrepancies between catheter and Doppler estimates of valve effective orifice area can be predicted from the pressure recovery phenomenon: practical implications with regard to quantification of aortic stenosis severity. J Am Coll Cardiol 2003; 41: 435–42.
7. Zile MR, Gaasch WH. Heart failure in aortic stenosis: improving diagnosis and treatment. N Engl J Med 2003; 348: 1735–6.
8. Nishimura RA, Grantham A, Connoly HM, et al. Low-output, low-gradient aortic stenosis in patients with depressed left ventricular systolic function. Circulation 2002; 106: 809–13.
9. Khot UN, Novaro GM, Popovic ZB, et al. Nitroprusside in critically ill patients with left ventricular dysfunction and aortic stenosis. N Engl J Med 2003; 348: 1756–63.
10. Ford LE, Feldman T, Carroll JD. Valve resistance. Circulation 194; 89: 893–5.
11. Levine RA, Schwammenthal E. Stenosis is in the eye of the observer: Impact of pressure recovery on assessing aortic valve area. J Am Coll Cardiol 2003; 41: 443–4.
12. Ford LE, Feldman T, Chiu YC, Carroll JD. Hemodynamic resistance as a measure of functional impairment in aortic valvular stenosis. Circ Res 1990; 66: 1–7.
13. Voelker W, Reul H, Nienhaus G, et al. Comparison of valvular resistance, stroke work loss, and Gorlin valve area for quantification of aortic stenosis. Circulation 1995; 91: 1196.
14. Feldman T, Ford LE, Chui YC, Carroll JD. Changes in valvular resistance, power dissipation, and myocardial reserve with aortic valvuloplasty. J Heart Valve Dis 1992; 1: 55–64.
15. Jiang L, de Prada JA, Lee MY, et al. Quantitative assessment of stenotic aortic valve area by using intracardiac echocardiography: in vitro validation and initial in vivo illustration. Am Heart J 1996; 132: 137–44.
16. Foster GP, Weissman NJ, Picard MH, et al. Determination of aortic valve area in valvular aortic stenosis by direct measurement using intracardiac echocardiography: a comparison with the Gorlin and continuity equations. J Am Coll Cardiol 1996; 27: 392–8.
17. Gilon D, Cape EG, Handschumacher MD, et al. Effect of three-dimensional valve shape on the hemodynamics of aortic stenosis: three-dimensional echocardiographic stereolithography and patient studies. J Am Coll Cardiol 2002; 40: 1479–86.
18. Carroll JD, Carroll EP, Feldman T, et al. Sex-associated differences in left ventricular function in aortic stenosis of the elderly. Circulation 1992; 86: 1099–107.
19. Carroll JD, Hellman K, Feldman T. Systolic hypertension complicating aortic stenosis: the double-loaded ventricle. Circulation 1993; 88: I-102.
20. Malouf JF, Enriquez-Sarano M, Pellikka PA, et al. Severe pulmonary hypertension in patients with severe aortic stenosis: clinical profile and prognostic implications. J Am Coll Cardiol 2002; 40: 789–95.
21. ACC/AHA Guidelines for the Management of Patients with Valvular Heart Disease. A report of the American College of Cardiology/American

Heart Association. Task Force on Practice Guidelines (Committee on Management of Patients with Valvular Heart Disease). J Am Coll Cardiol 1998; 32: 1486–588.

22. Grossman W, Jones D, McLaurin LP. Wall stress and patterns of hypertrophy in the human left ventricle. J Clin Invest 1975; 56: 56–64.

23. Wisenbaugh T, Spann JF, Carabello BA. Differences in myocardial performance and load between patients with similar amounts of chronic aortic versus chronic mitral regurgitation. J Am Coll Cardiol 1984; 3: 916–23.

24. Olson LJ, Subramanian R, Edwards WD. Surgical pathology of pure aortic insufficiency: a study of 225 cases. Mayo Clin Proc 1984; 59: 835–41.

25. Faggiano P, Aurigemma GP, Rusconi C, Gaasch WH. Progression of valvular aortic stenosis in adults: literature review and clinical implications. Am Heart J 1996; 132: 408–17.

26. Dodge HT, Sandler H, Ballew DW, Lord JD Jr. The use of biplane angiocardigraphy for the measurement of left ventricular volume in man. Am Heart J 1960; 60: 762–76.

27. Sandler H, Dodge HT. The use of single plane angiocardiograms for the calculation of left ventricular volume in man. Am Heart J 1968; 75: 325–34.

28. Croft CH, Lipscomb K, Mathis K, et al. Limitations of qualitative angiographic grading in aortic or mitral regurgitation. Am J Cardiol 1984; 53: 1593–8.

29. Hunt D, Baxley WA, Kennedy JW, et al. Quantitative evaluation of cineaortography in the assessment of aortic regurgitation. Am J Cardiol 1973; 31: 696–700.

30. Fioretti P, Roelandt J, Tirtaman C, et al. Value of the regurgitant volume to end diastolic volume ratio to predict the regression of left ventricular dimensions after valve replacement in aortic insufficiency. Eur Heart J 1987; 8(Suppl C): 15–20.

31. Cohn LH, Mason DT, Ross J Jr, et al. Preoperative assessment of aortic regurgitation in patients with mitral valve disease. Am J Cardiol 1967; 19: 177–82.

32. Goldschlager N, Pfeifer J, Cohn K, et al. The natural history of aortic regurgitation. A clinical and hemodynamic study. Am J Med 1973; 54: 577–88.

33. Hirshfeld JW Jr, Epstein SE, Roberts AJ, et al. Indices predicting long-term survival after valve replacement in patients with aortic regurgitation and patients with aortic stenosis. Circulation 1974; 50: 1190–9.

34. Bonow RO, Lakatos E, Maron BJ, Epstein SE. Serial long-term assessment of the natural history of asymptomatic patients with chronic aortic regurgitation and normal left ventricular systolic function. Circulation 1991; 84: 1625–35.

35. Carabello BA, Williams H, Gash AK, et al. Hemodynamic predictors of outcome in patients undergoing valve replacement. Circulation 1986; 74: 1309–16.

36. Tornos MP, Olona M, Permanyer-Miralda G, et al. Clinical outcome of severe asymptomatic chronic aortic regurgitation: a long-term prospective follow-up study. Am Heart J 1995; 130: 333 9.

37. Bonow RO, Rosing DR, Maron BJ, et al. Reversal of left ventricular dysfunction after aortic valve replacement for chronic aortic regurgitation: influence of duration of preoperative left ventricular dysfunction. Circulation 1984; 70: 570–9.

38. Greenberg B, Massie B, Bristow JD, et al. Long-term vasodilator therapy of chronic aortic insufficiency. A randomized double-blinded, placebo-controlled clinical trial. Circulation 1988; 78: 92–103.

39. Lin M, Chiang HT, Lin SL, et al. Vasodilator therapy in chronic asymptomatic aortic regurgitation. enalapril versus hydralazine therapy. J Am Coll Cardiol 1994; 24: 1046–53.

40. Scognamiglio R, Fasoli G, Ponchia A, Dalla-Volta S. Long-term nifedipine unloading therapy in asymptomatic patients with chronic severe aortic regurgitation. J Am Coll Cardiol 1990; 16: 424–9.

14

Impact of new percutaneous techniques of aortic valve replacement on cardiology/cardiac surgical practice

Saibal Kar, Prediman K Shah

Introduction

Aortic valve disease (stenosis and/or regurgitation) is a common clinical problem and is likely to continue to increase in frequency with aging of the population. The traditional therapeutic approach to symptomatic and severe aortic valve disease has largely revolved around surgical replacement of the aortic valve, although infrequently reconstruction and surgical valvulotomy, especially in children, have also been among the options. The outcome of patients undergoing aortic valve replacement surgery has in general ranged from good to excellent, often even in very elderly patients, especially when stenosis is the predominant lesion and despite left ventricular dysfunction. However, there are many clinical circumstances where surgical intervention in patients with significant aortic valvular disease poses a relatively high risk of morbidity and mortality. Therefore, recent attempts at percutaneous aortic valve replacement have aroused considerable enthusiasm. In this chapter, we will briefly review the implications of this developing approach on the surgical management of aortic valve disease.

Surgical management of aortic valve disease

The two major categories of aortic valve disease are aortic stenosis and aortic regurgitation. Aortic valve stenosis is the most common cardiac valve disorder in the Western world. Two factors account for its common occurrence: roughly 1–2% of the population is born with a bicuspid aortic valve, which is prone to develop stenosis with age, and calcific and degenerative aortic valve stenosis occurs with advanced age and is bound to increase in frequency with the increased life expectancy in modern times.[1]

The first attempt to correct aortic valve disease via surgery was reported in 1954 by Charles Hufnagel, Proctor Harvey, and colleagues in their groundbreaking publication on the effective surgical treatment of end-stage aortic insufficiency.[2] Their challenge with this procedure was to interrupt aortic outflow without the benefit of circulatory support machinery. They devised a clever method of interrupting the aorta just distal to the subclavian artery, and then suturing a ball cage valve into the distal aorta. The obvious uninterrupted blood flow to the arch vessels allowed the patient to successfully tolerate the surgical procedure. The relief of regurgitation was thus only partial, but proved sufficient to provide meaningful palliation. In fact, the first patient survived for 7 years. This first attempt, although successful, led to only partial relief of aortic regurgitation, and was not useful for patients with aortic valve stenosis.

Advances during the next two decades brought refinements to the cardiopulmonary bypass system and the creation of various metallic and bioprosthetic valves. By placing the patient on cardiopulmonary bypass, the surgeon could expose the aortic valve, excise it, and replace the diseased valve with a prosthetic valve of suitable size. Significant improvements in cardiac protection and development of lower-profile valves led to significant improvements during hospitalization and in long-term outcomes of these patients. Aortic valve replacement therefore became the treatment of choice in most cases of symptomatic aortic valve disease (Table 14.1).[3]

Despite these successes, aortic valve replacement (AVR) through open-heart surgery has its limitations. The surgical 30-day mortality rate for isolated AVR is around 3.4% (3.1% risk-adjusted) and the actuarial survival rate at 5 years is around 78%.[4,5] At follow-up, there are important valve-related complications, including thromboembolism, bleeding from anticoagulation, reoperation, and prosthetic valve endocarditis (Table 14.2).[5] Additionally, most cases of severe aortic stenosis occur in elderly patients, who often have other comorbid conditions that increase surgical risk: these include age over 80 years, left ventricular failure, and associated need for coronary artery bypass surgery.[6–8] Young patients with aortic valve disease often outlive the bioprosthetic valve, requiring second or even third reoperation. Finally, although there is evidence that AVR in symptomatic patients is associated with a significant increase in life expectancy as compared with those who refused surgery (Figure 14.1), the role of cardiac valve replacement in patients with asymptomatic severe aortic valve stenosis is still controversial.[9]

Patients with asymptomatic severe aortic valve stenosis have a good prognosis, although up to 2% can develop sudden cardiac death as their first clinical manifestation. Yet, the risk of cardiac surgery often outweighs the benefits in this group, and they are frequently treated conservatively with careful sequential follow-up. The current guidelines of the American College of Cardiology/Amercian Heart Association recommend intense follow-up and risk stratification of patients with asymptomatic severe aortic valve stenosis as an alternative to AVR.[3] Only patients who fail exercise testing are recommended for AVR. The limitations of surgery for aortic valve disease patients dictate the need for low-risk, minimally invasive surgical procedures, or percutaneous techniques for valve repair/replacement.

Table 14.1 Recommendations for aortic valve replacement in aortic stenosis and aortic regurgitation[a]

Indication	Class[b]
Aortic valve stenosis (AS)	
1. Symptomatic patients with AS	I
2. Patients with severe AS undergoing surgery for coronary artery disease or other valve disease	I
3. Patients with moderate AS undergoing coronary artery bypass surgery or surgery on the aorta or other valves	IIa
4. Asymptomatic patients with severe AS and left ventricular (LV) dysfunction or abnormal response to exercise (hypotension)	IIa
Aortic regurgitation (severe) (AR)	
1. Patients with NYHA functional class III and IV symptoms and preserved LV systolic function, Defined as normal ejection fraction at rest (>50)	I
2. Patients with NYHA functional class II symptoms and preserved LV function, but with progressive LV dilatation or declining ejection fraction at rest on serial studies	I
3. Asymptomatic or symptomatic patients with mild to moderate LV dysfunction at rest (ejection fraction 0.25–0.49) or severe LV dilatation (end-diastolic dimension >75 mm or end-systolic dimension >55 mm)	IIa

[a]Modified from the ACC/AHA Guidelines for the Management of Patients with Valvular Heart Disease: a report of the American College of Cardiology/American Heart Association Task Force on Practice Guidelines (Committee on Management of Valvular Heart Disease). J Am Coll Cardiol 1998; 82: 1486–588.[3]
[b]Level of evidence: class I are conditions for which there is evidence of and/or general agreement that a given procedure or treatment is useful and effective; class IIa are conditions for which there is conflicting evidence, though the weight of evidence/opinion is in favor of usefulness/efficacy.

Table 14.2 Results following aortic valve replacement

Variable	
Hospital mortality rate (risk-adjusted)	3.1%
Actuarial survival rate at 5 years	80%
Thromboembolic events	2.3%/patient-year
Anticoagulant-induced bleeding	2.7%/patient-year
Prosthetic valve endocarditis	1.0%/patient-year

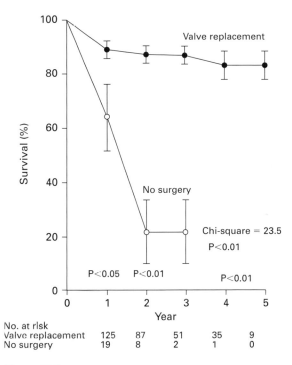

Figure 14.1

Survival among patients with severe symptomatic aortic stenosis who underwent valve replacement and similar patients who declined to undergo surgery. (Reproduced from Schwarz et al. Circulation 1982; 66: 1105–10[9] with permission from Lippincott Williams & Wilkins.)

Balloon valvuloplasty for aortic stenosis

The development of balloon angioplasty brought forth interventional cardiology, and the 1990s saw advances, including the use of metallic stents, which at present has become the preferred treatment for symptomatic coronary artery disease. In just a few years, percutaneous coronary interventions have surpassed coronary artery bypass surgery as the best choice for most coronary artery disease patients in North America.

Initially encouraged by the successes of coronary angioplasty, physicians used the same technique to dilate stenosed aortic, pulmonary, and mitral valves. Aortic valvuloplasty is successful for children and adolescents with congenital aortic valve stenosis. Most elderly and adult patients suffer from degenerative calcific aortic stenosis. This often makes successful aortic valve dilata-

tion difficult, and, despite initial improvement, recurrent stenosis remains as high as 60% within 6–12 months.[10] Furthermore, it is uncommon to achieve substantial increases in valve area with balloon valvuloplasty, and the patient is often left with a significant residual aortic stenosis.[10–12] In addition, balloon aortic valvuloplasty is not an option when significant aortic regurgitation is present. So, despite early enthusiasm, balloon aortic valvuloplasty in adults and older subjects is performed infrequently and is often only attempted for short-term palliation and more recently as part of percutaneous AVR.

Percutaneous aortic valve replacement

The maturation of interventional cardiology with the refinement of balloons and the development of stents led to the impetus for the development of a percutaneous approach to AVR. The late 1980s saw the birth of the stent, a metallic scaffold that could be used in various vascular structures. The stent was originally perceived as a platform from which drugs, or a valve, could be applied. In 1992, Andersen et al[13] reported the first case of a porcine valve mounted on a stent and implanted in the aorta of an animal model.

Bonhoeffer and his colleagues described a technique of mounting a jugular venous valve in a stent, then using it successfully to treat patients with severe pulmonary regurgitation due to graft failure in the pulmonary valve position. This group reported the first series of patients who underwent percutaneous valve replacement for incompetence or stenosis of right ventricular-to-pulmonary artery conduits.[14] At a follow-up of 10 months, all patients were found to be hemodynamically stable. These same investigators have developed a bovine jugular valve mounted in a double stent for potential use in AVR. This technique was successful in an animal model and will be tried in humans in the near future.[15]

Encouraged by these results, Alan Cribier, the pioneering cardiologist who had also introduced balloon aortic valvuloplasty several years before, and his associates reported the first successful implantation of a stent-mounted biologic membrane valve in a patient with critical aortic valve stenosis in April 2002.[16] Following this initial success, the Percutaneous Heart Valve (PHV) as designed by Percutaneous Valve Technologies (Edwards Life Sciences, Fort Lee, NJ) underwent modifications. The new PHV is composed of three equine pericardial leaflets mounted within a reinforced stent frame. These changes were made to increase the strength and durability of the valve. Using this new PHV, the same group reported their early experience in the first six patients with critical end-stage calcific aortic stenosis deemed too sick to undergo surgery (Table 14.3).[17] In this early experience in extremely sick patients, there was one procedure-related death. There was hemodynamic improvement in surviving patients, although all patients were left with varying degrees of aortic regurgitation due to paravalvular leak. This early experience demonstrated that PHV implantation in the aortic valve position is feasible without interfering with the origin of the coronary arteries. Designs to improve the anchorage, stability, and paravalvular leak will further improve its success. A pilot clinical study (I-REVIVE) has been completed in the same center and reports are forthcoming. A similar single-center study safety review in the USA, using the same valve, has received conditional approval from the Food and Drug Administration (FDA). While these studies are ongoing, several other companies have developed different types of PHV, which are undergoing clinical evaluation in human subjects.

Implications of percutaneous aortic valve replacement

In its current design, percutaneous AVR is not an acceptable substitute for aortic valve surgery for patients with significant aortic stenosis who are otherwise good-risk candidates, because of serious limitations, which are summarized in Table 14.4.[18] Surgical treatment therefore remains the treatment of choice. However, severely symptomatic patients considered too high risk to undergo surgery because of comorbidity or very poor ventricular function may be considered potential candidates for a palliative percutaneous approach as part of ongoing investigational protocols, since the procedure is not approved for general use. Notwithstanding these limitations, it is conceivable that, with further refinements in valve design, delivery, deployment technology, and attendant reductions in procedural risk and postprocedure complications and improvement in longevity of the valves, the percutaneous approach may well develop into a viable alternative to surgery even in average- to low-risk patients.

This exciting new technology is likely to have the same impact on clinical practice as that of percutaneous coronary intervention. The acceptance of this innovative technology will take place in stages.

Although percutaneous valve replacement technology holds great promise, prior to its acceptance several current limitations and chal-

Table 14.3 Early results using the Percutaneous Heart Valve (Percutaneous Valve Technologies) for patients with severe inoperable calcific aortic valve stenosis

Clinical variable	
Number of patients	6
Age	75±12 years (range 51–91 years)
Functional class (NYHA):	
Class IV	6
Cardiogenic shock	3
Successful deployment	5/6
Death:	
Acute procedure-related	1
Late deaths due to non-cardiac cause	3
Pre-implantation aortic valve area	0.49±0.08 cm^2
Aortic valve area at follow-up	1.63±0.05 cm^2
Post-procedure aortic regurgitation:	
Grade 3	2
Grade 1	3

Table 14.4 Limitations of the first-generation Percutaneous Heart Valve for aortic valve disease[4,5]

- The valve needs a large-diameter delivery catheter for successful deployment
- Accurate and secure deployment is often a challenge
- Post-deployment perivalvular leak is common
- Interference of the coronary ostium might be an issue in patients with severe aortic regurgitation
- There might be a need for temporary circulatory support to assure careful and accurate deployment of the valve
- The durability of the valve is unknown
- If an aortic valve is implanted percutaneously, subsequent surgical replacement of a malfunctioning valve could be challenging

lenges must be resolved. Such refinements will likely include:

- It must be assured that the valve can be delivered through a slender catheter, in the exact aortic valve position, without affecting coronary circulation, or causing significant paravalvular leaks.
- Once deployed, the valve must be shown to be at least as durable as surgically implanted biologic valves.
- Additionally, a need may arise to develop effective percutaneous circulatory assist devices to improve the safety of this technology in very sick patients.
- Large-scale clinical trials comparing this technology with conventional open-heart surgical procedures will be necessary to demonstrate equivalence or superiority to surgery.
- Currently, aortic valve replacement is only recommended for symptomatic patients with severe aortic stenosis; the risks of death outweigh the risks of surgery in asymptomatic severe aortic valve disease and preclude procedures. It is quite conceivable that if and when the percutaneous valve is proven to be safe and effective, it may be considered even for asymptomatic aortic stenosis patients. Treatment for this patient group could reduce the incidence of sudden cardiac death and/or help preserve left ventricular function.

Conclusions

The future of interventional cardiology and cardiac surgery appears highly energized. Engineers, cardiologists, and surgeons are working together to develop safe effective percutaneous or other minimally invasive methods to treat a multiplicity of valvular heart diseases. It is hoped that over time, repair/replacement of a valve via a midline sternotomy will become a rare occurrence, reserved for extreme cases only.

References

1. Carabello BA. Clinical practice: aortic stenosis. N Engl J Med 2002; 346: 677–82.
2. Hufnagel CA, Harvey PW, Rabil PJ, et al. Surgical correction of aortic insufficiency. Surgery 1954; 20: 673–83.
3. ACC/AHA Guidelines for the Management of Patients with Valvular Heart Disease: a report of the American College of Cardiology/American Heart Association Task Force on Practice Guidelines (Committee on Management of Valvular Heart Disease). J Am Coll Cardiol 1998; 82: 1486–588.
4. Aortic valve disease. In: Kouchoukos NT, Blackstone EH, Doty DB, Hanley FL, Karp RB (eds). Kirklin–Barrat–Boyes Cardiac Surgery, 3rd edn. Philadelphia: Churchill Livingstone, 2003: 554–656.
5. Zellner JL, Kratz JM, Crumbley AJ 3rd, et al. Long term experience with the St. Jude's medical prosthesis. Ann Thorac Surg 1999; 68: 1210.
6. Alexander K, Ansstrom K, Muhlbaier L, et al. Outcomes in cardiac surgery in patients ≥ 80 years: results from the National Cardiovascular Network. J Am Coll Cardiol 2000; 35: 731–8.
7. Powell DE, Turick PA, Rosenzweig BP, et al. Aortic valve replacement in patients with aortic stenosis and severe left ventricular dysfunction. Arch Intern Med 2000; 160: 1337–441.
8. Jamieson WRE, Edwards FH, Schwartz M, et al. Risk stratification for cardiac valve replacement. National Cardiac Surgery Database. Ann Thorac Surg 1999; 67: 943–51.
9. Schwarz E, Baumann P, Manthey J, et al. The effects of aortic valve replacement on survival. Circulation 1982; 66: 1105–10.
10. Bashmore TM, Davidson CJ, and the Mansfield Scientific Aortic Valvuloplasty Registry Investigators. Follow up recatheterization after balloon aortic valvuloplasty. J Am Coll Cardiol 1991; 17: 1168–95.
11. Litvack F, Jacobowski A, Buchbinder N, Eigler N. Lack of sustained clinical improvement in an elderly population after percutaneous aortic valvuloplasty. Am J Cardiol 1988; 62: 270–5.
12. McKay RG. The Mansfield Scientific Aortic Valvuloplasty Registry; overview of acute hemodynamic results and procedural complications. J Am Coll Cardiol 1991; 17: 485–91.
13. Andersen HR, Knudsen LL, Hasekam JM. Transluminal implantation of artificial valves: description of an expandable aortic valve: initial results with implantation by catheter technique in closed chest pigs. Eur Heart J 1992; 87: 704–8.
14. Bonhoeffer P, Boudjemline Y, Qureshi SA, et al. Percutaneous insertion of the pulmonary valve. J Am Coll Cardiol 2002; 39: 1644–9.
15. Boudjemline Y, Bonhoeffer P. Steps toward percutaneous aortic valve replacement. Circulation 2002; 105: 775–8.
16. Cribier A, Eltchaninoff H, Bash A, et al. Percutaneous transcatheter implantation of an aortic

valve prosthesis for calcific aortic stenosis. First human experience. Circulation 2002; 106: 3006–8.

17. Cribier A, Eltchaninoff H, Tron C, et al. Early experience with percutaneous transcatheter implantation of heart valve prosthesis for the treatment of end-stage inoperable patients with calcific aortic stenosis. J Am Coll Cardiol 2004; 43: 693–703.

18. Fish RD. Percutaneous heart valve replacement: enthusiasm tempered. Circulation 2004; 110: 1876–8.

15

Established methods of aortic valve repair and replacement

Prem S Shekar, Edward G Soltesz, Lawrence H Cohn

Introduction

The aortic valve is a trileaflet valve situated at the junction of the left ventricular (LV) outflow tract (LVOT) and the ascending aorta. This valve plays a critical role in maintaining efficient cardiac function. A variety of pathophysiologic conditions can affect this valve, producing a variety of disease patterns. Aortic valve disease is one of the more common pathologies that cardiologists and cardiac surgeons encounter in daily practice, because of its prevalence in elderly populations. Surgical repair or excisional replacement is the standard of care for severe aortic valve disease. Standard surgical therapy includes aortic valve repair, aortic valve-sparing procedures, and aortic valve replacement. This chapter provides an overview of the standard and established methods of aortic valve surgery that represent the gold standard against which all future therapies will be tested and tried.

Indications for aortic valve surgery

In 1998, the American College of Cardiology and the American Heart Association published consensus guidelines for managing patients with heart valve disease.[1] These guidelines delineate three classes of indications for surgical intervention of valvular disease. Class I is recommended; class IIa,b is recommended but less well established, and class III is not recommended.

Aortic valve stenosis

Class I indications for aortic valve surgery include both symptomatic patients with severe aortic stenosis and asymptomatic patients with severe aortic stenosis undergoing other cardiac surgeries, including coronary artery bypass graft, other aortic surgery, or surgery on other valves. Class IIa indications for aortic valve surgery include patients with moderate aortic stenosis undergoing other cardiac surgeries, or with LV dysfunction, or with abnormal response to exercise (hypotension).[1] The distinction between mild, moderate, and severe aortic stenosis is summarized in Table 15.1.

Aortic valve regurgitation

Class I indications for patients with aortic valve regurgitation include all patients with chronic severe regurgitation of the aortic valve with class III or IV New York Heart Association (NYHA) symptoms who have preserved LV function at

Table 15.1 Aortic stenosis: level of severity

	Area (cm²)	Mean gradient (mmHg)
Mild	>1.5	<25
Moderate	1.0–1.5	25–50
Severe	<1.0	>50

rest; patients with class II NYHA symptoms but progressive LV dilatation and declining ejection fraction; patients with Canadian Cardiovascular Society functional class II or greater angina (with or without coronary artery disease); and patients with mild to moderate LV dysfunction at rest. Patients undergoing coronary artery bypass surgery, or surgery on the aorta and other heart valves with moderate to severe aortic regurgitation are also included in class I. However, patients with functional NYHA class II symptoms with preserved LV function and a stable LV size and systolic function, as well as asymptomatic patients with normal LV systolic function but severe LV dilatation, comprise class IIa indications for aortic valve surgery.[1]

Other indications for aortic valve surgery

Patients undergoing surgery of the aortic root or for ascending aortic aneurysms who have aortic valve insufficiency or stenosis may also benefit from a concomitant aortic valve procedure. Patients with infective endocarditis of the aortic valve will require valve replacement for control of sepsis, heart failure, or both.

Techniques for aortic valve surgery

The techniques used in aortic valve surgery can be broadly divided into two categories: (1) aortic valve repair and (2) aortic valve replacement. A wide range of aortic valve replacements are available, including mechanical, bioprosthetic, homograft, and autograft. Aortic valve repair is also possible in a select set of patients.

Basic surgical procedure

Aortic valve surgery is usually performed through a midline sternotomy incision. Isolated aortic valve surgery and reoperations can be performed using a minimal-access upper hemisternotomy incision, which has recently gained popularity.[2] In isolated instances, aortic valve replacement can be performed via a right anterolateral thoracotomy through the second rib interspace. The essential steps of aortic valve replacement are depicted in Figure 15.1. All operations on the aortic valve are performed on cardiopulmonary bypass after systemic heparinization and cannulation of the ascending aorta and right atrium. Diastolic arrest of the heart is achieved with cardioplegia. The aorta is cross-clamped and a transverse aortotomy is made to expose the aortic valve (Figure 15.1A). The procedure is then tailored according to the plan.

For patients requiring mechanical or stented bioprosthetic valve replacement, the aortic valve is excised and the aortic valve annulus is carefully debrided of all calcific fragments (Figure 15.1B). Valve sizers provided by the manufacturer are used to ensure that the prosthesis is a proper fit (Figure 15.1C). The standard technique for implanting the prosthesis is to place multiple pledgeted vertical everting/inverting mattress sutures of 2–0 Ethibond into the annulus of the aortic valve and then onto the sewing ring of the prosthetic valve (Figure 15.1D). The valve is lowered into position, and the sutures are tied and cut (Figure 15.1E). The aortotomy is closed only after ensuring that the valve is well seated on the annulus and that the coronary arteries lie truly above the level of the sewing ring.

For cases that require stentless bioprosthetic valves, the procedure is essentially the same. In addition to being anchored at the level of the annulus and the sewing ring, this valve will also require a running suture of 4–0 polypropylene along the commissural posts and the edge of the valve to secure it to the wall of the aortic root.

In biological aortic valve replacements, such as the aortic valve homograft or pulmonary valve autograft technique (Ross procedure), the aortic valve is completely excised along with the aortic root, and, at the same time, coronary 'buttons' are created. The homograft or autograft is then debrided to size and sewn into position at the level of the aortic valve annulus. Another anastomosis is created at the level of the proximal-to-mid ascending aorta. The coronary buttons are then reimplanted into this new aorta. In the Ross procedure, a homograft is used to replace the excised pulmonary valve.

The minimal-access upper hemisternotomy approach to aortic valve surgery is rapidly becoming the procedure of choice for patients

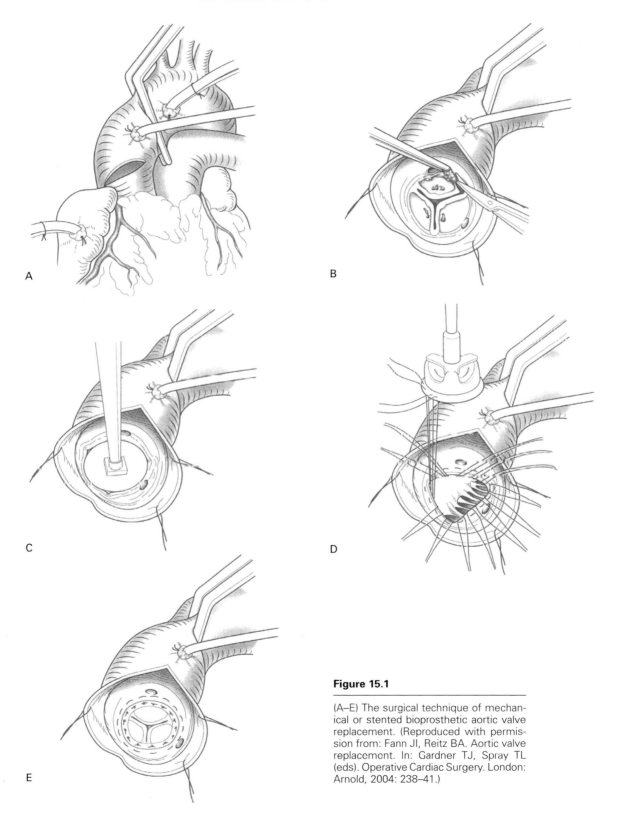

A

B

C

D

E

Figure 15.1

(A–E) The surgical technique of mechanical or stented bioprosthetic aortic valve replacement. (Reproduced with permission from: Fann JI, Reitz BA. Aortic valve replacement. In: Gardner TJ, Spray TL (eds). Operative Cardiac Surgery. London: Arnold, 2004: 238–41.)

with isolated aortic valve disease. The benefits of this approach, aside from cosmesis, include reduced pain, trauma, transfusion requirements, and cost, while maintaining a qualitative surgical result. All of the above have greatly improved patient satisfaction.[2] Over the last decade, we have performed over 700 aortic valve replacements and repairs at the Brigham and Women's Hospital through the upper hemisternotomy approach. Of these, 89 (13%) have been aortic valve reoperations, which have been performed with an operative mortality rate of 2%.[3–5]

Techniques for aortic valve repair

Few aortic valves are amenable to repair in adult patients 65 years of age or older, because of the incidence of calcific degeneration. However, certain instances warrant the reparative approach in selected patients.

Aortic valve debridement

In cases of mild to moderate aortic stenosis in patients undergoing other cardiac surgical procedures, mechanical or chemical debridement of the valve can be performed to improve the mobility of the aortic valve cusps and reduce the degree of stenosis.[6–8]

Perforated valve

Aortic valve cusp perforation can cause aortic insufficiency secondary to endocarditis or iatrogenic perforation. A simple patch of fresh or glutaraldehyde-fixed pericardium will correct this problem.[9]

Deformed valve

Various disease processes of the aortic valve, especially rheumatic fever, can cause shortening or deformity of the aortic valve cusp. Pericardium may be used to extend these deformed cusps.[10]

Prolapsing cusp

Although this is a rare cause, aortic regurgitation can be due to prolapse of a single cusp of the aortic valve. This can be repaired by plicating the free margin of the cusp. Subcommissural plication may also be required in addition to plication of the free wall of the cusp, itself.

Valve-sparing operations on the aortic root and ascending aorta

Aortic valve-sparing operations are used in patients who have aneurysms of the ascending aorta or the aortic root that are associated with aortic insufficiency. In patients with ascending aortic aneurysm and aortic valve insufficiency, there is usually distraction of the three commissural posts of the aortic valve due to the large aneurysm. Transecting the aneurysm at its base just above the sinotubular junction and remodeling the junction using a prosthetic graft usually corrects this condition. Sparing the otherwise functional valve can have a significant impact on long-term survival. The use of a prosthetic graft of appropriate size will return the relationship of the three commissural posts of the aortic valve to normal, thereby correcting the aortic insufficiency.[11]

Tirone David and Magdi Yacoub have developed a number of valve-sparing procedures to remodel aortic roots in the setting of aortic root aneurysms.[12,13] All of these procedures entail a complete excision of the aneurysm and the aortic root, as well as creation of coronary 'buttons', leaving only a small sliver of tissue along the commissural posts and the base of the aortic valve. A regular Dacron tube graft or a specially created sinus of Valsalva graft can be used to remodel the aortic root. Depending on the technique used – either the Yacoub technique or the David technique – the commissural post of the aortic valve is either part of the reconstruction or is completely deployed within the Dacron tube graft. After completion of these anastomoses, the coronary buttons are reimplanted onto the new aorta (Figure 15.2).

The Cleveland Clinic reported a large series of 94 patients who underwent repair of a bicuspid aortic valve.[14] The freedom from reoperation in this series was about 84% at 7 years. For patients who have aortic insufficiency with ascending aor-

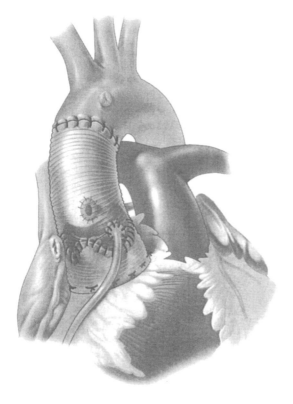

Figure 15.2

Illustration of aortic root remodeling – a valve-sparing procedure – showing the completed repair with three commissures suspended inside the graft. The aortic sinus remnants are secured to the Dacron graft with coronary artery buttons reimplanted in the remnant. (Reproduced with permission from: David TE. Aortic valve repair and aortic valve sparing operations. In: Cohn LH, Edmunds LH Jr (eds). Cardiac Surgery in the Adult. New York: McGraw-Hill, 2003: 811–23.[6])

tic aneurysm that requires just an adjustment of the sinotubular junction with a Dacron tube graft, the freedom from aortic valve replacement at 5 years was 97% in one study. The freedom from moderate to severe aortic insufficiency at 5 years was about 98%.[15]

Because of the complexity of the procedure, the experience with aortic root remodeling with the Yacoub or the David technique is mainly limited to the institutions where these operations originated. Yacoub et al reported an 89% freedom from aortic valve replacement at 10 years in his series of 158 patients.[13] David, in his series, reported a freedom of aortic valve replacement of 99% at 10 years.[16] In this series, late echocardiographic studies showed the freedom from moderate aortic insufficiency at 10 years to be about 83%.

Techniques for aortic valve replacement

Aortic valve replacement is one of the oldest operations performed in cardiac surgery. In 1958, Hufnagel et al replaced the aortic valve with a Lucite ball valve in the descending thoracic aorta in a patient who had severe aortic insufficiency, with excellent results.[17] This was probably the first report of a successful aortic valve replacement. From the earliest operations to today, aortic valve replacement has remained a commonly performed and extremely successful procedure in cardiac surgery. At the Brigham and Women's Hospital, we performed 3791 aortic valve replacements between 1992 and 2004, averaging 292 a year – or about 4 aortic valve replacements every 5 days.

Aortic valve replacement can be subdivided into three categories: (1) mechanical valve replacement; (2) bioprosthetic valve replacement; and (3) biological valve replacement (Figure 15.3). The ideal aortic prosthesis should be widely available, easy to implant, durable, non-thrombogenic, and hemodynamically equivalent to a normal native valve.

Choice of aortic valve prosthesis

For patients needing aortic valve replacement, the choice of valves revolves primarily around the following issues:

- age of the patient
- lifestyle
- reoperation.

Mechanical aortic valves demonstrate excellent results in terms of long-term freedom from reoperation. In most cases, the valve will outlive the average adult cardiac surgery patient. This good result comes with the disadvantages of anticoagulation, which is required for the life of the mechanical valve. Moreover, long-term anticoagulation

Bioprosthetic valves   Prosthetic valves

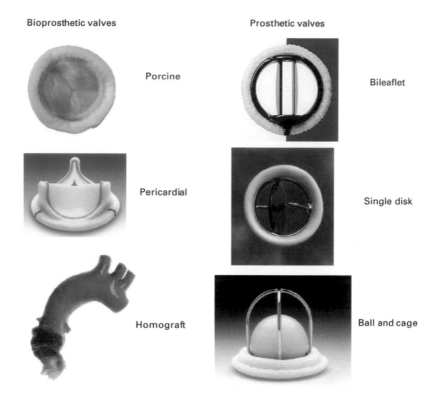

Porcine

Bileaflet

Pericardial

Single disk

Homograft

Ball and cage

Figure 15.3

Bioprosthetic and mechanical valves.

carries a significant risk of thromboembolism and hemorrhage. For patients who lead a very active lifestyle, such as those involved in contact sports or those with occupations that can render them to easy injury/bruising, anticoagulation may be an unacceptable choice.

Bioprosthetic valves, which do not require anticoagulation, can be a viable option for older patients and for those who wish to preserve lifestyle. These valves currently last in excess of 15 years and have a reduced risk of anticoagulation-associated complications. Stented bioprosthetic valves have a risk of thromboembolism of 0.5–1% per year. After 15 years or more, however, a reoperation may be required to replace a failing bioprosthetic valve. Modern technology and surgical techniques permit reoperative aortic valve replacement to be done with a reasonably low risk of morbidity and mortality. Therefore, this may be a better choice for patients who are older

and need to be free from the constraints of chronic anticoagulation medication.

The biological valves, such as the aortic homograft, although not requiring anticoagulation, have well-documented long-term problems with calcification. Homografts are slowly falling into disfavor, as they are relatively harder to reoperate upon and do not come with a great degree of benefit over the standard stented bioprosthetic valve. The pulmonary autograft may be appropriate for select young patients, but some surgical groups believe that this is a double-valve operation for a single-valve disease with relatively little benefit.

Today, bioprosthetic aortic valve replacement is recommended to most patients over 65 years of age. Others, especially those between 50 and 64 years old, are apprised of the benefits and disadvantages of each and permitted to make a personal choice.

Prosthetic valves for replacement in the aortic position

Mechanical valves

There are three types of mechanical valve: ball and cage, monoleaflet tilting disk, and bileaflet tilting disk mechanical valves (Figure 15.3). All mechanical valves require formal anticoagulation with warfarin, and studies have confirmed an overall risk of thromboembolism in patients on warfarin therapy of 1–2% per year.

The classic example of the ball and cage mechanical valve is the Starr–Edwards valve, which was one of the first mechanical valves developed for cardiac use.[18] It has undergone very little change since 1965 and continues to be used sporadically around the world for aortic valve replacement. The Starr–Edwards valve has a higher profile compared with other available valves, as well as a higher risk for thromboembolism, although it has proven its value with a low level of mechanical failure.

The classic example of the monoleaflet tilting disk valve, the Björk–Shiley valve, is no longer manufactured. Currently, the few monoleaflet valves used are the Medtronic Hall valve (Medtronic, Inc., Minneapolis, MN), the Omni-Carbon valve (Medical Inc., Inver Grover Heights, MN), and the All-Carbon monodisk valve (Sorin Biomedica, Saluggia, Italy).

The bileaflet mechanical valve, which is now considered the gold standard for aortic valve replacement, is the third category of mechanical valve design. These valves have an extremely low profile and very low complication and thromboembolism rates. The St Jude Medical valve (St Jude Medical, Inc., St Paul, MN) is the classic example of the standard bileaflet valve and is used worldwide. Other bileaflet tilting disk valves include the CarboMedics valve (CarboMedics Inc., Austin, TX), and the On-X valve (Medical Carbon Research Institute (MCRI), Austin, TX).

Stented bioprosthetic valves

The stented bioprosthetic valves are xenografts derived from animal tissues that have been stented on a semirigid sewing ring for ease of application. The animal tissue in all xenograft valves is chemically treated or 'fixed' with glutaraldehyde, which crosslinks the collagen fibers and reduces antigenicity. Glutaraldehyde fixation is, unfortunately, the Achilles' heel of the xenograft, as calcification is prone to occur in non-viable tissue. There have been three generations of stented bioprosthetic valves, distinguished by improvements in the nature of the treatment process. The first-generation bioprosthetic valves are high-pressure pre-fixation valves, such as the Medtronic Hancock I. The second-generation bioprosthetic valves are treated with low- or zero-pressure fixation and include the Medtronic Hancock II valve and the Carpentier–Edwards Supra-Annular valve (Edwards Life Sciences, Irvine, CA). Third-generation prosthetic valves are subjected to an antimineralization process, in addition to zero- or low-pressure fixation. This process is designed to reduce material fatigue and calcification. An example of a third-generation prosthetic valve is the Medtronic Mosaic Porcine valve.

Stentless bioprosthetic valves

The stentless bioprosthetic valve represents a newer generation of the xenograft valve. These valves lack the semirigid ring that supports the valvular tissue of the stented bioprosthetic valves described above. Commonly, these are porcine aortic valves that are supported by a film of Dacron along the periphery. The stentless valve can be implanted in the subcoronary position or as a full or hemi-root. Examples of this type of valve are the Toronto Stentless Porcine (SPV) (St Jude Medical, Inc., St Paul, MN), the Edwards Prima, and the Medtronic Freestyle. Theoretically, the stentless porcine valve has a lower gradient at smaller sizes, and therefore should aid in reducing afterload on the LV and assist with LV remodeling. In some prospective randomized studies, however, these valves do not appear to be better than the third-generation stented valves.[19]

Aortic valve homografts

Aortic valve homografts are harvested from human cadavers and then cryopreserved. Homograft aortic valves went through a period of intense popularity, but their use is now declining.

Durability is the primary shortcoming of the homograft valve, with a freedom from reoperation at 20 years of 38–50% and a freedom from structural valve failure at 20 years of 18–32%.[20,21] While the longevity of the homograft may be comparable to that of the current generation of bioprosthetic valves, the operation required to place the homograft aortic valve is complex and involves excision of the entire aortic root and the creation of coronary buttons. The valve has to be sewn into position at the aortic annulus and attached to the mid or ascending aorta, after which the coronary buttons are reimplanted. This is a technically more complex operation for aortic valve replacement. Although the homograft aortic valve lasts about 15 years and does not necessitate anticoagulation, reoperation involving the aortic valve homograft can be difficult because of the tendency of the treated homograft valve to calcify. Re-replacement of this calcified homograft is usually tedious and increases the perioperative mortality significantly. Currently, homografts are reserved for certain indications, the most important being endocarditis of the aortic valve.

Pulmonary autografts

Placement of a pulmonary autograft is commonly known as the Ross operation. In this procedure, the diseased aortic valve is removed and replaced with a pulmonary autograft, and the pulmonary valve is replaced by a homograft. The advantages of this operation include freedom from thromboembolism, improved hemodynamics through use of a native autograft valve, ability of the autograft to grow as the patient grows, and use of living autologous tissue. The pulmonary autograft procedures have had the best results in institutions where large volumes of these cases are routinely performed. Many hold the view that this is a complex operation for a simple disease process. Indications for this procedure are currently limited to young patients who have a small aorta, a small aortic annulus, and a life expectancy greater than 20 years. The autograft, when used as a root replacement, has good longevity. Hence, it is now a very selective operation that is rarely performed outside of experienced centers. Use of the Ross procedure has decreased since its peak in the late 1990s.

Antithrombotic therapy for valves

All patients who receive mechanical valves require anticoagulation.[1] The recommended target international normalized ratio (INR) is between 2 and 3. Some recommend an INR range of 2.5–3.5 for higher-risk patients with mechanical valves along with low-dose aspirin therapy, and an INR range of 2–3 for lower-risk patients. Caged ball valves will require a higher degree of anticoagulation, with INR in excess of 3.5.

Bioprosthetic and biological valves do not require anticoagulation. Although the AHA guidelines recommend anticoagulation for the first 3 months after bioprosthetic valve replacement in the aortic position,[1] most centers do not use any anticoagulation. Most centers discharge and maintain patients on low-dose aspirin therapy.

Outcomes of aortic valve replacements

Early outcomes

The operative mortality rate from aortic valve replacements accomplished with a mechanical or a stented bioprosthetic valve ranges between 1% and 4%.[22] The factors that influence mortality from aortic valve replacement are advancing patient age, LV function, heart failure symptoms, other cardiac diseases, renal failure, active endocarditis, emergent operations, and reoperations. Long-term survival with mechanical versus bioprosthetic valves is equivalent. In most published series, the expected survival rate from aortic valve replacement is about 80–85% at 5 years, 65–75% at 10 years, and 45–55% at 15 years.[22]

Mortality related to bioprosthetic and mechanical valves

Mortality attributable to bioprosthetic or mechanical valve failure is defined as any death caused by structural valve deterioration, non-structural valve deterioration, valve thrombosis, embolism, bleeding, prosthetic valve endocarditis, and reoperation. The valve-related mortality rate has been reported between 37% for mechanical valves and 41% for bioprosthetic valves at 15 years. Non-valvular deaths accounted for about 17% with mechanical valves and 21% with bioprosthetic valves at 15 years.[23]

Valve-related morbidity

The morbidity attributable to bioprosthetic or mechanical valve replacement basically includes the same conditions detailed above for valve-related mortality. In addition, however, one has also to consider cerebral thromboembolic events, such as transient ischemic attacks (TIA), neurologic deficits, and stroke.

Structural valve deterioration

The currently available mechanical prostheses, for example, the St Jude Medical bileaflet valve, are extremely resilient to structural valve deterioration. Currently available stented bioprosthetic valves, however, have a 10–15% rate of structural valve deterioration in patients over 60 years of age at 10 years. The freedom from reoperation for aortic valve replacement should be at least 95% at 10 years and about 90% or more at 15 years with mechanical valves. With bioprosthetic valves, freedom from reoperation is about 95% at 5 years, 90% at 10 years, and about 70% at 15 years with the current generation of valves. Farivar and Cohn[24] showed that hypercholesterolemia is an important risk factor for bioprosthetic valve calcification, failure, and reoperation.

Prosthetic valve thrombosis

Thrombosis is a very rare but devastating complication of mechanical aortic valve replacement. This complication occurs in less than 0.2% of cases per year. It is usually related to non-compliance with anticoagulation management. This is a terminal and fatal event in most cases. In a very few instances, the patient will reach the hospital with a stuck valve, with high gradients across the valve, or with severe acute aortic insufficiency. Most of these cases have a very high mortality at reoperation.

Prosthetic valve endocarditis

Endocarditis of the prosthetic valve is categorized as early (occurring within 60 days of implantation) and late (occurring after 60 days of implantation). The bacteriologic make-up of early and late endocarditis is different, as is the source of inoculation. The annual risk of prosthetic valve endocarditis is about 0.6–0.9% per patient per year. Mechanical valves seem to have a slightly higher incidence of early endocarditis than stented bioprosthetic valves. Prosthetic valve endocarditis requires reoperation more often than not. The indications for operation are early endocarditis, heart failure, valve dysfunction, paravalvular leaks, conduction defects, and abscess. Development of persistent bacteremia with antibiotic therapy and large vegetations with systemic emboli are also indications for operation. Paravalvular leak with evolving hemolysis constitutes another indication for reoperation on a mechanical or stented bioprosthetic valve.

Mortality for homograft valves

The operative mortality for homograft valves is about 1–5%. The mortality is higher when the operation is performed on patients in cardiogenic shock or in patients with prosthetic valve endocarditis as compared with elective procedures.

At the Brigham and Women's Hospital, we performed a total of 248 homograft valve replacements in the 17-year period between 1987 and 2004, with a 2% mortality rate in non-endocarditic patients and a 13% mortality rate in patients with infective endocarditis.[25]

Mortality for pulmonary autograft valves

The Brigham and Women's experience with the pulmonary autograft has comprised 40 cases with an operative mortality rate of 2.5% (1/40). The reported pulmonary homograft failure and stenosis rate is about 10% at 7 years.[26]

Conclusion

Aortic valve disease is a common cardiac pathology in surgical practice today – more so because of our aging population. Numerous options are still available for valve repair or replacement. The decision as to which type of valve best suits the individual patient can be complex and warrants a thorough understanding of current technology. Recommendations are made in consideration of a host of factors, including pathophysiologic conditions, age of the patient, and patient lifestyle and preference. For severe aortic valve disease, surgical repair or replacement remains the standard of care.

Acknowledgment

The authors wish to acknowledge the technical assistance of Michelle Pokorny, PA-C, and Ann S Adams for medical editing.

References

1. Bonow RO, Carabello B, de Leon AC, et al. ACC/AHA Guidelines for the Management of Patients with Valvular Heart Disease. Executive Summary. A report of the American College of Cardiology/American Heart Association Task Force on Practice Guidelines (Committee on Management of Patients with Valvular Heart Disease). J Heart Valve Dis 1998; 7: 672–707.
2. Byrne JG, Hsin MK, Adams DH, et al. Minimally invasive direct access heart valve surgery. J Card Surg 2000; 15: 21–34.
3. Byrne JG, Aranki SF, Couper GS, et al. Reoperative aortic valve replacement: partial upper hemisternotomy versus conventional full sternotomy. J Thorac Cardiovasc Surg 1999; 118: 991–7.
4. Byrne JG, Karavas AN, Adams DH, et al. Partial upper re-sternotomy for aortic valve replacement or re-replacement after previous cardiac surgery. Eur J Cardiothorac Surg 2000; 18: 282–6.
5. Cohn LH. Minimally invasive valve surgery. J Card Surg 2001; 16: 260–5.
6. David TE. Aortic valve repair and aortic valve sparing operations. In: Cohn LH, Edmunds LH Jr (eds). Cardiac Surgery in the Adult. New York: McGraw-Hill, 2003: 811–23.
7. Desai N, Christakis G. Stented mechanical/bioprosthetic aortic valve replacement. In: Cohn LH, Edmunds LH Jr (eds). Cardiac Surgery in the Adult. New York: McGraw-Hill, 2003: 825–55.
8. Otaki M. A new modification of debridement valvuloplasty for acquired aortic valve disease. J Card Surg 1994; 9: 103–8.
9. Denyer MH, Elliott CM, Robicsek F. Pericardial patch repair of aortic cusp perforation caused by cardiac catheterization. J Card Surg 1988; 3: 155–7.
10. Duran CM, Gometza B, Shahid M, Al-Halees Z. Treated bovine and autologous pericardium for aortic valve reconstruction. Ann Thorac Surg 1998; 66: S166–9.
11. David TE, Feindel CM. An aortic valve-sparing operation for patients with aortic incompetence and aneurysm of the ascending aorta. J Thorac Cardiovasc Surg 1992; 103: 617–21; discussion 622.
12. David TE, Feindel CM, Bos J. Repair of the aortic valve in patients with aortic insufficiency and aortic root aneurysm. J Thorac Cardiovasc Surg 1995; 109: 345–51; discussion 351–2.
13. Yacoub MH, Gehle P, Chandrasekaran V, et al. Late results of a valve-preserving operation in patients with aneurysms of the ascending aorta and root. J Thorac Cardiovasc Surg 1998; 115: 1080–90.
14. Casselman FP, Gillinov AM, Akhrass R, et al. Intermediate-term durability of bicuspid aortic valve repair for prolapsing leaflet. Eur J Cardiothorac Surg 1999; 15: 302–8.
15. David TE, Ivanov J, Armstrong S, et al. Aortic valve-sparing operations in patients with aneurysms of the aortic root or ascending aorta. Ann Thorac Surg 2002; 74: S1758–61; discussion S1792–9.
16. David TE. Aortic valve-sparing operations for aortic root aneurysm. Semin Thorac Cardiovasc Surg 2001; 13: 291–6.
17. Hufnagel C, Vilkgas P, Nahas H. Experiences with new types of aortic valvular prothesis. Ann Surg 1958; 147: 636–45.
18. Starr A, Edwards M. Mitral replacement: clinical experience with a ball valve prosthesis. Am Surg 1961; 154: 726.
19. Cohen G, Christakis GT, Joyner CD, et al. Are stentless valves hemodynamically superior to stented valves? A prospective randomized trial. Ann Thorac Surg 2002; 73: 767–75; discussion 775–8.
20. O'Brien MF, Harrocks S, Stafford EG, et al. The homograft aortic valve: a 29-year, 99.3% follow up of 1,022 valve replacements. J Heart Valve Dis 2001; 10: 334–44; discussion 335.
21. Langley SM, McGuirk SP, Chaudhry MA, et al. Twenty-year follow-up of aortic valve replacement with antibiotic sterilized homografts in 200 patients. Semin Thorac Cardiovasc Surg 1999; 11: 28–34.
22. Edwards FH, Peterson ED, Coombs LP, et al. Prediction of operative mortality after valve replacement surgery. J Am Coll Cardiol 2001; 37: 885–92.
23. Hammermeister K, Sethi GK, Henderson WG, et al. Outcomes 15 years after valve replacement with a

mechanical versus a bioprosthetic valve: final report of the Veterans Affairs randomized trial. J Am Coll Cardiol 2000; 36: 1152–8.

24. Farivar RS, Cohn LH. Hypercholesterolemia is a risk factor for bioprosthetic valve calcification and explantation. J Thorac Cardiovasc Surg 2003; 26: 969–75.

25. Byrne JG, Gudbjartsson T, Karavas AN, et al. Biological vs. mechanical aortic root replacement. Eur J Cardiothorac Surg 2003; 23: 305–10.

26. Linden PA, Cohn LH. Medium-term follow up of pulmonary autograft aortic valve replacement: technical advances and echocardiographic follow up. J Heart Valve Dis 2001; 10: 35–42.

16

Non-surgical aortic valve replacement: History, present, and future perspectives

Younes Boudjemline, Sachin Khambadkone, Philipp Bonhoeffer

Introduction

Leonardo da Vinci described the anatomy of the aortic valve in great detail. But it was not until the 1950s that advances were made in the field of surgical treatment for patients with valve diseases. In 1951, Hufnagel and colleagues developed a ball valve prosthesis for 'off-pump' insertion into the descending aorta to treat patients with severe chronic aortic valve insufficiency.[1] A few years later, more effective approaches began with the availability of cardiopulmonary bypass. In the early 1960s, the introduction of the ball valve prosthesis by Harken and Starr in orthotopic position established the basis of aortic valve surgery.[2,3] In the following years, many more advances were made to improve the outcomes of patients with aortic valve disease, making this surgery a low-risk procedure in most instances. Later, in the field of cardiology, physicians were able to shift from invasive treatment to less invasive procedures to limit patient discomfort, cost, morbidity, and mortality. Thus, closure of heart defects and relief of vascular or valvular stenosis are now performed without surgery, using a transcatheter technique. Despite transcatheter treatment of valvular diseases being well established for obstructive lesions, cardiac valve replacement has remained until recently entirely in the surgical field. Since 1981, when Charles Dotter in a review paper[4] first suggested the possibility of transcatheter placement of prosthetic valves, tremendous developments have made percutaneous valve replacement a reality. This chapter focuses on transcatheter valve replacement of the aortic valve, discussing anatomic considerations with regard to percutaneous valve placement, the various devices and approaches developed over the past few years, and the future prospects for these procedures.

Anatomic considerations regarding transcatheter replacement of the aortic valve

The development of transcatheter techniques for aortic valve replacement requires detailed knowledge of the area of the aortic valve. We will rapidly review the various anatomic considerations to be taken into account to develop such devices.

Vascular access

The first limitation is access to the diseased valve. Current valves for transcatheter insertion require large sheaths for their insertion and delivery. Therefore, the retrograde approach via a femoral artery can be problematic in children and adults who have additional vascular diseases. However, large vascular access has been used without major problems for the treatment of aortic aneurysms. Through a retrograde approach, access to the diseased valve can be difficult, in particular, in the case of a heavily calcified valve. Another possible access is via an anterograde approach. The femoral vein is first punctured and the left atrium is entered trans-septaly, as performed for mitral valve dilatation. To facilitate advancement of the delivery system into the area of the valve to be replaced, a loop between the femoral vein and the contralateral artery can be created.

Implantation site and adjacent structures

An arterial access used to inject contrast dye can also be helpful for precise placement of the device during its deployment. It is, indeed, very important to locate the position of the native valve, the sinus, the sinotubular junction, and the ascending aorta giving rise to the coronary arteries. One should, moreover, remember that coronary anatomy might differ from one individual to another. Two additional anatomic factors are important when considering a way to anchor the device. The existence of a fibrous continuity between leaflets of the mitral and aortic valves and the contractility of the subaortic area make anchorage below the aortic valve difficult. Placement of a device in that region might lead to iatrogenic mitral insufficiency or secondary fracture of the implanted device. In our opinion, anchorage is preferable using the native leaflets, the sinus, the sinotubular junction, and the ascending aorta.

Pressure regimen

The systemic blood pressure complicates anchorage of the device. During systole, blood is ejected at high pressure through the opened valve. During diastole, when the valve is closed, there is a large pressure gradient between the aorta and the left ventricle, where the pressure is close to zero. During the cardiac cycle, particularly at closure and opening of the valve, there is a high risk of dislodgement.

Considerations regarding underlined diseases

As well as these anatomic considerations, the underlying disease is important to consider in order to develop a suitable device. In the case of aortic stenosis with highly calcified leaflets, the stent needs high radial forces, and a balloon-expandable stent seems to be preferable. As mentioned previously, consideration of the relationship between diseased leaflets and coronary orifices is important in order to avoid accidental occlusion of the coronary ostia during deployment of the device. The irregular structure of this calcified region increases the risk for paravalvular leak, since the device, even if opened in a circular manner, would not make contact with the whole surface of the diseased valve. Impairment of coronary artery circulation by the device or the native valve reclined by the implanted valve would lead to death if normal circulation were not re-established rapidly. This is particularly important in the presence of heavily calcified valves (aortic valve stenosis) or dysplastic valves with supplementary tissue (aortic valve insufficiency). This abnormal tissue, either calcific or dysplastic, might obstruct the coronary ostia when pushed against the wall by the newly implanted valve. Embolization of calcium deposits during placement of the device is a possible complication that should be prevented. Percutaneously implantable temporary filters can play a role during valve insertion. In the case of long-standing aortic valve insufficiency, the aortic valve and the proximal aortic root are usually dilated. In these patients, large valve implants are required and special precautions need to be taken in respect of anchorage and position, since no calcifications are present to help in positioning and prevent dislodgement.

History of percutaneous valve replacement

In 1992, Andersen and colleagues introduced the idea of a valve supported by a stent.[5] They reported for the first time that implantation of an artificial valve was possible transluminally in closed-chest animals. The valve, taken from an aortic valve of a pig, was sutured onto a balloon-expandable homemade stent. The external diameter of the device was 32 mm when fully expanded and 12 mm when manually collapsed over the balloon catheter. Because of this overall diameter, its insertion into peripheral vessels was impossible. The system was inserted into a 41 Fr flexible introducer sheath advanced retrogradely in the aorta after puncture of the abdominal aorta, which had been surgically isolated. The device was delivered in various sites into the descending and ascending aorta. This valved stent was implanted successfully into nine pigs. All of the animals survived the postimplantation period. The implanted valves were all functional, with only trivial regurgitation in two pigs. Left ventricular end-diastolic pressure was unchanged in all pigs where implantation was made in the ascending aorta. Subcoronary implantation was attempted in two animals and resulted in restriction of coronary blood flow. In those animals, small movements of the delivery sheath occurred during inflation of the balloon, leading to suboptimal positioning of the valved stent. In the same year, Pavcnik and colleagues developed a caged-ball mechanical valve in dogs.[6] The cage was a barbed Gianturco self-expanding stainless steel stent consisting of four to six flat, flexible 3 cm long stainless steel wires attached at the cranial end to form the top of the cage. The ring was constructed of two stainless steel wires coiled together in a springlike configuration and covered with an expandable nylon mesh. The ring was attached to the cage assembly with a length of stainless steel tubing. The ball was a detachable latex balloon placed at the tip of a 60 cm long 5 Fr catheter. It was filled either with air ($n = 3$), contrast medium ($n = 6$), or a liquid silicone material ($n = 3$) that polymerized within 25 minutes after mixing. The device was delivered successfully through an 11 or 12 Fr PTFE sheath below the coronary arteries in 12 dogs. The native valve was trapped between the ring and the aortic wall. The ring and the cage were easily positioned. Once in position, the ball was inserted, inflated, and released within the previously positioned cage. In the early follow-up, all implanted ball valves were functioning with normally 'filled' coronary arteries. However, the ball escaped into the aorta within 3 hours following its implantation.

These studies showed that the development of a mechanical or biological aortic valve for transcatheter implantation was feasible, but because of either the size of the vascular access required for its delivery or early prosthetic dysfunction,

none of these devices had clinical application. It was not until early 2000 that this idea re-emerged and had a human prospect. During that year, we and others successfully developed valved devices for transcatheter replacement of semilunar valves.

Peschel and colleagues (personal communication, 2000) developed a porcine aortic or pericardial valve mounted in a self-expandable stent that requires a 24 Fr delivery sheath for its deployment. A feasibility test on animals was reported in 1996.

In the same year, Sochman and colleagues described a mechanical disk valve.[7] The device consisted of a Z-stent-based valve cage with a locking mechanism and a prosthetic tilting disk. The flexible disk was made of a 0.010-inch nitinol wire braided into the shape of an ellipse and covered by a 0.1 mm thick PTFE membrane. The valve cage was delivered first, followed by the disk, through a 10–12 Fr catheter. This device was tested in four dogs. The implanted valve functioned well for up to 3 hours. No mid-term or long-term studies were performed.

Following successful transcatheter implantations of a valved stent in the pulmonary position in animals as well as in humans, we investigated the possibility of implanting a valve in the aortic position. The device comprised a glutaraldehyde-fixed bovine jugular vein valve sewn into a balloon expandable stent. Because the assembly consisted of a valved venous segment with a length of approximately 2.5 cm, this assembly, in the case of orthotopic placement, would lead to coronary artery obstruction. Moreover, despite very interesting properties in vitro, where the valve supported up to 100 mmHg of back-pressure, no in vivo data were available on venous valve function submitted to systemic pressures. Our first implantation was, therefore, attempted in a heterotopic position, i.e in the descending aorta ($n = 3$) and/or the brachiocephalic trunk ($n = 3$) in animals with traumatically created massive aortic insufficiency.[8]

All animals were successfully implanted. Four of the six valved stents implanted in the descending aorta were competent on hemodynamic and angiographic evaluations. One of the implanted valves showed a slight insufficiency, which was considered to be negligible angiographically and hemodynamically. The remaining deficient valve occurred in one sheep that had a large descending aorta due to overdilatation of an 18 mm valve. The insufficiency was central and related to non-coaptation of the valvular leaflets. Another valved stent was successfully implanted inside the first, impinging on the function of the old valve. This new stent was expanded with a 20 mm balloon catheter, and was competent and non-stenotic. All three valved stents implanted in the brachiocephalic trunk were competent.

Despite successful implantation and perfectly functioning valves, none of the animals survived longer than 24 hours. The control sheep died less than 2 hours after the aortic valve insufficiency was created. The animals in the one-stent and two-stent groups died within 24 hours after the procedure. At autopsy, macroscopic examination confirmed good function of all implanted valves, and showed normal left ventricular volume. One aortic leaflet was completely torn in all of the sheep, explaining the severity of the insufficiency. The death was related to the severity of the insufficiency and the acute rather than chronic pattern of its creation. The experiments, however, confirmed good function of the venous valve and encouraged us to continue to develop a valved stent for aortic valve replacement using this valve.

As a second step, in order to approach the native aortic valve, we repeated these experiments after cutting off the venous wall located between the commissures in a group of animals with mild and severe aortic insufficiency. We hypothesized and demonstrated that this cutoff was not altering the function of the venous valve.[9] Because the created spaces allowed for coronary artery perfusion, we attempted to implant this device in a native aortic valve. Although implantation was successful, all experiments failed as a result of coronary artery obstruction, impairment of the mitral valve, acute embolization in the ascending aorta, or paraprosthetic leak.[10] We designed a framework to overcome these drawbacks. A two-step strategy was developed. The first step was intended to ensure the orientation and locking of the device in the aortic orifice. The second step acted as a supporting structure for the heterograft. To guarantee precise orientation of this device with regard to the coronary orifices, we fixed three self-expandable nitinol hooks onto a previously prepared valved stent. These hooks were engineered to fit into the three native aortic leaflets. Modified devices were successfully implanted in vivo. The coronary arteries remained unobstructed. There was no stent migration or mitral insufficiency during the early follow-up and up to 2 months.[11]

In 2002, Lutter and colleagues reported the results of successful animal studies.[12] A valved stent made of a porcine aortic valve mounted into a self-expandable nitinol stent containing barbs for anchorage was deployed through a 22 Fr sheath in the ascending ($n = 8$) and descending ($n = 6$) aorta via the infrarenal aorta or iliac artery after a surgical cutdown. Technical problems with the stent twisting in the aorta were encountered in two pigs in the early phase of the experiment. The length of the stent was increased from 21 to 28 mm to overcome this problem. One animal died of intractable ventricular fibrillation during positioning of the guidewire in the left ventricle. Eleven animals had successful implants, with satisfactory hemodynamics in eight. Three had mild valvular or paravalvular regurgitation. Good positioning of the valved stent was reached in 8 of 11 pigs. Three animals implanted in the ascending aorta had stent misplacement at a distance of 2–10 mm from the desired position. Findings at autopsy demonstrated that the anchoring barbs of all stents were sufficiently embedded into the aortic wall in the descending aorta group. In the ascending aorta group, in two cases out of eight, the valved stent was sufficiently anchored in the aortic wall or the left ventricular outflow tract, whereas two of the supracoronary group were not fully embedded because of a minimal shift in the lumen. In the subcoronary group ($n = 2$), in one animal only the distal barbs were anchored, whereas the proximal barbs did not reach the wall of the left ventricular outflow tract because of the positioning of the stent. Morphologic aortic damage did not occur in any of the placed stent assemblies.

A number of companies are working on new devices. All are based on the same concepts as presented above. The results of these studies will become available in the near future.

Present status

Based on in vitro and in vivo studies in animals, Alain Cribier and his team have been able to insert a biological valve via a percutaneous technique in patients with end-stage aortic valve stenosis.[13–16] The percutaneous heart valve that they developed in collaboration with Percutaneous Valve Technology (PVT) Inc. is based on a balloon-expandable stainless steel stent (316LVM) in which a trileaflet valve made of equine pericardium (3F Inc.) has been sutured. The valved stents have a height of 14.5 mm and are available in two diameters: 21 mm and 23 mm. The first human implantation was performed in April 2002 on a compassionate basis in moribund patients with severely calcific aortic stenosis and major cardiac and non-cardiac associated diseases. To our knowledge, 18 patients have been included in the study so far (I-REVIVE study) (A Cribier, personal communication, 2004). During a meeting in Frankfurt in June 2004, Cribier presented the acute and midterm follow-up results on the initial 18 implantations. As an inclusion criterion, all included patients had been denied surgical valve replacement by at least two surgeons (not involved in the study) due to unstable hemodynamics and/or multiple comorbidities. All procedures were performed under local anesthesia and mild sedation. A trans-septal antegrade or retrograde approach was used for aortic valve insertion in 13 and 5 cases, respectively. All patients had an aortic valve balloon predilatation with a 23 mm balloon catheter. The device was then mechanically crimped over a 22 mm diameter balloon catheter and advanced over a guidewire through a 24 Fr sheath to the aortic valve. Valves were delivered in a subcoronary position by balloon inflation using calcification as a radio-opaque marker to position the device precisely. The device was successfully delivered in 88.9% of cases. Acute hemodynamic and angiographic results after valve implantation showed no residual gradient. Valve area increased significantly to 1.70±0.1 cm^2. Procedural complications (31.25%) included stroke ($n = 1$), pericardial tamponade ($n = 1$), and deaths ($n = 3$) related to valve embolization, and intractable cardiogenic shock after predilatation of the valve and after relief of severe ischemia of the leg. Moderate to severe paraprosthetic regurgitation was observed in five cases (31.25%). Marked and sustained hemodynamic, echocardiographic, and clinical improvement was observed after all successful valvular implants. Left ventricular end-diastolic volume remained unchanged, whereas left ventricular ejection fraction increased significantly. Ten non-cardiac deaths occurred during follow-up. To date, only one patient has survived for more than 6 months after valve implantation, the other survivors ($n = 2$) having less than 6 months of follow-up.

This preliminary experience showed the feasibility and effectiveness of the technique. The severity of the cases included in the study explained the number of complications. However, it seems obvious that there is still some place for further technical developments and refinements of the device.

Future perspectives on approaches to the aortic valve

Conventional surgery for aortic valve replacement requires extracorporeal circulation. In the future, the approaches to the aortic valve will tend to limit surgical access but also the length and the need for extracorporeal circulation. Sutureless aortic valve replacement is one example of this. The use of these devices, eliminating the time taken to suture the new aortic valve, will reduce the time under bypass and surgery and hopefully the morbidity/mortality linked to the technique.

Another step forward will be 'off-pump' aortic valve replacement. In this regard, two approaches can be considered. The first and most attractive in the short term is to approach the aortic valve with the collaborative expertise of both cardiac surgeons and interventionists. The device and its delivery system would be inserted through a central vascular access or via the left ventricular apex exposed by the surgeon. Implantation would be performed using external direct vision or using intracardiac, epicardial, and/or transesophageal echocardiography. Such a hybrid approach will provide greater safety for patients, allowing for example a better orientation of the device with respect to the coronary arteries and surrounding structures. This technique also allows the device to be secured after its implantation by suturing it to the aortic wall to avoid early and late dislodgements. Moreover, conversion to the standard technique with extracorporeal circulation could be undertaken rapidly in the case of any life-threatening events during implantation. Finally, the use of this technique will enlarge the number of devices, since their use will not be limited by the size of vascular access. Any valve substitutes mounted on any vascular stent may be used, with much less limitation in terms of size. However, anatomic considerations will always need to be taken into account to match the valved stent to the anatomy of the patients and the particular hemodynamic pattern of the aortic root. Huber et al[17] have recently investigated this approach with success in animals with normal aortic valves. One important drawback of this technique in comparison with sutureless and conventional surgeries is the inability to retrieve the abnormal aortic valve. Indeed, in the case of aortic valve stenosis, this might be a problem for adequate relief of stenosis and to avoid paravalvular leak, which has been linked to the irregular geometry of the calcified aortic valve. A complete percutaneous valve replacement also allows for an 'off-pump' replacement of the aortic valve. This technique has been applied with success in animals as well as in humans, as mentioned previously, completely avoiding cardiopulmonary bypass and extending the indications for aortic valve replacement to previously inoperable patients.

Future developments are needed to lower the incidence of paravalvular leak and device/calcium embolization and reduce the risk of mitral damage and coronary blood flow impairment. Smaller and better adapted delivery systems will, for example, be required in order to simplify access to the diseased aortic valve. Research on other valves and stent technologies will be necessary to refine the design of the ideal device. This is obviously the ultimate goal; however, the safety of these procedures will need to be increased through technical improvements. Many groups are currently working in this field. Besides these technological advances, other collaborative approaches can be envisaged. One approach that we are presently investigating is the possibility of using the frame of a surgically implanted biological aortic valve as a support for a valved stent. Such a frame, using radio-opaque markers, will also provide an orientation for the valve to be implanted percutaneously with respect to the position of the coronary artery ostia and mitral valve. If the feasibility and the efficacy of this type of technique can be demonstrated, this will lead to the consideration of biological valves as first-line substitutes even in young patients, for whom mechanical valves are usually favored. The possi-

bility of easily inserting, at low risk, a new valve using a transcatheter technique might change this latter view. This approach will, however, require modifications of the current biological valves or surgical strategy in order to increase, for example, the radio-opacity of the valve frame. As mentioned previously, all of these 'off-pump techniques' leave the abnormal aortic valve in place. Several teams are trying to develop devices and techniques capable of retrieving calcifications of a stenotic aortic valve using catheters. It is difficult to believe that this will not create massive aortic insufficiency, which might make transcatheter valve replacement more difficult in the context of acute aortic regurgitation with a failing left ventricle.

Conclusion

There has been intensive work in the field of percutaneous aortic valve replacement over the last few years. Initially considered impossible, it has become a reality. Human applications have recently begun with various devices. New devices are about to be introduced and begin clinical trials. Most clinicians are still skeptical about the technique. However, looking at the number of teams working on the subject, it is likely that replacement of the aortic valve will be feasible in a large proportion of patients with aortic valve disease. All of the questions regarding the feasibility, safety, and efficacy of the technique are being addressed. Careful preclinical evaluation must be the rule, and animal experiments are difficult because of the lack of good models to properly evaluate percutaneous valve implantations. If we are careful, percutaneous or minimally invasive valve replacement will open a new chapter in interventional and surgical cardiology and become a conventional procedure.

References

1. Hufnagel CA, Harvey WP, Rabil P, McDermott TF. Surgical correction of aortic valve insufficiency. Surgery 1954; 35: 673–80.
2. Starr A, Edwards ML. Mitral replacement: the shielded ball valve prosthesis. J Thorac Cardiovasc Surg 1961; 42: 673–82.

3. Harken DE, Taylor WJ, Lefemine AA, et al. Aortic valve replacement with a caged ball valve. Am J Cardiol 1962; 9: 292–9.

4. Dotter CT. Interventional radiology – review of an emerging field. Semin Roentgenol 1981; 16: 7–12.

5. Andersen HR, Knudsen LL, Hasenkam JM. Transluminal implantation of artificial heart valves. Description of a new expandable aortic valve and initial results with implantation by catheter technique in closed chest pigs. Eur Heart J 1992; 13: 704–8.

6. Pavcnik D, Wright KC, Wallace S. Development and initial experimental evaluation of a prosthetic aortic valve for transcatheter placement. Work in progress. Radiology 1992; 183: 151–4.

7. Sochman J, Peregrin JH, Pavcnik D, et al. Percutaneous transcatheter aortic disc valve prosthesis implantation: a feasibility study. Cardiovasc Intervent Radiol 2000; 23: 384–8.

8. Boudjemline Y, Bonnet D, Sidi D, Bonhoeffer P. Percutaneous implantation of a biological valve in the aorta to treat aortic valve insufficiency: a sheep study. Med Sci Monit 2002; 8: BR113–BR116.

9. Boudjemline Y, Bonhoeffer P. Percutaneous implantation of a valve in the descending aorta in lambs. Eur Heart J 2002; 23: 1045–9.

10. Boudjemline Y, Bonhoeffer P. Steps toward percutaneous aortic valve replacement. Circulation 2002; 105: 775–8.

11. Boudjemline Y, Bonhoeffer P. Percutaneous aortic valve replacement: Will we get there? Heart 2001; 86: 705–6.

12. Lutter G, Kuklinski D, Berg G, et al. Percutaneous aortic valve replacement: an experimental study. I. Studies on implantation. J Thorac Cardiovasc Surg 2002; 123: 768–76.

13. Cribier A, Eltchaninoff H, Bash A, et al. Percutaneous transcatheter implantation of an aortic valve prosthesis for calcific aortic stenosis: first human case description. Circulation 2002; 106: 3006–8.

14. Cribier A, Eltchaninoff H, Tron C, et al. Early experience with percutaneous transcatheter implantation of heart valve prosthesis for the treatment of endstage inoperable patients with calcific aortic stenosis. J Am Coll Cardiol 2004; 43: 698–703.

15. Eltchaninoff H, Tron C, Cribier A. Percutaneous implantation of aortic valve prosthesis in patients with calcific aortic stenosis: technical aspects. J Interv Cardiol 2003; 16: 515–21.

16. Bauer F, Eltchaninoff H, Tron C, et al. Acute improvement in global and regional left ventricular systolic function after percutaneous heart valve implantation in patients with symptomatic aortic stenosis. Circulation 2004; 110: 1473–6.

17. Huber CH, Tozzi P, Corno AF, et al. Do valved stents compromise coronary flow? Eur J Cardiothorac Surg 2004; 25: 754–9.

17

Clinical experience with the Percutaneous Heart Valve for treatment of degenerative aortic stenosis

Alain Cribier, Helene Eltchaninoff, Christophe Tron, Fabrice Bauer, Deborah Nercolini, Carla Agatiello, Vasilis Babaliaros

Introduction

Whereas tens of thousands of patients with valvular disease can benefit every year from surgical valve replacement, a number of patients are excluded from this cohort. This subset includes a large number of high-risk or terminal patients considered unacceptable for surgery, and, in many parts of the world, indigent patients who cannot afford extensive thoracic operations. Offering an optimal therapeutic solution to this group of patients is the primary goal of the recently developed percutaneous aortic valve.

In 1986, balloon aortic valvuloplasty (BAV) was introduced by our group as an option for non-surgical or high-risk patients with degenerative aortic stenosis (mainly elderly patients with multiple comorbidities).[1] Until recently, BAV remained the only percutaneous intervention for this subset of patients. The procedure has been shown to effectively palliate the symptoms of congestive heart failure and diminish the rate of rehospitalization. However, the duration of benefits remains unpredictable, rarely lasting more than 1 year and leading to multiple redo procedures in selected cases.[2–5] In light of the aging population and the marked improvements in technique and safety, BAV has recently attracted renewed interest. It is considered a class IIb indication for patients with serious comorbid conditions accord-ing to American College of Cardiology/American Heart Association (ACC/AHA) guidelines.[6]

The development of stent technology opened a new era in the field of non-surgical treatment of valvular heart disease. In 1992, Andersen et al[7] reported the first experiment in which a stent-mounted pig valve could be successfully implanted at various places in the aorta; technical limitations, however, precluded human application. In 2000, Bonhoeffer et al,[8] using a bovine jugular vein mounted in a platinium–iridium stent, reported successful pulmonary valve implantation in a lamb model and subsequently in the incompetent pulmonary artery conduit of children and young adults.[9–11] This group was the first to demonstrate the applicability of percutaneous stent–valve technology in humans.

For our group, the concept of percutaneous valve replacement in degenerative aortic stenosis emerged in the early 1990s as a way to overcome the limitations of BAV. In 1993, personal unpublished autopsy studies in patients with calcific aortic stenosis confirmed that a Palmaz–Shatz stent, 23 mm in diameter, could open the native diseased valve regardless of the amount of calcification, and securely remain in position without impeding the coronary ostia or the mitral valve. In 1999, Percutaneous Valve Technology, a company based in Ft Lee, NJ, USA, helped us develop an original stent-mounted Percutaneous Heart Valve

(PHV); the valve was extensively tested ex vivo and in more than 100 animals.[12] In April 2002, the first PHV was implanted in a patient with cardiogenic shock and inoperable aortic stenosis.[13] Since this landmark case, improvements in procedural technique and in the design of the PHV prompted a feasibility study at our institution. PHV implantation was attempted in a series of 20 profoundly ill patients on a compassionate basis. The results obtained in the first patients of this series have been reported.[14] This chapter will describe in detail the techniques used for PHV implantation, and summarize the preliminary results to date.

Device description

The PHV

This consists of a radio-opaque balloon-expandable stainless steel stent, 23 mm in maximal diameter, with an integrated unidirectional trileaflet tissue valve and a polyethylene cuff (Figure 17.1). The tissue valve is firmly sutured to the frame and attachment bars. The tissue valve is fabricated from three sections of equine pericardium that has been preserved in low concentrations of buffered glutaraldehyde.

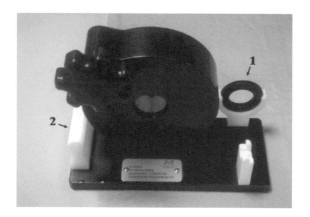

Figure 17.2

The crimping tool allows a symmetrical reduction of the PHV diameter from its expanded size to its collapsed size by turning the rotary knob. The black ring (1) allows measurement of the delivery balloon. If the balloon/PHV assembly can pass through the sizing tube (2), it will also pass through the 24 Fr sheath.

The crimping tool

This is a compression device that symmetrically reduces the overall diameter of the PHV from its expanded size to its collapsed size over the delivery balloon catheter (Figure 17.2). The crimper

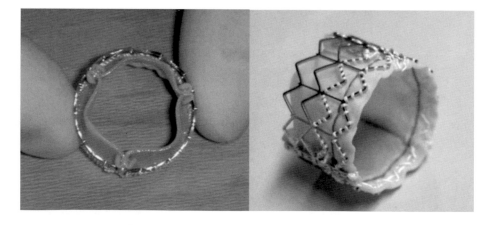

Figure 17.1

Top and side views of the three-leaflet equine pericardial valve attached to the stainless steel stent.

comprises a metal housing and a compression mechanism that is closed manually by means of a rotary knob located on the housing. The crimper is equipped with two gauges: a 24 Fr check gauge that is used to verify that the balloon/PHV assembly has been suitably collapsed to allow introduction through a 24 Fr introducer (COOK, Bjaeverskov, Denmark), and a 22 mm check gauge, which verifies the delivery balloon diameter at full inflation.

The delivery balloon catheter

This is a commercially available Z-MED II (NuMED, Inc., Hopkinton, NY) percutaneous transluminal balloon catheter (22 mm × 3 cm), 120 cm in length. The balloon catheter is purged of air before mounting the stent. A 20 ml syringe is used to determine the exact amount of solution (1:9 contrast/saline) necessary to obtain a 22 mm balloon diameter.

Preprocedural evaluation

Complete clinical evaluation with transthoracic (TTE) and transesophageal (TEE) echocardiography, and cardiac cathoterization with left ventriculography and coronary and aortic angiography, is used to select patients. The technique was approved for use on a compassionate basis in patients declined for surgical valve replacement by two surgeons. A surgical risk scoring system (Parsonnet's Score) based on age, left ventricular function, coronary disease and coexisting medical conditions is used to estimate the extent of high-risk comorbidities.[15] We included patients above 70 years of age, in New York Heart Association (NYHA) functional class IV or cardiogenic shock, and a baseline valve area <0.7 cm². Patients with a native aortic valve annulus size >25 mm or <19 mm, evidence of bacterial endocarditis or other infection, intracardiac thrombus seen by TEE, or coagulopathy were excluded.

Techniques of PHV implantation

The PHV can be implanted using either the antegrade trans-septal or the retrograde approach,

each having advantages and limitations. The antegrade approach was used in the first case of PHV implantation in a patient who presented without femoro-iliac arterial access.[13] This approach was repeated thereafter since it appeared to be feasible and well adapted for insertion of a large 24 Fr introducer into the femoral vein. Since mid-2003, however, the retrograde approach has also been successfully attempted in selected patients with relatively healthy, straight, and large (>7 mm in diameter) femoro-iliac arteries.

Regardless of the technique used, the procedure requires local anesthesia and mild sedation. Aspirin (160 mg) and a loading dose of clopidogrel (300 mg) are administered 24 hours before the procedure. Antibiotics for bacterial endocarditis prophylaxis are given just before the procedure.

In all cases, the procedure starts with reassessment of baseline parameters (right- and left-sided pressures, transvalvular aortic gradient, and aortic valve area using the Gorlin formula). These same measurements are obtained after PHV implantation. Supra-aortic angiograms are performed in order to select the optimal view showing the aortic valvular apparatus perpendicular to the screen and the coronary ostia clearly visible. The anteroposterior view is generally selected, and a frame frozen on another screen will be one of the markers used at the time of PHV implantation.

A 5 Fr pacemaker lead is placed into the right ventricle. The stimulation parameters are controlled, and the pacemaker is set on demand at 80 beats/min. Temporary pacing is mandatory, not only to treat the possible occurrence of complete heart block during the intracardiac maneuvers, but also to provide transient rapid pacing at a rate of 200–220 beats/min. At this rate, cardiac output is immediately diminished, and the balloon is perfectly stabilized during inflation across the diseased valve, allowing effective valve predilatation and precise PHV delivery. The pacemaker lead should be tested before balloon inflation, and the demand rate of 80 beats/min should prevent episodes of significant bradycardia.

Antegrade trans-septal approach

The antegrade trans-septal approach has been the primary mode of valve delivery. Although more technically demanding, the advantages of this approach are the facilitated implantation of the device in heavily diseased valves and the lower risk of inserting a 24 Fr sheath in the femoral vein rather than the femoral artery.

Trans-septal catheterization

Trans-septal catheterization should be performed using a standard technique. To review, an 8 Fr Mullins sheath, dilator, and Brockenbrough needle is advanced to the level of the superior vena cava from the right common femoral vein. After pulling back the assembly into the right atrium in the anteroposterior projection, we prefer to cross the septum in the left lateral view, at the distal third of a virtual line connecting the aortic valve (the distal tip of the pigtail catheter) to the posterior border of the heart (Figure 17.3). After completion of the trans-septal puncture, 5000 IU of heparin are administered intravenously. Through the Mullins sheath in the left atrium, a 7 Fr Swan–Ganz catheter (Edwards Lifesciences, Irvine, CA, compatible with 0.035 inch guidewires) is advanced across the mitral valve and

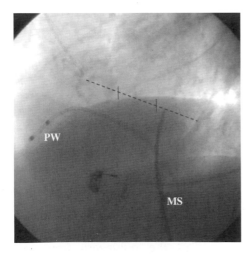

Figure 17.3

Technique of trans-septal puncture. In the lateral view, the septum is crossed at the distal third of an imaginary line between the aortic valve (pigtail catheter) and the posterior border of the heart. PW, pacing wire; MS, Mullins sheath with dilator and Brockenbrough needle.

into the left ventricle. Using a pigtail catheter in the ascending aorta as reference, the aortic transvalvular gradient is recorded.

Guidewire placement

While in the left ventricle, the Swan–Ganz catheter is advanced until the distal tip faces the left ventricular outflow tract (Figure 17.4A). Subsequently, a 0.032 inch straight guidewire can be directed through the catheter and across the aortic valve. With the balloon deflated, the Swan–Ganz catheter is pushed over the wire and into the ascending aorta. The balloon is then re-inflated, the catheter is advanced in the descending aorta (Figure 17.4B), and the guidewire is removed.

A 0.035 inch 360 cm stiff guidewire (Amplatz, Extra Stiff, COOK) is advanced through the Swan–Ganz catheter into the descending aorta, to the level of the common iliac bifurcation. The Swan–Ganz catheter is removed, and the guidewire is snared (Microvena, Amplatz Goose Neck, GN 2500, White Bear Lake, MN) through an 8 Fr sheath in the left common femoral artery (Figure 17.4C). The guidewire is externalized while close attention is paid to maintain a large loop of wire in the left ventricle and prevent traction on the mitral valve. Under fluoroscopic visualization, the second operator must push the guidewire forward from the right femoral vein while the first operator pulls on the wire from the left femoral artery. If this maneuver is not done carefully, the guidewire loop will be straightened, causing severe mitral regurgitation and subsequent hemodynamic collapse. The externalized parts of the wire should be equivalent on both sides (approximately 100 cm).

Dilatation of the interatrial septum

A 10 mm balloon septostomy catheter (Owens, Boston-Scientific Scimed, Inc., Maple Grove, MN) is advanced over the stiff guidewire (compatible with a 10 Fr sheath) in the right femoral vein, and positioned within the interatrial septum. A 30:70 contrast/saline solution in a 10 ml syringe is used for balloon inflation (Figure 17.4D). At least two balloon inflations are performed and held for 30 s. The balloon catheter is then removed.

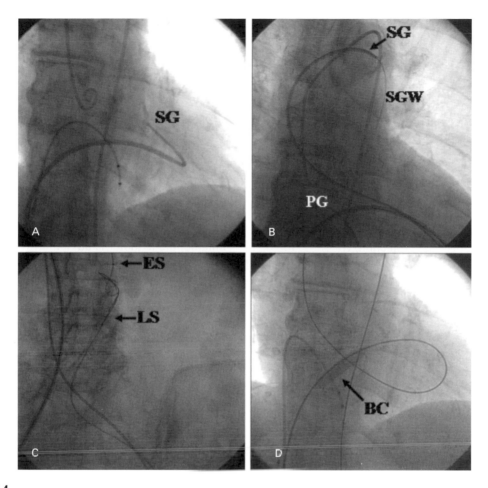

Figure 17.4

(A) The Swan–Ganz catheter (SG) is advanced into the left ventricle until the distal tip faces the left ventricular outflow tract before crossing with the 0.032 inch straight guidewire. (B) The 0.032 inch straight guidewire (SGW) is pushed through the Swan–Ganz catheter in the descending aorta. PG, pigtail catheter. (C) The 360 cm long 0.035 inch extrastiff guidewire (ES) is externalized through the left femoral artery after being snared. LS, lasso. (D) Interatrial septal dilatation using a 10 cm diameter balloon catheter (BC).

Predilatation of the aortic valve

The native valve must be predilated before PHV implantation. We use a 23 mm balloon valvuloplasty catheter, 30 mm long (Z-Med II, NuMED Canada Inc., Cornwall, Ontario), carefully purged of air and inflated with a 1:9 contrast/saline solution in a 20 ml syringe. In the 40° right anterior oblique view, the balloon is advanced over the stiff guidewire through a 14 Fr sheath (COOK) in the right femoral vein, and positioned across the native aortic valve.

Immediately prior to inflation, rapid right ventricular pacing is performed. The balloon is then immediately inflated (Figure 17.5), deflated, and withdrawn from the outflow tract. While withdrawing the catheter, the second operator must push forward the guidewire from the right femoral artery in order to maintain the guidewire loop unchanged in the left ventricle. Two or three balloon inflations are normally performed for effective predilatation. The persistence of a waist on the fully inflated balloon is a contraindication to PHV implantation.

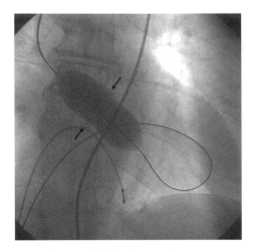

Figure 17.5

Predilatation of the native aortic valve using a 23 mm diameter balloon catheter advanced over the extrastiff guidewire through the right femoral vein (black arrows indicate aortic valve calcification).

PHV implantation

The 14 Fr sheath in the right femoral vein is exchanged for a 24 Fr introducer (COOK). From the left femoral artery, a 7 Fr Sones (B-type)

catheter is advanced over the stiff guidewire until its distal tip is positioned approximately 2 cm above the aortic valve. The PHV/balloon assembly is then introduced from the 24 Fr sheath, over the guidewire, and across the interatrial septum. The PHV should advance easily through the left atrium, across the mitral valve, and into the left ventricle until its distal tip faces the native aortic valve.

Careful positioning of the PHV/balloon assembly across the native diseased valve is then performed. Positioning is facilitated by the use of the Sones catheter, which is in contact with the distal tip of the Z-MED II balloon. The device can be advanced or pushed back across the native valve by applying pressure on the balloon or the Sones catheter. Using the calcification of the native valve and the reference image obtained during supra-aortic angiography as markers, the center of the PHV is accurately positioned in the middle of the aortic valve.

Immediately prior to delivery, rapid pacing is performed. A 20 ml syringe is used to quickly inflate the balloon with the entire amount of pre-measured contrast/media solution. After complete expansion (Figure 17.6A), the balloon should be immediately deflated, and the fast pacing interrupted. The total duration of rapid pacing and balloon inflation should not exceed a few

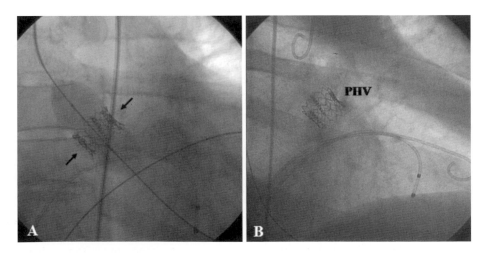

Figure 17.6

(A) Delivery of the PHV. The balloon is inflated after the PHV is positioned in the center of the aortic valve calcifications (black arrows). (B) The PHV in place within the native aortic valve in the anteroposterior view. The pigtail catheter in the left ventricle is used to protect the mitral valve during guidewire removal.

seconds. The deflated balloon is quickly withdrawn, leaving the guidewire in place across the PHV.

A 6 Fr pigtail catheter is pushed over the guidewire from the right femoral vein and advanced into the mid-left ventricle. With the pigtail catheter in place, the guidewire can be safely removed from the femoral vein (Figure 17.6B) without injury to the mitral valve apparatus. Transvalvular pressure gradients can then be measured across the newly implanted valve.

Retrograde approach

In the course of our experience, the retrograde approach appeared as a possible alternative to the antegrade route. The most attractive advantage of this approach was the simplicity and speed with which it could be performed. Because the femoral artery is cannulated by the 24 Fr delivery sheath, this approach should be limited to patients with femoral and iliac vessels that are adequate in size (inner diameter >7 mm) and without significant tortuosity or disease. Preclosure of the femoral puncture site is performed at the beginning of the procedure using two 10 Fr Perclose devices (Abbots Vascular, Redwood City, CA).[16,17]

Crossing the native valve

After initial baseline measurements, the aortic valve must be crossed with a guidewire. Proper technique permits negotiation of the stenotic aortic valve in all cases within a few minutes. We use a 0.035 inch straight-tip guidewire and a 7 Fr Sones (B-type) catheter to facilitate passage or, in cases of enlarged ascending aorta, an Amplatz left coronary artery catheter. In the 40° left anterior oblique view, the catheter tip is pointed posteriorly and positioned at the upper border of the valve. The catheter is then slowly pulled back with strong clockwise rotation, and the guidewire is used to repeatedly probe the aortic valve. After the valve has been crossed with the wire, the catheter is advanced into the left ventricle. The transvalvular gradient is obtained using aortic pressure measured from the 8 Fr arterial sheath as reference.

Guidewire placement

A 0.035 inch, 270 cm long, extrastiff guidewire (Amplatz, Extra Stiff, COOK) is inserted into the Sones (or Amplatz) catheter, and the diagnostic catheter is removed. Before use, the flexible end of this wire must be reshaped into an exaggerated pigtail curve to decrease the risk of left ventricular trauma or arrhythmia. The 8 Fr arterial sheath is removed and replaced by a 14 Fr sheath.

Predilatation of the aortic valve

As in the anterograde approach, a Z-Med II balloon catheter (NuMed Canada, Inc.), is prepared and purged of air. The 23 mm balloon is advanced from the common femoral artery, over the stiff guidewire, into the proximal aorta. Using the calcifications of the leaflets as a landmark, the balloon is positioned across the aortic valve. Two or three balloon inflations are usually needed for adequate predilatation. Each inflation should be performed during rapid cardiac pacing to prevent ejection of the balloon.

Percutaneous insertion of the 24 Fr sheath

The balloon catheter is withdrawn while leaving the stiff guidewire in the left ventricle. The 14 Fr sheath is then removed while hemostasis is obtained with manual compression. Additional local anesthesia is administered, and the femoro-iliac axis is carefully predilated using three polyethylene dilators (18, 20, and 22 Fr). Predilatation should be cautiously performed under fluoroscopic visualization. After successful dilatation, the 24 Fr sheath can be introduced into the femoro-iliac arteries.

PHV implantation

The PHV/balloon assembly is prepared as previously described. Through the 24 Fr sheath, this device is advanced over the guidewire, and pushed across the aortic valve. Using the calcification of the leaflets and the reference image obtained during thoracic aortography as markers, the PHV is accurately positioned in the native

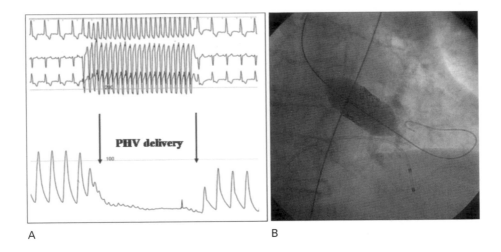

A   B

Figure 17.7

(A) The aortic blood pressure recording during rapid right ventricular pacing (arrows), demonstrating the effect of a sudden drop in cardiac output. (B) Retrograde delivery of the PHV.

valve. During rapid cardiac pacing (Figure 17.7A), a 20 ml syringe is used to quickly inflate the delivery balloon (Figure 17.7B). The balloon is then deflated, and the catheter is rapidly withdrawn, leaving the guidewire in place across the PHV. A pigtail catheter can be advanced over this guidewire to measure the trans-PHV gradient, using the sidearm of the sheath as a measure of central aortic pressure.

Final measurements and long-term follow-up

Following implantation of the valve, right and left heart catheterization is performed to reassess baseline parameters. Transvalvular gradient and cardiac outputs are measured, and the new aortic valve area is calculated as previously described. Blood samples are collected for measurement of oxygen saturation and assessment of interatrial shunting. If the patient does not have renal insufficiency, a left ventriculogram is done to document left ventricular function and the degree of mitral regurgitation. Also depending upon the renal status, an angiogram of the thoracic aorta and the coronary arteries can be performed to assess the amount of residual aortic regurgitation and the relation of the stent valve to the coronary ostia (Figure 17.8). All catheters are subsequently

removed, leaving vascular access sites for closure. If the retrograde approach has been used, the femoral artery entry site is closed using the predelivered Perclose sutures, or a surgical repair in case of failure. A pneumatic compression device or hand pressure is applied to venous entry sites.

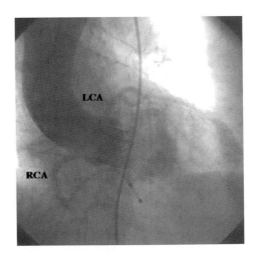

Figure 17.8

Post PHV implantation, the supra-aortic angiogram confirms the patency of the coronary ostia and the absence of aortic regurgitation. LCA, left coronary artery; RCA, right coronary artery.

The patients are closely monitored during follow-up. Clinical evaluation and echocardiographic examination are performed immediately post procedure, at day 1, day 7, 1 month, and every 3 months thereafter (TTE and TEE at day 1, TTE thereafter). Postprocedural treatment includes 75 mg of clopidogrel daily for 1 month and 160 mg of daily aspirin indefinitely. Subcutaneous low-molecular-weight heparin is administered during the hospitalization stay. Oral anticoagulants are given only in patients with chronic atrial fibrillation, starting 2 days before discharge.

Clinical experience

In our institution, PHV implantation has been performed on a compassionate basis in 20 end-stage patients with severe calcific aortic stenosis (transvalvular gradient 43 ± 12 mmHg, aortic valve area 0.56 ± 0.06 cm^2). These patients were advanced in age (78 ± 10 years) and had multiple life-threatening comorbidities (Parsonnet Score 52 ± 7). The most frequent cardiovascular comorbidities were severe left ventricular dysfunction, cardiogenic shock, extensive coronary atherosclerosis, porcelain aorta, and carotid artery disease. The most frequent non-cardiac comorbidities were cancer, chronic obstructive lung disease, and end-stage renal failure.

The detailed results obtained in this first series of patients will be published later and have been partially reported.[14] Briefly, PHV implantation was attempted using the antegrade approach in 12 patients (one failure) and the retrograde approach in 6 (two failures, with subsequent successful trans-septal implantation in one case during the same session). The PHV was successfully and accurately implanted in 15 patients, with a final valve area of 1.70 ± 0.1 cm^2. In all cases, the device was without significant transvalvular gradient and did not impinge on the coronary ostia. Periprocedural complications included one stroke (during aortic valve predilatation), one episode of pericardial tamponade (during pacing lead placement), and three deaths. Procedural deaths occurred in two patients in cardiogenic shock (one during predilatation of the aortic valve and one after immediate PHV migration in a patient who presented with grade IV aortic regurgitation after complicated balloon valvuloplasty). The third death occurred in a patient after removal of the arterial 24 Fr sheath following a successful procedure (no cause was found at autopsy; death was attributed to a crush-type syndrome). In four patients in whom the antegrade approach was used, a brief period of hemodynamic collapse occurred during guidewire-induced mitral regurgitation. Postimplantation perivalvular aortic regurgitation was noted in a few cases (grade III in four patients, and grade II in one patient), but was of no consequence clinically. Seven days post procedure, all patients with successful PHV implantation had dramatic amelioration of symptoms, and increased left ventricular function ($42 \pm 18\%$ to $55 \pm 12\%$).

Ten non-cardiac-related deaths have occurred during follow-up (between 1 and 5 months) due to the inevitable progression of pre-existing comorbidities or complications after non-cardiac surgery. There has been no evidence of PHV dislodgement or deterioration of function observed by echocardiography thus far. To date, the longest follow-ups are 10, 13, and 14 months. In these patients, the PHV function remains unchanged. They continue to experience remarkable clinical improvement.

Future directions

Our preliminary clinical experience in patients with severe calcific aortic stenosis confirms the feasibility of PHV implantation. In patients with a successful procedure, a valve area of 1.7 cm^2 was consistently achieved, with minimal transvalvular gradient and no impingement of the coronary ostia. These benefits remain unchanged during follow-up and are associated with dramatic relief of heart failure. Some degree of perivalvular leak has been observed due to imperfect apposition of the stent frame within the asymmetric calcified native valve. Further improvements in stent size and design should address this problem.

In this subset of elderly patients without surgical options, successful PHV implantation is already superior to balloon aortic valvuloplasty. At our institution, we are examining the impact of valve implantation in patients with less significant comorbidities. In this cohort, we hope to study the long-term performance of the PHV and the continuing clinical benefits of this technique. Other pilot trials are expected to start in the near future in European and American centers. Ultimately, multicenter pivotal trials will be required to determine the role of this promising therapeutic approach in patients with non-operable aortic stenosis.

References

1. Cribier A, Savin T, Saoudi N, et al. Percutaneous transluminal valvuloplasy of acquired aortic stenosis in elderly patients: an alternative to valve replacement. Lancet 1986; 1: 63–7.

2. Safian RD, Berman AD, Diver DJ, et al. Balloon aortic valvuloplasty in 170 consecutive patients. N Engl J Med 1988; 319: 125–30.

3. The NHLBI Participants. Percutaneous balloon aortic valvuloplasty. Acute and 30-day follow-up results in 674 patients from the NHLBI Balloon Valvuloplasty Registry. Circulation 1991; 84: 2383–97.

4. Otto CM, Mickel MS, Kennedy W, et al. Three-year outcome after balloon aortic valvuloplasty. Insights into prognosis of valvular aortic stenosis. Circulation 1994; 89: 642–50.

5. Lieberman EB, Bashore TM, Hermiller JB, et al. Balloon aortic valvuloplasty in adults: failure of procedure to improve long term survival. J Am Coll Cardiol 1995; 26: 1522–8.

6. ACC/AHA Guidelines for the Management of Patients with Valvular Heart Disease. A report from the American College of Cardiology/American Heart Association Task Force on Practice Guidelines (Committee on Management of Patients with Valvular Disease). J Am Coll Cardiol 1998; 32: 1486–588.

7. Andersen HR, Knudsen LL, Hasemkam JM. Transluminal implantation of artificial heart valves: description of a new expandable aortic valve and initial results with implantation by catheter techniques in closed chest pigs. Eur Heart J 1992; 13: 704–8.

8. Bonhoeffer P, Boudjemline Y, Saliba Z, et al. Transcatheter implantation of a bovine valve in pulmonary position: a lamb study. Circulation 2000; 102: 813–16.

9. Bonhoeffer P, Boudjemline Y, Saliba Z, et al. Percutaneous replacement of pulmonary valve in a right-ventricle to pulmonary-artery conduit with valve dysfunction. Lancet 2000; 356: 1403–5.

10. Bonhoeffer P, Boudjemline Y, Qureshi SA, et al. Percutaneous insertion of the pulmonary valve. J Am Coll Cardiol 2002; 39: 1664–9.

11. Boudjemline Y, Agnoletti G, Piechaud JF, et al. [Percutaneous pulmonary valve replacement: towards a modification of the prosthesis]. Arch Mal Coeur Vaiss 2003; 96: 461–6.

12. Cribier A, Eltchaninoff H, Borenstein N, et al. Transcatheter implantation of balloon expandable prosthetic heart valves: early results in an animal model. Circulation 2001; 104(Suppl II): II-552 (abst).

13. Cribier A, Eltchaninoff H, Bash A, et al. Percutaneous transcatheter implantation of an aortic valve prosthesis for calcific aortic stenosis: first human case description. Circulation 2002; 106: 3006–8.

14. Cribier A, Eltchaninoff H, Tron C, et al. Early experience with percutaneous transcatheter implantation of heart valve prosthesis for the treatment of end-stage inoperable patients with calcific aortic stenosis. J Am Coll Cardiol 2004; 43: 698–703.

15. Parsonnet V, Dean D, Bernstein AD. A method of uniform stratification of risk for evaluating the results of surgery in acquired adult heart disease. Circulation 1989; 79(Suppl I): I-3–I-12.

16. Feldman T. Percutaneous suture closure for management of large French size arterial and venous puncture. J Interv Cardiol 2000; 13: 237–42.

17. Solomon LW, Fusman B, Jolly N, et al. Percutaneous suture closure for management of large French size in aortic valvuloplasty. J Invasive Cardiol 2001; 13: 592–6.

18

The CoreValve in the aortic position

Jean-Claude Laborde, Eberhard Grube, Denis Tixier, Raoul Bonan

Introduction

Aortic valve diseases comprise aortic stenosis or aortic regurgitation, which most of the time are associated. Accounting for the vast majority of aortic valve disease, aortic stenosis has a prevalence of around 1–2% in those aged over 65 and 4% in those over 85. It is mainly due to calcific stenosis on the bicuspid valve, senile degeneration, or rheumatic disease. Aortic valve regurgitation affects approximately 5 out of every 10 000 people. Common etiologies includes acute rheumatic fever, dystrophic lesions of the ascending aorta, and infectious endocarditis.

The inevitable progress of the disease leads to surgical valve replacement, which consists of implantation of either a mechanical or a biological prosthesis (heterograft or allograft) via thoracotomy.[1–7] This requires both general anesthesia and cardiopulmonary bypass, which can lead, in the aging population, to disorders in vital functions (heart, brain, and kidneys). Moreover, due to the high complication rate and discomfort to the patient, and to frequent associated polyvisceral illnesses, there are still some patients who are not suitable candidates for an open-heart procedure and hence are not treated.

These are the reasons why other less invasive techniques have been tried for several years. Percutaneous procedures commonly performed for peripheral and coronary angioplasties for several decades have been used in valve disease management; balloon mitral or aortic valvuloplasties are performed as 'salvage' procedures in non-operable patients with acute heart failure.[8–10]

Several companies are now developing devices that could allow percutaneous treatment of mitral (valve repair and annuloplasty), pulmonary, and aortic (bioprosthetic implant) valves, avoiding open-heart surgery.[11–15]

CoreValve has developed a device consisting of a bioprosthetic valve made of pericardial tissue mounted and sutured in a self-expanding nitinol frame. The CoreValve aortic valve prosthesis is delivered percutaneously via a specific catheter-based technique and implanted within the diseased aortic valve. The procedure is performed under local (or general) anesthesia and with femoro-femoral cardiac assistance.

Material

The CoreValve aortic valve prosthesis (AVP) consists of a self-expanding heart valve frame designed for the replacement of a native valve or an in-place bioprosthetic aortic heart valve. Once deployed, the prosthesis is not retrievable from the site of expansion.

The procedure is performed under general anesthesia and femoro-femoral left ventricular assistance. Vascular access is via surgical cut-down with angiography and potentially transesophageal echocardiography for proper positioning of the heart valve. Because the procedure does not remove the native valve leaflets, the term 'ReValving' (a trade-mark) has been applied so as to differentiate it from the surgical technique that removes leaflets and local calcifications.

The CoreValve frame

The CoreValve self-expanding frame is a three device frame made from laser-cut nitinol tubing (Figures 18.1 and 18.2). Each level carries out a particular function:

- The upper part (*aortic level*) of the frame increases the prosthesis fixation to the aortic wall and aligns the system parallel to the blood flow.
- The middle part (*commissural level*) carries the valve. It is constrained to a given diameter corresponding to the optimal diameter of the tissue valve. It holds the valve leaflets in their functional position. The convex shape of this level is opposed to the concavity of the coronary sinus to preserve the natural hemodynamic flow.
- The lower conical part (*annulus level*) firmly anchors the prosthesis to the aortic annulus, preventing any migration and paravalvular leaks thanks to its high radial force.

Because of the self-expanding nature of the frame, it can adapt to non-circular local anatomies and does not recoil following expansion.

The CoreValve frame has been submitted to various studies:

- *Finite element analysis.* This method simulates in a model the behavior of the ReValving frame and highlights the zones of mechanical effort. This study shows that the stress of the valve functioning is concentrated at the commissural level. The current frame design is compatible with long-term mechanical durability (Figure 18.3).
- *Fatigue testing.* Fatigue tests are conducted on the frame alone and on the valve–frame combination using a durability tester. In this test, the ReValving undergoes accelerated aging (4×10^8 cycles). A comparison with

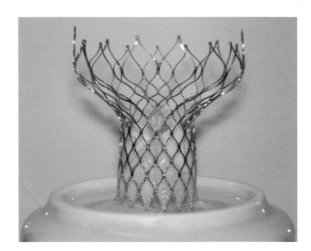

Figure 18.2

The P15.2 prosthesis.

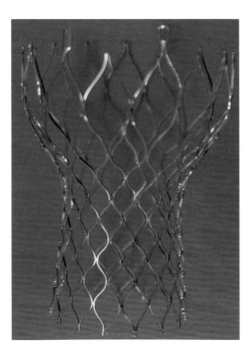

Figure 18.1

CoreValve self-expanding frame made from laser-cut nitinol tubing.

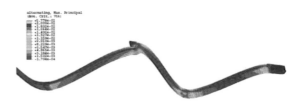

Figure 18.3

Finite element analysis.

US Food and Drug Administration (FDA)-approved valves showed equivalent durability (Figure 18.4).

- *Pulse duplicator test.* The functioning of the valve–frame combination is evaluated with the same test. It shows that the leaflets do not touch the frame while opening. The opening area is very satisfactory and the flow pattern is adequate. Compared with other FDA-approved valves, the gradient is low.

The CoreValve valve

The replacement tissue heart valve received special attention from the CoreValve team when designing the ReValving technology. The valve has to be both functional and durable. The key to this challenge is to design an optimal frame-to-valve integration. The valve is made of a standard biological tissue (animal pericardium). It is fixed to the frame in a surgical manner using monofilament sutures. The valve is mounted on the middle part (commissural level) of the frame. The lower conical part of the frame is covered by pericardium. The design and the mounting on the frame are based on the goal of reducing local stress and therefore enhancing durability.

Design and mounting also take into consideration the goal of reducing the overall size and improving the quality of folding when compressed for implantation. An in vitro test showed that the CoreValve frame with mounted valve could be compressed in a 21 Fr outer-diameter catheter.

Histologic studies

Histologic studies to validate the integrity of the tissue valve following compression and decompression prior to implantation showed no trauma to the valve.

The CoreValve catheter

The catheter carries the heart valve prosthesis and delivers it at the deployment site. It has the flexibility, tractability, and rigidity that are required to navigate to the aortic annulus. The sheath and pusher antagonistic movements, carried out using the handle, allow the prosthesis to be loaded and released (Figure 18.5). For a simpler and safer procedure, the proximal PTFE–Pebax sheath diameter is reduced to 14 Fr. The space required by the compressed prosthesis is more important: the working Rilsan–Pebax distal end has a 21 Fr diameter (Figure 18.6A). The inner pusher is a plastic and metal element.

Two ways of delivering the prosthesis (controlled expansion and high-speed expansion) can be carried out thanks to an easy-to-use PVC handle (Figure 18.6B). The different components are:

- a thumbwheel to carry out the controlled expansion
- a threaded button to activate the high-speed expansion.

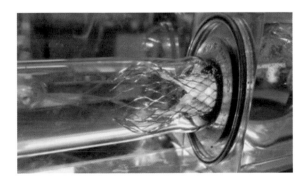

Figure 18.4

Fatigue testing.

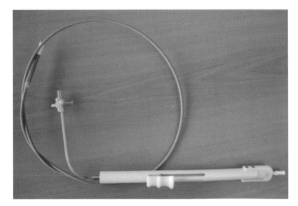

Figure 18.5

Delivery catheter.

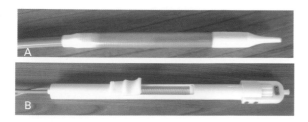

Figure 18.6

(A) Distal end of the delivery catheter (Rilsan–Pebax). (B) Easy-to-use PVC handle.

Reversed movements have to be executed to close the catheter by pushing the sheath out of the handle.

Control of prosthesis expansion using the thumbwheel is very precise. It is possible to pass from one mode of expansion to the other as frequently as required.

The CoreValve loading tool

The loading system is used to collapse the framed valve into the catheter just before introducing it into the patient. The framed tissue valve is stored in its naturally expanded position to prevent any damage to the tissue of the valve. A few minutes before implantation, the framed valve is rinsed per standard bioprosthesis protocol and cooled so as to render the nitinol frame deformable and collapsible.

The CoreValve loading tool concept corresponds to the compression cone. The prosthesis is firstly pushed through a precompression cone. The catheter is then introduced in a way that does not damage the valve. The attached prosthesis is pulled into the catheter sheath using another compression cone and the catheter thumbwheel.

In vitro studies

Human explanted heart with calcified aortic stenosis

Human hearts were explanted, including the ascending aorta up to the root of the brachiocephalic arterial trunk. After immobilizing the

hearts, the distance between the arteriotomy and the aortic annulus was measured. The left atrium was opened, the mitral valve visualized, and its effective orifice area (EOA) measured. The prosthesis was loaded into the delivery catheter previously used during the animal study and the prosthesis was implanted.

The following analysis was then carried out:

- through the left atrium, verification of the mitral valve, determination of the mobility of the two mitral leaflets, and measurement of the mitral EOA
- cut-down of the aorta to the distal end of the prosthesis
- verification that the left and right coronary arteries ostia stayed uncovered and were perfectly free with the help of a 1 mm coronary guide
- search for paravalvular leaks with a 1 mm metal tip inserted between the aortic wall and the external rim of the frame
- further dissection of the aorta to the annulus, and verification of the adequate positioning of the prosthesis relative to the annulus and the subannular zone.

Results

The CoreValve delivery was event-free each time.

The P6.2 prosthesis (first-generation prosthesis) frequently interfered with the mitral valve leaflet. The P12.1 prosthesis (first-generation prosthesis), lacking the subannular frame, was never in contact with the mitral valve more than 3 mm, while the leaflet complete length was measured at 30 mm. With the P12.1 prosthesis, no reduction of the EOA was noted and there was no reduction in mobility of the anterior and posterior leaflets.

The implantation of the CoreValve prosthesis left a free passage to both coronary orifices. On one occasion the prosthesis partially obstructed the passage. This happened with the P6.2 prosthesis, which did not have a commissural diameter limited in expansion. The P12.1 prosthesis has a constraint on the upper layer of the frame that allows for optimal valve prosthesis function and also prevents the frame from interfering in any way with the coronary ostia.

The P6.2 prosthesis exhibited minor paravalvular leaks. Two possible causes were identified: the distance between two adjacent stitches on the valve (3–5 mm) left passage for leakage; and the implanted prostheses were undersized relative to the anatomy, thus having limited radial force.

The assembly of the P12.1 prosthesis (mounting the valve on the frame) was changed to a running suture, thus limiting leaks between pericardium tissue and frame.

On three implantations, balloon expansion following the implantation was shown to reduce the leaks by pushing the frame further inside the aortic wall. Leaks of a lesser diameter were still observed, but were minimal, meaning that the 1 mm probe could be pushed in these leaks with repeated strong applications. Since these leaks have not been significant in animal implantations, the model of cadaver hearts, which of course lack blood pressure to extend the vessel and anatomy, can be questioned.

Cadaver studies

Access was carried out via the right femoral artery/external iliac artery and left subclavian artery. An extrastiff guidewire was inserted up to the aortic valve. The ascending aorta was opened for visualization. The delivery catheter was pushed on the wire, and after delivery of the prosthesis, the following analysis was carried out: after cut-down of the aorta to the distal end of the prosthesis, verification that the left and right coronary artery ostia remained uncovered and were perfectly free with the help of a 1 mm coronary guide, a search for paravalvular leaks with a 1 mm metal tip inserted between the aortic wall and the external rim of the frame, further dissection of the aorta to the annulus, and verification of the adequate positioning of the prosthesis relative to the annulus and the subannular zone.

With the described elements, two human cadavers were implanted using the P15.2 prosthesis and the C4.2 catheter (actual design). The first implantation was done in a 76-year-old male cadaver, 4 days after death.

The external iliac artery was measured at an external diameter of >12 mm, compatible with access of the CoreValve delivery catheter. An Amplatz 0.038 inch extrastiff guidewire was advanced up to the abdominal artery. No further progression was possible.

A retroperitoneal approach was then made in order to gain access to the external iliac artery. Severe calcifications were noticed, which explained the difficulty in advancing the guidewire. The guidewire was introduced through the abdominal aorta and advanced up to the aortic valve. A visualization opening was made in the ascending aorta in order to see the progression of the catheter.

The CoreValve delivery catheter was advanced over the guidewire. Progression was difficult. Possible causes were calcifications in the thoracic aorta, blood clots, and a non-cylindrical shape. Nevertheless, the catheter took the bending of the aortic arch following the guidewire. In this position, the frame could be expanded in a controlled manner at the level of the valve annulus but outside the anatomy because of the lack of precise visualization.

The heart was then explanted for a better view of the implantation site.

The second implantation was made on a 78-year-old male cadaver 4 days postmortem. A retroperitoneal approach was made in order to gain access to the external iliac artery. The guidewire was introduced through the abdominal aorta and advanced up to the aortic valve. A visualization opening was made in the ascending aorta in order to see the progression of the catheter.

The CoreValve delivery catheter was advanced over the guidewire. Progression was easy and uneventful. The catheter slid over the bending of the aortic arch, following the guidewire. In this position, the frame could be expanded in a controlled manner at the level of the valve annulus but outside the anatomy because of the lack of precise visualization.

Implantation with the CoreValve delivery catheter was possible through a retroperitoneal access. Access through the external iliac artery seems possible, but can be rendered difficult or impossible in the event of a calcified abdominal aorta. The flexibility of the CoreValve delivery catheter is compatible with access over the subclavian artery.

The observations were as follows: absence of interference with the mitral valve was confirmed with this new prosthesis (Figure 18.7); the coronary ostia were unchanged and the coronary arteries were free from any obstruction (Figure 18.8); the radial force of the frame was sufficient to maintain the expected opening, even through a heavily calcified valve, and no paravalvular leaks were observed around the frame (Figure 18.9). The flexibility of the CoreValve delivery catheter is compatible with access over the subclavian artery.

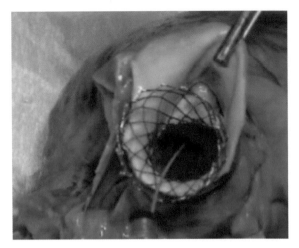

Figure 18.9

Adequate radial force without paravalvular leak in a cadaver experiment.

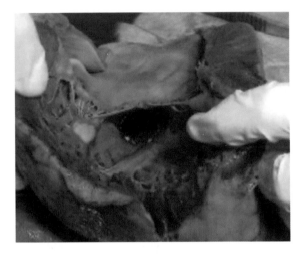

Figure 18.7

No impairment of the mitral valve is seen in this cadaver experiment.

Animal studies

Objective

The objective of this study was to confirm the feasibility of percutaneous heart valve replacement in a beating heart in a sheep model using aortic implantation with a self-expandable cardiac tissue valve prosthesis. We monitored security and efficacy during and after implantation by studying:

- control of the delivery of the prosthesis
- precision of implantation on the aortic valve annulus
- quality of fixation of the prosthesis to the surrounding tissue
- absence of migration of the prosthesis
- correct perfusion of the coronary arteries.

Animal model

The animal model chosen was the sheep.[16–22] According to the literature, this model is the only one accepted as such for valve testing in the orthotopic position. The anatomy above the valve annulus and especially the coronary sinuses are

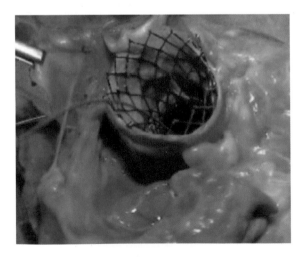

Figure 18.8

Free coronary ostium in a cadaver experiment.

close to the human equivalents. The CoreValve frame, with one part located in the vicinity of these sinuses and bridging the coronary sinuses with an 'ascending aorta segment', could therefore reproduce the advantage envisioned in humans.

However, one major difference from human anatomy described in the literature (and also encountered by other teams) was confirmed. In the sheep model, there is no space between the aortic and mitral valve annuli (the so-called inter-aortico-mitral ridge) as is well described in humans and noted by all surgeons performing heart valve replacements. Therefore, since the CoreValve frame has an element that covers the subannular space and the inter-aortico-mitral ridge, this causes various degrees of mitral regurgitation.

Conventional anesthesia with Pentothal (thiopental) 10 mg/kg intravenously and isoflurane 2% in 100% O_2 was used on these sheep.

Arterial access was obtained through the femoral arteries and the brachiocephalic trunk for the prosthesis implantation. Angiographies of the ascending aorta and the left ventricle were performed before implantation for aortic ring measurement, and after implantation for aortic valve or paravalvular leakage evaluation.

Implantations

With the first-generation prosthesis, 35 animals were implanted. Modifications of the prostheses and delivery catheters derived from an internal development program.

Precise implantation

The CoreValve heart valve was delivered each time with total accuracy, except for the very first implant (23-Oct-02). On that occasion, the self-expandable prosthesis jumped out of the delivery system. Since then, a technique (CoreValve retaining hooks) has been applied to withhold the prosthesis until the external sheath is fully pulled back.

Absence of migration

After complete implantation, the prosthesis migrated six times. The reasons were well understood in each case. A proper solution was also found when needed and underlines the fact that this complication is well controlled by the prosthesis design. The six cases were as follows:

- 05-Nov-02: The catheter tip, insufficiently smooth, hooked the prosthesis upon retrieval. This problem was never encountered after modification of the tip.
- 12-Nov-02: The prosthesis was made out of a metal wire that was smaller (0.014 inch diameter) and therefore supplied insufficient radial force. Following this encounter, frames with at least one element with a thicker wire (0.016 inch diameter), and therefore a higher radial force, were used.
- 25-Nov-02: The part of the prosthesis intended to anchor on the valve annulus was made of a smaller wire (0.014 inch diameter). After this implantation, the whole frame was made with thicker wire (0.016 inch diameter).
- 6-Dec-02 and 14-Oct-03: Measurements of the valve annulus (25 mm) and the ascending aorta (30 mm) showed that the prosthesis that was available would be significantly undersized. No other CoreValve prosthesis was then available. It was nonetheless decided to implant in order to document the consequences of the anticipated migration.
- 11-Jun-03 AM: The prosthesis was precisely implanted under echocardiographic guidance, but migrated upon return to normal blood flow. This was due to insufficient radial force.
- 26-Jun-03 and 22-Jul-03: The angioplasty procedure combined with blood pressure over the balloon led to migration of the prosthesis.

Free coronary flow

Ninety-four percent of implanted prostheses showed free coronary blood flow. This was assessed by free coronary flow at the angiography and no persistent ECG modification. We can conclude that our prosthesis design does not alter the coronary perfusion following delivery and in the hours after implantation.

Only two cases exhibited obstruction of blood flow:

- 13-May-03: The leaflet level is offset.
- 11-Jun-03 AM: The angioplasty balloon used to reposition the prosthesis occluded the coronary arteries.

More recently, animal experiments with the latest-generation prosthesis, with ReValving technology (actual design), involving 21 animals, have been performed to validate the system prior to the clinical studies. In brief, using the same protocol, 17 animals were euthanized early and showed good adhesion, no impairment of coronary flow, no prosthesis migration, and no valvular or para-valvular leaks. Two 10-day and two 6-week follow-ups confirmed the intimate adhesion of the frame to the local tissue and persistent good valvular function, with absence of valve tear, calcification, and impairment.

Conclusions from animal studies

- The CoreValve heart valve can be loaded into a delivery system and delivered to the animal's valvular site through an endovascular approach on a beating heart.
- The prosthesis can be precisely implanted on the animal's valve annulus. The added features of the frame's ultimate design gives the device in this animal model controlled delivery, precise implantation, satisfactory attachment to the adjacent tissues and absence of migration.

Human studies

After successful cadaver and animal studies, a human feasibility and safety study has been planned.[23] The objectives of the investigation are to demonstrate the safety and feasibility of percutaneous implantation of the CoreValve prosthetic valve in patients requiring replacement of their native or bioprosthetic aortic valve. That study will be carried out as a prospective, single-arm feasibility study, which will be conducted in accordance with the Standard EN-ISO 14155:

2003 on clinical investigations with medical devices on compassionate-use patients and in accordance with recommendations guiding physicians in biomedical research involving human subjects adopted by the 18th World Medical Assembly, Helsinki, Finland, 1964 and later revisions.

The inclusion criteria are as follows:

- age ⩾18 years
- native or bioprosthetic aortic valve disease of either endocarditic or non-endocarditic origin, defined as valve regurgitation ⩾3 and/or valve stenosis with an aortic valve area <1 cm^2 by echocardiographic measure
- aortic valve annulus diameter ⩾20 mm and ⩽23 mm by echocardiographic measure
- eligibility for an open-heart surgical aortic valve replacement
- documented left ventricular ejection fraction ⩾30%.
- signed informed consent.

The exclusion criteria are as follows:

- known hypersensitivity or contraindication to aspirin, heparin, ticlopidine, clopidogrel, or nitinol, or sensitivity to contrast media that cannot be adequately premedicated
- any sepsis, including active endocarditis
- uncontrolled atrial fibrillation
- any condition considered as a contraindication for extracorporeal assistance
- any femoral, iliac, or aortic vascular condition (stenosis or tortuosity) that precludes insertion and endovascular access to the aortic valve
- symptomatic carotid or vertebral artery narrowing disease
- abdominal or thoracic aortic aneurysm
- bleeding diathesis or coagulopathy, or refusal of blood transfusion
- severe renal failure (creatinine ⩾2.5 mg/dl)
- pregnancy
- enrolment in another investigational device study.

Primary endpoints are safety and feasibility. Safety is determined in terms of clinical outcome: composite major adverse cardiac, cerebral, and vascular events (MACCVE) and death at discharge. MACCVE include:

- major arrhythmia
- myocardial infarction
- cardiac tamponade
- valve non-structural dysfunction or structural deterioration
- emergent aortic valve replacement surgery, coronary bypass surgery, or percutaneous coronary intervention
- cardiogenic shock
- endocarditis
- stroke or transient ischemic attacks (TIAs)
- aortic dissection
- access site vessel dissection
- vessel perforation
- acute vessel occlusion
- major bleeding.

Procedure feasibility is defined by device functionality based on an investigator evaluation rating and the rate of procedural success at discharge:

- The rating will evaluate the system's ability to:
  - load the valve on the delivery catheter, using the loading system
  - access the aortic valve with the delivery catheter
  - deploy the valve accurately across the aortic native or bioprosthetic valve
  - remove the intact delivery system.
- The rate of procedural success at discharge is defined as valve success without MACCVE or death at discharge. Valve success is defined as adequate device placement and functionality as assessed by angiography at the end of the procedure.

Secondary endpoints are defined as:

- patient's functional status evaluated by NYHA functional class at 15 days, 30 days, and 3 months
- patient's left ventricular ejection fraction measured by Doppler echocardiography at 15 days, 30 days, and 3 months
- valve performance (including valve surface area, transvalvular gradient, and valve regurgitation grade) measured by control Doppler echocardiography at 15 days, 30 days, and 3 months

- incidence of valve migration at 15 days, 30 days, and 3 months, as demonstrated by echocardiography
- incidence of paravalvular leak at 15 days, 30 days, and 3 months, as measured by Doppler echocardiography
- incidence of composite MACCVE and death at discharge, 15 days, and 3 months
- incidence of valve endocarditis at 15 days and 3 months
- rate of access site complications requiring treatment
- incidence of surgical cardiovascular intervention
- incidence of overall adverse events.

Clinical experience to date

The first human implantations were conducted with success in early summer 2004. The first patient was a 62-year-old male with terminal inoperable lung cancer and with severe calcified stenosis and regurgitation of the aortic valve (Figure 18.10). The implantation was uneventful, through a right inferior limb artery cut-down. Post implantation, no valvular gradient and no significant paravalvular or centrovalvular leaks were recognized, and an improved cardiac function was maintained until his death due to respiratory insufficiency at day 6.

The second patient was a 30-year-old male with severe aortic regurgitation (Figure 18.11). Again, implantation through a right inferior limb artery cut-down was easy. Post implantation, no paravalvular or valvular regurgitation were documented, and selective cannulation of the left coronary ostium confirmed the freedom of the coronary ostium and the feasibility of a selective approach to the coronary artery. Ultrasonic evaluation at 48 hours showed less than 3 mmHg of transvalvular gradient and a significant improvement in left ventricular function. This patient died at day 10 with no valvular or heart dysfunction from a 'crush syndrome' complication from the lengthy arterial cross-clamping (a right inferior limb artery approach for the introduction of the catheter and a left femoral approach for femoro-femoral circulatory assistance).

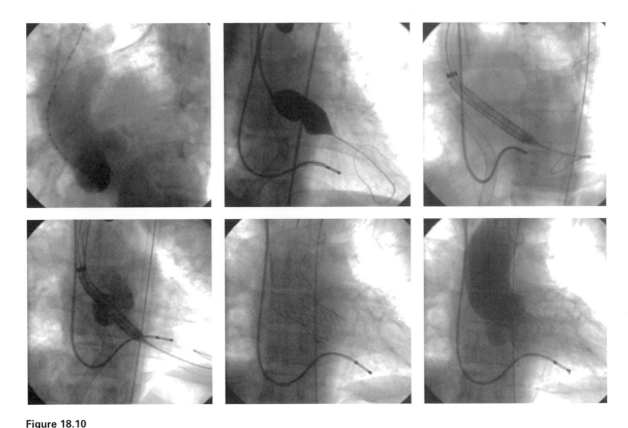

Figure 18.10

First human implantation, in a 62-year-old patient.

In February 2005, a 60-year-old female with severe aortic regurgitation received a revalving procedure through a right inferior limb artery cut-down. The first implant was implanted too low, showing significant aortic regurgitation. A second implant was implanted successfully, with no documented post implantation paravalvular or valvular regurgitation. The patient returned home on day 7 after an uneventful hospital stay. Control echocardiography showed 15 mmHg of trans-valvular gradient and no valvular regurgitation, centro- or paravalvular.

In February 2005, a 68-year-old female with severe aortic calcified stenosis received a revalv-ing procedure through a right inferior limb artery cut-down. The patient was able to walk to her postoperative day 2 control echocardiogram, which showed low transvalvular gradient and no

valvular regurgitation, centro- or paravalvular. The patient returned home after an uneventful hospital stay.

Conclusion

The CoreValve ReValving system presents a self-expanding multisegment frame prosthesis for percutaneous aortic valve replacement. This concept has a number of benefits: avoiding balloon damage to the pericardial leaflets at the time of implantation, providing improved radial force for better anchorage on the annulus, preventing periprosthesis leak and migration, and permitting self-orientation in the ascending aorta as much as a supplementary anchorage. The retrograde approach proposed with the actual catheter size

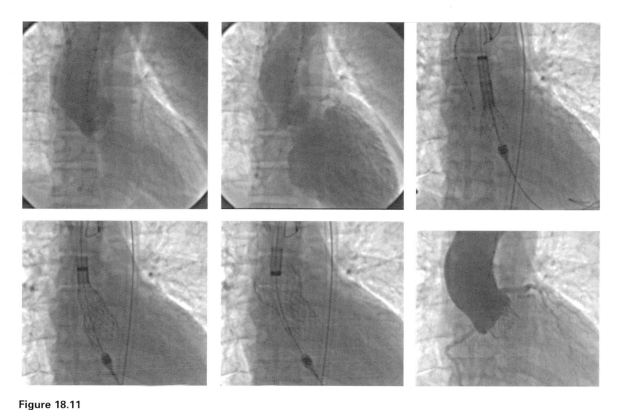

Figure 18.11

Second human implantation, in a 30-year-old patient.

tracking over the wire may encounter some difficulties in small and diseased arteries, but avoids further damage to the mitral anterior leaflet.

The concept has been validated in the first four human implants, and clinical studies are ongoing.

References

1. Otto CM, Kuusisto J, Reichenbach DD, et al. Characterization of the early lesion of 'degenerative' valvular aortic stenosis: histological and immunohistochemical studies. Circulation 1994; 90: 844–53.

2. Otto CM, Lind BK, Kitzman DW, et al. Association of aortic-valve stenosis with cardiovascular mortality and morbidity in the elderly. N Engl J Med 1999; 341: 142–7.

3. Novaro GM, Tiong IY, Pearce GL, et al. Effect of hydroxymethylglutaryl coenzyme A reductase inhibitors on the progression of calcific aortic stenosis. Circulation 2001; 104: 2205–9.

4. Ross J Jr, Braunwald E. Aortic stenosis. Circulation 1968; 38(Suppl V): V61–V67.

5. Bonow RO, Rosing DR, Maron BJ, et al. Reversal of left ventricular dysfunction after aortic valve replacement for chronic aortic regurgitation: influence of duration of preoperative left ventricular dysfunction. Circulation 1984; 70: 570–9.

6. Klodas E, Enriquez-Sarano M, Tajik AJ, et al. Surgery for aortic regurgitation in women: contrasting indications and outcomes compared with men. Circulation 1996; 94: 2472–8.

7. Carabello BA, DeLeon AC, Edmunds LH, et al. ACC/AHA Guidelines for the Management of Patients with Valvular Heart Disease (Committee on Management of Patients with Valvular Heart Disease). J Am Coll Cardiol 1998; 32: 1486–588.

8. Letac B, Cribier A, Koning R, Lefebvre E. Aortic

stenosis in elderly patients aged 80 or older: treatment by percutaneous balloon valvuloplasty in a series of 92 cases. Circulation 1989: 80: 1514–20.

9. Percutaneous balloon aortic valvuloplasty: acute and 30-day follow-up results in 674 patients from the NHLBI Balloon Valvuloplasty Registry. Circulation 1991: 84; 2383–97.

10. Cribier A, Remadi F, Koning R, et al. Emergency balloon valvuloplasty as initial treatment of patients with aortic stenosis and cardiogenic shock. N Engl J Med 1992; 323: 646.

11. Cribier A, Eltchaninoff H, Bash A, et al. Percutaneous transcatheter implantation of an aortic valve prosthesis for calcific aortic stenosis: first human case description. Circulation 2002; 106: 3006–8.

12. Boudjemline Y, Bonhoeffer P. Steps toward percutaneous aortic valve replacement. Circulation 2002; 105: 775–8.

13. Cribier A, Eltchaninoff H, Tron C, et al. Early experience with percutaneous transcatheter implantation of heart valve prosthesis for the treatment of end-stage inoperable patients with calcific aortic stenosis. J Am Coll Cardiol 2004; 43: 698–703.

14. van Herwerden LA, Serruys PW. Percutaneous valve implantation: back to the future? Eur Heart J 2002; 23: 1415–16.

15. Boudjemline Y, Bonhoeffer P. Percutaneous valve insertion: a new approach? J Thorac Cardiovasc Surg 2003; 125: 741–2.

16. Cribier A, Eltchaninoff H, Tron C, et al. Percutaneous artificial cardiac valves: from animal experimentation to the first human implantation in a case of calcified aortic stenosis. Arch Mal Coeur Vaiss 2003; 96: 645–52.

17. Boudjemline Y, Bonhoeffer P. Percutaneous implantation of a valve in the descending aorta in lambs. Eur Heart J 2002; 23: 1045–9.

18. Boudjemline Y, Bonnet D, Sidi D, Bonhoeffer P. Percutaneous implantation of a biological valve in the aorta to treat aortic valve insufficiency – a sheep study. Med Sci Monit 2002; 8: BR113–BR116.

19. Andersen HR, Knudsen L, Hasenkam JM. Transluminal implantation of artificial heart valves. Description of a new expandable aortic valve and initial results with implantation by catheter technique in closed chest pigs. Eur Heart J 1992; 13: 704–8.

20. Lutter G, Matern U, Berg G, et al. Percutaneous transluminal implantation of an aortic valve in aortic position: a porcine study. Thorac Cardiovasc Surg 2001; 49(Suppl 1): 67.

21. Lutter G, Kuklinski D, Berg G, et al. Percutaneous aortic valve replacement: an experimental study. I. Studies on implantation. J Thorac Cardiovasc Surg 2002; 123: 768–76.

22. Ferrari M, Hellige G, Schlosser M, et al. Percutaneous aortic valve replacement with a self-expanding stent – first animal results. Eur Heart J 2002 (Suppl): 156.

23. Mitka M. Trials planned for testing nonsurgical approach to replacing heart valves. JAMA 2003; 289: 1366–7.

19

Development of a nanosynthesized metallic percutaneous aortic valve

Steven R Bailey

Introduction

Senile degenerative aortic stenosis is an increasingly frequent cause of pulmonary edema or heart failure, often requiring repeat and prolonged hospitalization. Unfortunately, many of these patients are aged and/or suffer from comorbid conditions, placing them at high surgical risk.[1-4] The current American College of Cardiology/American Heart Association (ACC/AHA) guidelines[5] state that aortic valve replacement is the only effective treatment for severe aortic stenosis. These same guidelines state that percutaneous balloon valvotomy has a limited role in older adults and that it is not a substitute for valve replacement but may be used as a bridge to subsequent therapy, including valve replacement. The technique of percutaneous balloon aortic valvuloplasty may result in improved symptoms if performed successfully, but has a high risk of periprocedural complications. Percutaneous balloon valvotomy also has a high recurrence rate, with renarrowing rates reported to be as high as 50% at 6 months.[6]

Mechanical aortic valve replacements have had the longest durability, but there are associated problems of a larger residual gradient post implantation and a higher risk of thromboembolism compared with biological valves. Surgically implanted biological valves have an increased risk of degeneration due to inflammation/rejection (xenografts) and a shorter life span, but they have fewer thromboembolic events and a decreased need for anticoagulation and offer the opportunity to achieve larger effective valve areas after implantation.[7]

Percutaneous implantation of an aortic heart valve offers the possibility of adapting the techniques learned from percutaneous balloon aortic valvuloplasty in high-risk patients to allow permanent implantation of a therapeutic artificial valve. Because solid metal leaflets could not be compressed to a small enough size to allow a percutaneous approach, investigations to date have focused upon the incorporation of tissue valve leaflets upon a stent scaffold for percutaneous implantations.

We report the development of an ultrapure nanosynthesized nitinol microporous leaflet, less than 10 μm in thickness, that has been incorporated in to an expandable nitinol cage for implantation into the aortic valve annulus.

Methods

The development of three-dimensional technologies for synthesis of metal has been pioneered by scientists at Advanced Bioprosthetic Materials Inc (ABPS). Using a novel technique and a specialized chamber, pure metal ions of nickel and titanium are placed into a subatmospheric environment and exposed to a high voltage, resulting in time- and temperature-specific metal assembly of nitinol (Figure 19.1).

We have previously demonstrated that this metal has increased purity and strength compared with conventionally manufactured nitinol metals.[8] An important feature of this manufacturing process is the ability to synthesize ultrathin metal using selective ion deposition at thicknesses not achievable with conventional metal manufacturing processes that remove varying thicknesses of metal with each step. We have additionally developed a technique that allows

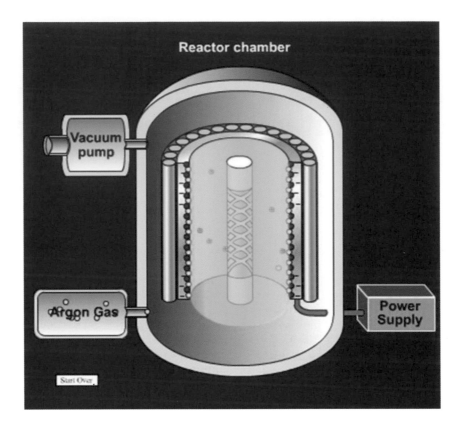

Figure 19.1

Cartoon illustrating the concept of a three-dimensional chamber for nanosynthesis of metals.

this metal to be microporous, improving its radial or longitudinal properties and resulting in greater flexibility. Additionally, the nitinol cage used to anchor the valve into the aortic annulus offers the opportunity to enlarge the aortic annulus after implantation.

Monolithic percutaneous heart valve prototypes (ABPS valves) have been manufactured using the process described above, as have composite valve (Figure 19.2). These prototype aortic valves have demonstrated the ability to be compressed into a 10 Fr introducer system (Figure 19.3). Currently, other percutaneous aortic valve implants under investigation require introducers larger than 20 Fr in order to allow implantation.

In vitro analysis of the ABPS valve in a flow chamber demonstrated low opening and closing pressures with full leaflet excursion.

Prototype ABPS percutaneous aortic heart valves, with an unconstrained expanded diameter of 20 mm, have been acutely implanted into the aortic annulus of pigs to demonstrate the feasibility of implantation. The implantation was performed using a protocol approved by the University of Texas Health Sciences Center at San Antonio Animal Use Committee.

The implants were performed using a retrograde approach from the carotid and femoral arteries. The introducer sheath was advanced across the aortic valve over an extra support 0.035 inch wire and the distal segment of the valve was advanced into the left ventricular outflow tract to anchor the valve cage. The valve was implanted by withdrawing the sheath back across the valve to anchor it in place across the aortic annulus (Figure 19.4).

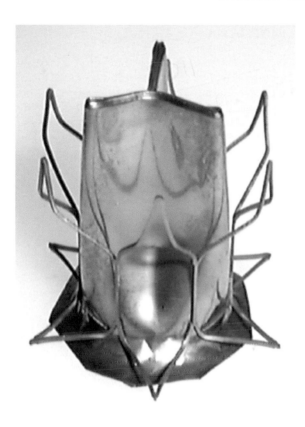

Figure 19.2

Prototype ABPS percutaneous aortic valve.

Results

This ultrapure microporous membrane, used as the valve leaflet for a percutaneous aortic metal valve, has been shown in vitro and in vivo in a stent cover model implanted into porcine carotid arteries to have 85% coverage at 3 days and 100% coverage at 10 days (Figure 19.5).

The percutaneous aortic valve implants were successful and did not dislodge during the short time of observation. The ABPS percutaneous aortic valves successfully expanded the aortic annulus and excluded the native aortic valve leaflets alongside the periphery of the valve. The coronary arteries were patent, without evidence of ostial compromise.

Discussion

Percutaneous aortic valve implantation represents a new opportunity to improve patient outcomes in a subgroup of patients who currently may not have treatment options. Percutaneous aortic heart valves, currently in phase I trials, utilize a biological tissue valve incorporated into a balloon-expandable or self-expanding stent platform.

We have presented the initial investigation of a new all-metal nanosynthesized valve designed to

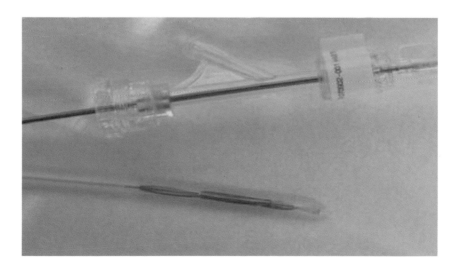

Figure 19.3

Percutaneous aortic valve compressed in a 10 Fr sheath.

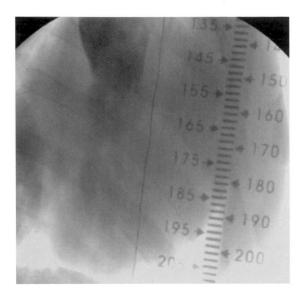

Figure 19.4

Fluoroscopic image post implantation of percutaneous

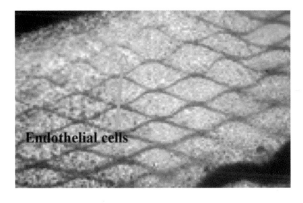

Figure 19.5

Endothelialization of microporous membrane.

be implanted into the aortic annulus to treat aortic stenosis. This ABPS valve utilizes ultrapure micron-thick metal valve leaflets attached to a self-expanding nitinol frame for percutaneous replacement of a diseased aortic valve.

We have demonstrated that such a valve can be delivered in a retrograde fashion via a peripheral artery using a 10 Fr introducer sheath and implanted across the aortic annulus. The valve did not compromise the coronary circulation after acute implantation.

Limitations

This chapter has detailed the early prototype development. Full characterization of the histologic and hemodynamic performance of this valve is not included here. Continued investigation into the healing process, including endothelialization, deposition of fibrin and thrombus, and the effectiveness of valve expansion, is required.

Subsequent long-term implant studies in animal models are currently being planned.

Conclusions

Senile degenerative aortic stenosis represents a complex high-risk subset of patients who currently have limited treatment options. New technologies for percutaneous heart valve implantation are being developed.

A new approach using a nanosynthesized all-metal expandable valve utilizing ultrathin microporous leaflets is being developed. The low profile of this prosthesis is attractive for percutaneous delivery. The properties of microporous nitinol allow the creation of flexible leaflets with mechanical properties that are well suited for a heart valve. We have presented the initial concept and supportive data for future investigations.

Acknowledgments

This study was supported in part by the Janey Briscoe Center for Excellence in Cardiovascular Research at the University of Texas Health Sciences Center at San Antonio and by Advanced Bioprosthetic Surfaces Inc., San Antonio, Texas. The authors have equity positions in Advanced Bioprosthetic Surfaces Inc.

The author would like to recognize Christopher Boyle for his important role in the valve development and construction.

References

1. Florath I, Rosendahl UP, Mortasawi A, et al. Current determinants of operative mortality in 1400

patients requiring aortic valve replacement. Ann Thorac Surg 2003; 76: 75–83.

2. Aksoyek A, Ulus AT, Tutun U, et al. Cardiac valve replacement with mechanical prostheses in patients aged 65 years and over. J Heart Valve Dis 2004; 13: 641–50.

3. Langanay T, De Latour B, Ligier K, et al. Surgery for aortic stenosis in octogenarians: influence of coronary disease and other comorbidities on hospital mortality. J Heart Valve Dis 2004; 13: 545–52.

4. Gehlot A, Mullany CJ, Ilstrup D, et al. Aortic valve replacement in patients aged eighty years and older: early and long-term results. J Thorac Cardiovasc Surg 1996; 111: 1026–36.

5. ACC/AHA Guidelines for the Management of Patients with Valvular Heart Disease. A Report of the American College of Cardiology/American Heart Association Task Force on Practice Guidelines (Committee on Management of Patients with Valvular Heart Disease). J Am Coll Cardiol 1998; 32: 1486–588.

6. Agarwal A, Kini AS, Attanti S, et al. Results of repeat balloon valvuloplasty for treatment of aortic stenosis in patients aged 59 to 104 years. Am J Cardiol 2005; 95: 43.

7. Akins CW, Hilgenberg AD, Vlahakes GJ, et al. Results of bioprosthetic versus mechanical aortic valve replacement performed with concomitant coronary artery bypass grafting. Ann Thorac Surg 2002; 74: 1098–106.

8. Palmaz JC, Bailey S, Marton D, Sprague EA. Influence of stent design and material composition on procedure outcome. J Vasc Surg 2002; 36: 1031–9.

Section 3

The mitral valve

20

Embryology of the mitral valve and pathology of mitral valve stenosis and regurgitation

Jack Titus, Shannon Mackey-Bojack

Mitral valve anatomy

Normal functioning of the mitral valve depends on the entire mitral valve apparatus, which includes the annulus fibrosus, leaflets, chordae tendinae, and papillary muscles. Factors essential for proper valve function are thin mobile leaflets, free unrestricted commissures, and appropriate length and position of chordae tendinae and papillary muscles.[1]

Annulus fibrosus

The annulus fibrosus is an incomplete connective tissue ring that is most easily demonstrated at the right and left trigones. The right trigone (central fibrous body) is located between the mitral valve, tricuspid valve, and aortic valve. The left trigone is between the mitral and aortic valves. A thin ring of connective tissue continues from the trigones posteriorly, but fades as it approaches the lateral one-half to one-third of the valve. This region, occupied by the posterior leaflet, is in direct connection with the left atrium and left ventricle. The ring is also incomplete between the two trigones; this area is occupied by the anterior mitral leaflet, which has fibrous continuity with the aortic valve.[2–4]

Leaflets

The mitral valve has two leaflets: anterior and posterior (Figure 20.1). The anterior leaflet occupies less of the annular circumference than the posterior leaflet; however, the basilar attachment

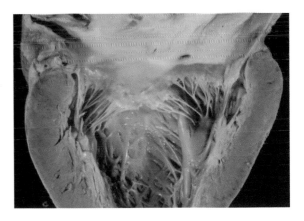

Figure 20.1

Normal mitral valve. The anterior leaflet is greater in length from base to free edge and the posterior leaflet occupies a greater circumference of the valve. The valve leaflets are thin and translucent. Thin, individual chordae tendinae insert into two papillary muscles.

to the free edge is larger. The anterior leaflet is responsible for most of the valve closure during systole. It is trapezoid in shape. Grossly, it has two zones: 'clear' and 'rough'. The 'clear' zone is the smooth, proximal atrial aspect of the valve. The 'rough' zone is at the free edge of the leaflet, and is usually the site of insertion of chordae tendinae.[5,6] The anterior leaflet does not attach to the annulus fibrosus, but is in direct continuity with the non-coronary and left cusps of the aortic valve.[2]

The posterior leaflet occupies the majority of the annular circumference of the mitral valve, but is much shorter from base to free edge. The posterior leaflet is subdivided into scallops designated anterior, middle (central), and posterior. The posterior leaflet, unlike the anterior leaflet, does not have distinct clear and rough zones, mainly because chordae tendinae insert into the entire ventricular surface of the leaflet.[3,5–7]

The anterior and posterior leaflets are separated by commissures, designated anterolateral and posteromedial. The commissures are morphologic regions of the valve that do not extend completely to the annulus; thus, the leaflet tissue is continuous about the valve annulus.[8]

Histologically, the leaflets have distinct layers (Figure 20.2). Both the atrial and ventricular surfaces have a thin endocardial layer composed of endothelial cells, elastic tissue, collagen, and occasional muscle cells (usually smooth muscle). The fibrosa of the valve is on the ventricular surface, and it is the main structural support of the valve. The fibrosa is composed of dense collagen tissue, elastic fibers, and occasional smooth muscle cells. The atrial aspect, the atrialis, has the same components, but in lesser degree. The middle layer, the spongiosa, consists of loose connective tissue in a background rich in proteoglycans. The spongiosa of the valve is thought to provide a cushioning support that absorbs the impact of the continual opening and closing of the valve. The valve leaflets are normally avascular.[9,10]

Chordae tendinae

The chordae tendinae derive from the left ventricle during absorption of the ventricular wall during embryogenesis.[10–15] They are normally

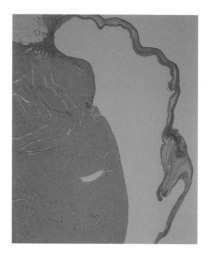

Figure 20.2

Photomicrograph of a normal mitral valve, stained with an elastic stain: section from posterior mitral valve and lateral wall of the left ventricle. The normal three layers of the valve are seen. The layer closest to the left atrium is the atrialis. This layer is in continuity with the endocardium of the left atrium. The layer closest to the ventricle is the fibrosa. This layer contains elastic and muscle cells and provides the major structural support for the valve. The middle layer, spongiosa, is rich in proteoglycans.

avascular fibrous strands that connect the papillary muscles to the leaflets. Chordae tendinae from both papillary muscles insert into both leaflets. Older terminology classifies chordae as first-, second-, and third-order chords.[8] Anatomically, this classification is as follows: first-order chords insert into the free edge of the leaflets, second-order chords insert into the ventricular surface of the leaflets, and third-order chords usually insert into the basal segment of the posterior leaflet.

A second classification scheme for chordae tendinae incorporates anatomic landmarks into the classification.[16] In this classification, there are also three main types of chordae, which are termed commissural chordae, anterior leaflet chordae, and posterior leaflet chordae. The commissural chordae, as the name indicates, insert in the region of valve commissures. Typically, a single chord arises from the papillary muscles, branches in a fan pattern, and inserts into the leaflets at the commissures. Anterior leaflet chordae are further subdivided into paramedial, central or strut, and paracommissural. These chordae insert into the rough zone of the anterior leaflet. The central or strut chordae are usually single, thick chordae that provide essential support to the anterior leaflet. Posterior leaflet chordae insert into both the rough zone of the leaflet and the basal portion of the leaflet. This group of chordae is further subdivided into basal chordae that arise from the ventricular wall and insert into the leaflet, and cleft chordae that extend from the papillary muscles to the scallops of the posterior leaflet.

Papillary muscles

The two papillary muscles in the left ventricle related to the mitral valve are the anterolateral and posteromedial papillary muscles. These papillary muscles arise from the upper apical third of the left ventricle, and are normally located beneath the corresponding commissures of the mitral valve. Both papillary muscles may have more than one head; the posteromedial papillary muscle most commonly has the greater number of heads.[2]

Mitral valve embryology

Formation of the atrioventricular valves occurs between the fifth and eighth weeks of development.[17] To understand the formation of the atrioventricular valves, it is necessary to discuss septation of the ventricles and the formation of the left ventricular outflow tract. Formation of the ventricular septum relies on the primary cardiac fold invaginating anterosuperiorly, fusion of the superior and inferior endocardial cushions, and the inlet septum invaginating inferiorly. Fusion of the endocardial cushions is required for the development of the mitral and tricuspid valvular orifices.[11,12]

Formation of the atrioventricular valves is mainly a process of invagination and myocardial undermining. As the heart is developing, sulcus tissue, which is extracardiac mediastinal mesenchymal tissue, protrudes into the atrioventricular sulcus between the developing atria and inlet ventricle, creating a flap. This flap is surrounded by atrial and ventricular tissue with sulcus tissue located in the middle, thus creating

three layers.[11,13] Undermining of the inlet portion of the ventricles forms the leaflet tissue, chordae tendinae, and papillary muscles.[10–15]

The development of the anterior leaflet is slightly more complex, as it is a major component of the left ventricular outflow tract. In addition to the sulcus tissue, protrusion of endocardial cushion tissue in the region of the future anterior leaflet becomes incorporated into the leaflet tissue. The amount of endocardial cushion tissue lessens as the heart grows.[12]

Congenital mitral valve abnormalities

Congenital abnormalities of the mitral valve may result in stenosis, insufficiency, or a combination of both. These abnormalities may result from a structural abnormality involving any portion of the mitral valve apparatus, or a combination of several components. Tables 20.1 and 20.2 list the more commonly encountered conditions causing congenital stenosis and insufficiency, respectively.

An important feature when considering treatment modalities for these conditions is the frequent concomitant occurrence of other congenital cardiac abnormalities. The presence and the type of the more frequent conditions is noted under each subheading.

The condition of mitral valve atresia is not discussed further as it is not amenable to transcatheter treatment.

Table 20.1   Congenital mitral valve stenosis
• Parachute mitral valve • Supravalvar ring of left atrium • Congenital commissural fusion • Obstruction by abnormal papillary muscles

Table 20.2   Congenital mitral valve insufficiency
• Cleft mitral leaflet • Accessory orifice of mitral valve • Anomalous mitral arcade • Short chordae tendinae

Congenital mitral valve stenosis

Congenital mitral stenosis (CMS) is an uncommon condition. It may result from an abnormality involving any part of the mitral valve apparatus and may be supravalvar, valvar, or subvalvar in position. Frequently, stenosis results from several processes occurring together.[18]

Parachute mitral valve

The original term 'parachute mitral valve' was first introduced in 1961 and was described in association with congenitally corrected transposition of the great arteries.[19] Parachute mitral valve is characterized by the presence of two normal leaflets and commissures, with the insertion of all chordae tendinae into a single papillary muscle – thus the resemblance to a parachute. Most commonly, one true papillary muscle exists; however, occasionally, there are two papillary muscles, one of which is often hypoplastic and frequently malpositioned.[20] The chordae are often shortened and thickened, resulting in decreased mobility of the leaflets; therefore, the combination of abnormal, shortened chordae and the attachment of chordae to a single papillary muscle lead to obstruction of blood flow into the left ventricle.

Parachute mitral valve is most often found in association with additional abnormalities.[1,18,21] In combination with other conditions causing left-sided obstruction, the term 'Shone syndrome' is often used;[18] the other types of left-sided obstruction are coarctation of the aorta, subaortic stenosis, and supravalvar ring of the left atrium.

Supravalvar ring of the left atrium

In this condition, a ring of dense fibrous tissue, often circumferential, is in the left atrium just above the mitral valve. This ring of fibrous tissue may protrude into the left atrium and, depending on its thickness, may decrease blood flow by creating an obstructing diaphragm.[18,22] As with parachute mitral valve, additional congenital anomalies are often present. Reported additional anomalies with supravalvar ring include ventricular septal defect, coarctation of the aorta, double-outlet right ventricle, parachute mitral valve, and subaortic stenosis.[1,18]

Congenital fusion of commissures, congenital mitral stenosis

A rare condition producing congenital mitral stenosis results from fusion of the valve commissures. In this condition, the leaflets are thickened and fibrotic, and the chordae tendinae frequently are shortened. The fusion of the commissures may create a 'funnel' appearance of the valve.[1] Grossly, this condition somewhat resembles rheumatic valvular disease. As with other conditions causing congenital mitral valve stenosis, additional cardiac abnormalities are common, especially those involving the aortic valve and aorta.[23]

Abnormalities of papillary muscles

Congenitally abnormally large papillary muscles may create mitral valve stenosis, either by obstruction of flow into the left ventricle or by malposition of the large papillary muscle just below the valve orifice.[1] Papillary muscles that are of normal size may also cause obstruction and stenosis when positioned high in the ventricle. Malformed or hypoplastic muscles when associated with shortened and thickened chordae tendinae may be another cause of mitral valve stenosis.[24]

Congenital mitral valve insufficiency

Cleft mitral valve

Cleft mitral valve is a condition frequently associated with atrioventricular canal (atrioventricular septal) defects. Cleft mitral valve as an isolated anomaly, or with cardiac anomalies other than atrioventricular canal defects, is rare.[25–27] In this condition, there is a 'cleft' in the anterior leaflet of the mitral valve. The cleft is typically shaped as an inverted 'V', with the wider portion of the cleft at the free edge of the leaflet; however, the cleft may have more of a rectangular shape. The cleft may either be located within the central portion of the leaflet or be eccentric (Figure 20.3). Over time, the free edges of the cleft may become fibrotically thickened and rolled, due to the turbulent flow through the defect. The chordae tendinae, which typically originate from the rough zone of the valve leaflet, often have anomalous insertions when they originate from the edges of the defect. In this condition, the chordae typically insert into the ventricular wall, commonly the septum, but also into the anterior wall. When the chordae insert into the ventricular septum, they typically do so in or near the region of the membranous septum.

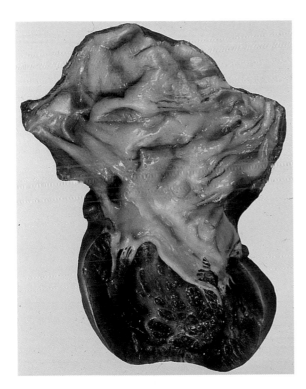

Figure 20.3

Isolated cleft in the anterior leaflet of the mitral vale. The cleft is eccentric in the anterior leaflet and has a slightly oval shape. The free edge of the anterior leaflet is fibrotically thickened and rolled, consistent with mitral valve insufficiency changes. Marked dilatation of the left atrium exists.

In a review of 20 cases with cleft mitral valve without atrioventricular canal defects, 9 cases had an isolated cleft mitral valve without any other significant cardiac abnormality and 11 had a cleft mitral valve with some other significant cardiac abnormality. In these cases, the additional conditions included ventricular septal defect, tricuspid valve atresia, complete transposition of the great arteries, corrected transposition of the great arteries, and aortic valve atresia. Down syndrome was present in 4 of the 20 cases.[26]

Cleft mitral valve may cause mitral valve insufficiency or subaortic stenosis. The degree of mitral valve insufficiency predominantly is related to the size of the cleft. Cleft mitral valve may cause subaortic stenosis by abundant, anomalous chordal insertions into the left ventricular outflow tract.

Anomalous mitral arcade

Layman and Edwards[14] first described anomalous mitral arcade in 1967. This condition is characterized by a fibrous bridge that extends between the two papillary muscles along the free edge of the anterior leaflet of the mitral valve. Commissures are often absent or poorly developed. Chordae tendinae may either be absent or very short and thickened. The papillary muscles are frequently large and may be obstructive. This condition is rare; it usually presents with mitral valve insufficiency.

Accessory orifice

Another condition that may cause mitral valve insufficiency is an accessory orifice of the mitral valve. In this condition, a separate ostium is present within the valve leaflet. This separate orifice in the valve tissue has separate chordae tendinae that arise from the free edges surrounding the ostium and insert independently into the papillary muscles.[1]

This condition can easily be distinguished from defects caused by infective endocarditis. With healed infective endocarditis, no separate chordae tendinae arise from the edges of any defect caused by the remodeling of the valve in the formerly infected area.

Short chordae tendinae

In this condition, the chordae tendinae are abnormally short, and as a result, the mobility of the leaflets is impaired.[28] This condition is rare and is usually associated with other abnormalities of the mitral valve apparatus, such as mitral valve arcade.[1]

Acquired mitral valve stenosis

Table 20.3 lists conditions associated with mitral valve stenosis.

Postinflammatory/rheumatic valvular disease

Once a frequently encountered condition in the USA, rheumatic valvular disease remains the most common cause of mitral valve stenosis in the world. In a single institutional review of surgical pathology valve specimens, postinflammatory/ rheumatic valve disease accounted for 99% of the specimens, with congenital valve diseases accounting for the other 1%.[29]

Rheumatic heart/valve disease results from an immune response to repeated exposure to group A β-hemolytic streptococci. The exact mechanism is not known, but there appears to be cross reactivity between bacterial antigens, specifically the streptococcal M protein, and the host tissues.

There are two main forms of the disease: an acute phase and a chronic phase. Acute rheumatic heart disease involves all layers of the heart – the pericardium, myocardium, and endocardium – and the cardiac valves.

The classic Aschoff nodule is the characteristic lesion of acute rheumatic heart disease. This lesion consists of areas of fibrinoid necrosis surrounded by lymphocytes, macrophages, plasma cells, and occasional giant cells. The 'caterpillar', or Anitschkow cell, is a macrophage with a wavy-appearing nucleus that is the characteristic cell of the Aschoff nodule. Acute rheumatic valve disease most commonly involves the mitral valve, followed distantly by the aortic, tricuspid, and pulmonary valves, in that order of occurrence. Wart-like vegetations that develop on valve leaflet or cusp surfaces characterize acute rheumatic valve disease. The vegetations are located on the atrial surface at the line of closure of the atrioventricular valves and the ventricular surface of the semilunar valves. Histologically, these vegetations consist of platelet and fibrin thrombi, which may overlie areas of fibrinoid necrosis and chronic inflammatory cells. The general concept is that damage to the endocardium leads to the formation of fibrin thrombi.[30] The vegetations are typically confined to the line of closure of the valves, but may rarely extend onto chordae. Acute rheumatic valve disease typically results in insufficiency of the valve, but stenosis alone or combined stenosis and insufficiency may be present.

Repeat infection with group A β-hemolytic streptococci may lead to chronic rheumatic valve disease. The gross morphologic findings of chronic rheumatic valve disease involve the leaflets, commissures, and chordae tendinae. The leaflets become fibrotically thickened, particularly along the line of closure, as a result of healing of vegetations during the acute phase. The characteristic changes of chronic rheumatic valve disease involve the commissures (Figure 20.4). The leaflets fuse together at the commissures, and the commissures become fibrotically thickened. Additional degenerative changes of calcification frequently occur. The fusion of the valve commissures with retraction of the leaflets creates the classic 'fish mouth' appearance of the orifice of

Table 20.3   Acquired mitral valve stenosis
Primary valvular abnormality
• Rheumatic/postinflammatory valve disease • Mitral valve annular calcification
Secondary conditions causing mitral valve stenosis

• Metabolic:
  – Mucopolysaccharidoses
  – Fabry's disease
  – Gout
• Autoimmune diseases:
  – Systemic lupus erythematosus (SLE)
  – Antiphospholipid antibody syndrome
  – Rheumatoid arthritis
• Whipple's disease
• Mediastinal irradiation

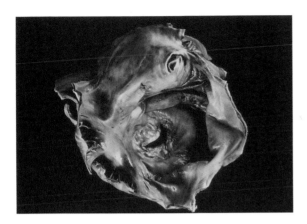

Figure 20.4

Mitral valve stenosis due to rheumatic/postinflammatory changes viewed from the left atrial aspect. The commissures are fused and the leaflets are fibrotically thickened, significantly narrowing the orifice and creating the classic 'fish mouth' appearance. The left atrium is markedly dilated.

the mitral valve when viewed from the left atrial aspect.[31,32]

Histologically, the abnormal valve has the normal three layers of atrialis, spongiosa, and fibrosa, but also has marked fibrous tissue deposition on the atrial surface. Initially, the fibrosis is an actively proliferating process, which eventually becomes dense fibrosis. Neovascularization of the normally avascular valve tissue occurs.

Once the valve reaches the stage of dense fibrosis or scarring, it is not possible to determine the exact underlying etiology of the disease, since other postinflammatory conditions can create similar gross and histologic findings. That is the reason that this condition, in patients without a clinical history of rheumatic fever, is best classified by the more generic term of postinflammatory valve disease.[30,33]

Non-postinflammatory/non-rheumatic acquired mitral valve stenosis

Few conditions other than postinflammatory states cause isolated mitral valve stenosis; more common is the combination of stenosis and

insufficiency. Other conditions that may cause stenosis are metabolic conditions, including mucopolysaccharidoses, Fabry's disease, and gout. The mucopolysaccharidoses are hereditary disorders of abnormal proteoglycan metabolism. The specific disorder depends on the underlying enzyme defect; examples of the mucopolysaccharidoses include Hurler syndrome, Hunter syndrome, and Sanfilippo syndrome. They are similar in that an enzyme deficiency results in accumulation of mucopolysaccharides. This material accumulates in many different organs, including the heart and cardiac valves. Grossly, the valve leaflets and occasionally the chordae tendinae are fibrotically thickened and shortened. Histologically, vacuolated, foamy cells that stain positively with Alcian Blue and periodic acid–Schiff (PAS) are present within the valves. Fabry's disease is an X-linked disease in which there is a deficiency in lysosomal hydrolase α-galactosidase resulting in deposition of trihexosylceramide in cardiac valves.[33] Deposition of this material may cause either stenosis or insufficiency.

Mediastinal irradiation may also cause valve stenosis by creating fibrotic thickening of the valve leaflets.[30]

Autoimmune diseases, including systemic lupus erythematosus (SLE), antiphospholipid antibody syndrome, and rheumatoid arthritis, may cause mitral valve stenosis. While insufficiency is the more common manifestation, it has been reported that 3% of patients with SLE will have mitral valve stenosis.[34] Stenosis is a result of fibrotic thickening of the valve leaflets. Rheumatoid arthritis may also cause mitral valve stenosis or insufficiency. Fibrinoid necrosis surrounded by chronic inflammatory cells may occur in the pericardium or myocardium or within cardiac valves in these conditions. Chronic inflammation may lead to fibrous thickening of the leaflets and mitral valve stenosis or insufficiency. SLE is further discussed in the following section on acquired mitral valve insufficiency.

Whipple's disease has been reported to cause mitral valve stenosis.[35] Whipple's disease causes weight loss, abdominal pain, arthritis, and lymphadenopathy. The causative agent of this disease is *Tropheryma whippelii*, a Gram-positive actinomycete.[36–38] The histologic finding diagnostic of Whipple's disease is PAS-positive foam cells in the jejunum. Similar findings may be found in cardiac valves. Chronic inflammation and fibrosis of the valve leaflets may lead to stenosis of the valve.[35,39]

Mitral valve annular calcification most commonly causes valvular insufficiency, but rarely may cause stenosis by preventing sufficient diastolic dilatation of the mitral valve annulus. Mitral annular calcification is more thoroughly described in the following section on acquired mitral valve insufficiency.

Acquired mitral valve insufficiency

Table 20.4 lists conditions associated with mitral valve insufficiency.

Table 20.4   Acquired mitral valve insufficiency

Primary valvular abnormality

- Mitral valve prolapse
- Mitral valve annular calcification
- Infective endocarditis
- Rheumatic/postinflammatory valve disease

Secondary cardiac conditions causing insufficiency

- Annular dilatation:
  - Atherosclerotic heart disease
  - Dilated cardiomyopathy
- Hypertrophic cardiomyopathy

Systemic conditions causing insufficiency

- Connective tissue disorders:
  - Marfan syndrome
  - Ehlers–Danlos syndrome
  - Osteogenesis imperfecta
- Systemic lupus erythematosus (SLE)
- Rheumatoid arthritis
- Amyloidosis
- Hypereosinophilic syndrome
- Carcinoid syndrome

Extrinsic causes

- Mediastinal radiation
- Medications
  - Methysergide
  - Ergotamine
  - Fenfluramine–phentermine
- Trauma
- Prior surgical procedure

Mitral valve prolapse

Mitral valve prolapse is a relatively common disorder; however, the term is often used to describe different conditions in which myxomatous change of the mitral valve occurs. Understanding of the disease entity mitral valve prolapse has developed and changed over time. It now appears that the disease is usually a genetic disorder, inherited in an autosomal dominant pattern. At this time, however, the exact gene abnormality has not been determined.[40–42] Based on current understanding of the disease, it appears that there are two groups of patients with this condition. In one group, which comprises the majority of patients, the disease more typically occurs in younger patients and is more common in females. In this group, the condition has a relatively benign course, and is often referred to as 'mitral valve prolapse syndrome'. The second group typically has a more severe course, and frequently requires surgical intervention; this patient population is often older and more commonly male.[40,43]

Mitral valve prolapse is a frequent finding in patients with connective tissue disorders, the most common of which is Marfan syndrome. Marfan syndrome results from a defect in the fibrillin gene; this abnormality leads to abnormal connective tissues.[44] Mitral valve prolapse is also encountered in patients with Ehlers–Danlos syndrome, osteogenesis imperfecta, and some other connective tissue disorders.

Mitral valve prolapse involves predominantly the posterior leaflet of the mitral valve. The central scallop of this leaflet is often the most severely affected.[45] The anterior leaflet may also be involved. When the anterior leaflet is involved, the posterior aspect of the anterior leaflet is more commonly affected. Grossly, involved leaflets are elongated and thickened, with a gray glistening appearance. The elongation and thickening of the leaflets may extend into chordae tendinae and weaken them structurally. These changes lead to billowing or interchordal hooding of the leaflets and protrusion (prolapse) of the leaflets into the left atrium during ventricular systole[9,46] (Figure 20.5). As a result of protrusion of the leaflets into the left atrium, the chordae tendinae are pulled taut and may rub against the endocardium of the left ventricle; over time, this leads to fibrotic thickening of the endocardium underlying the

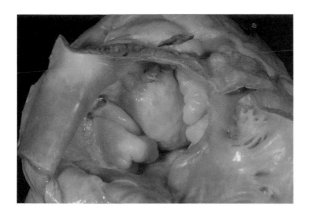

Figure 20.5

Mitral valve prolapse viewed from the left atrium. The valve leaflets are thickened and balloon into the left atrium. Fibrin thrombus is present on one of the protruding segments.

chordae, creating endocardial friction lesions, known as Salazar lesions[47] (Figure 20.6).

Structurally, marked expansion of the spongiosa layer of the valve results from increased deposition of mucopolysaccharides (Figure 20.7). This expansion of the spongiosa encroaches upon the valve fibrosa and disrupts the fibrous

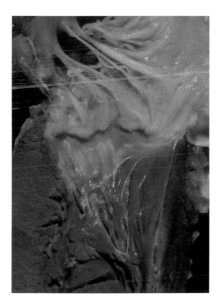

Figure 20.6

Salazar lesions. The prolapsed mitral valve leaflet is retracted upward, exposing fibrotic thickening of the left ventricular endocardium underlying the chordae tendinae of the posterior leaflet.

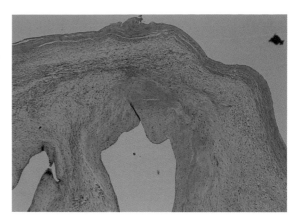

Figure 20.7

Photomicrograph of mitral valve prolapse. The atrial aspect is at the top of the figure. There is marked expansion of the spongiosa layer by increased deposition of proteoglycans, which disrupts the fibrosa. The expanded spongiosa encroaches upon the chordae tendinae, seen at the bottom of the figure.

and elastic fibers. This process may also extend into the chordae tendinae. These abnormalities lead to weakening of the major structural support of the valve, the fibrosa. Over time, fibrous plaques develop on both the ventricular and the atrial surfaces of the valve as a response to valvular dysfunction.[48,49]

Numerous complications are associated with mitral valve prolapse. In a review of chordae tendinae rupture, 88% of cases had underlying mitral valve prolapse change.[50] Other major complications of mitral valve prolapse include infective endocarditis, mitral insufficiency, arrhythmias,[51] and sudden death.[52–54]

Mitral valve annular calcification

Mitral valve annular calcification is a relatively common condition that most often occurs in elderly persons, more commonly women.[9,55] This condition may be associated with an increased risk of atherosclerotic cardiovascular disease.[56–59]

With annular calcification, dystrophic calcium deposition is present, mainly in the region of the annulus of the posterior leaflet of the valve (Figure 20.8). The calcium deposition may be minimal or quite pronounced, with protrusion into the left atrium, with or without adherence of the posterior leaflet to the ventricular wall. Most often, this process has no functional significance. If there is adherence of the leaflet to the ventricular wall or significant impediment of systolic contraction of the annular region, insufficiency of the valve may result. Infrequently, if diastolic relaxation of the annulus is impeded, valvular stenosis may occur.[60]

Histologically, amorphous collections of calcific material are present in the atrioventricular region of the left heart (Figure 20.9). The calcified material may extend into the myocardium at the base of the left ventricle. Chronic inflammatory cells and foreign body granulomatous reactions may be present as a reaction to the calcification.

The absence of commissural fusion and fibrotic thickening of the valve leaflets easily distinguish mitral valve annular calcification from rheumatic valvular disease. Rheumatic valvular disease uncommonly involves calcification within the annulus itself.

Complications of mitral valve annular calcification are rare. Annular calcific deposits may act as a nidus for the formation of thrombi, which may be a source of embolic events. Extremely uncom-

mon is encroachment and involvement of the calcific deposits on the cardiac conduction system.[40]

Pharmacologic agents

Several pharmacologic agents known to cause mitral valve insufficiency include methysergide, ergotamine, and the anorectic agents fenfluramine–phentermine. It is believed that, at least in part, serotonin and its metabolites are responsible for valvular changes associated with these drugs.[61–64] The pathologic features of this condition are remarkably similar to the valve changes seen in carcinoid syndrome. The difference is that drug-related abnormalities may involve either the left-sided or right-sided heart valves, whereas carcinoid syndrome typically affects the right-sided heart valves, unless there is an atrial septal defect. Valvular abnormalities associated with these agents appear to be related to length of use.[63]

Grossly, the valves are thickened and opalescent. Histologically, they maintain their underlying architecture, but develop 'stuck-on plaques' that encase the leaflets and occasionally the chordae tendinae. These plaques consist of myofibroblasts in a myxoid matrix. Initially, these plaques have a proliferative appearance, but, over time, the plaque becomes mainly dense

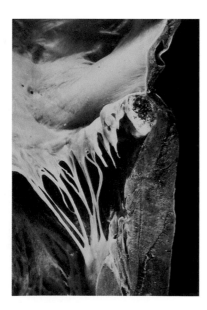

Figure 20.8

Annular calcification of the mitral valve: cross-section of left atrium, mitral valve, and left ventricle at the lateral wall. Calcified material is deposited, underlying the posterior leaflet and causing protrusion of the leaflet into the left atrium.

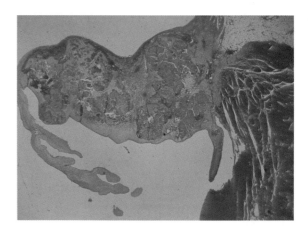

Figure 20.9

Photomicrograph of annular calcification of the mitral valve. Calcified nodules are deposited at the base of the leaflet. The distal leaflet and ventricular myocardium are not involved.

fibrous tissue. Chronic inflammatory cells and neovascularization may be present to variable degrees.[61]

Systemic lupus erythematosus

When SLE involves cardiac valves, insufficiency occurs more commonly than stenosis. Valves become thickened and may develop vegetations on their surfaces. Unlike most vegetations, the vegetations associated with SLE may form on either the atrial or the ventricular surfaces of the valve; these are termed Libman–Sacks vegetations.[65] Histologically, these vegetations consist of sterile platelet and fibrin thrombi; often, chronic inflammatory cells, myofibroblasts, and neovascularization also surround these vegetations. As the vegetations resolve, fibrosis and calcification on the valve surfaces result, and distortion of the valve leaflet architecture occurs.[66]

Healed infective endocarditis

Infective endocarditis frequently causes mitral valve insufficiency; since this process is not treated by percutaneous procedures, it is not further described herein. As infective vegetations heal, the involved valve leaflet may become fibrotically thickened and retracted, and may develop calcific deposits. Secondary orifices or fenestrations in the valve may develop due to remodeling of the valve by the healing process and/or destruction of tissues by the infection. Occasionally, when the vegetations involve the chordae tendinae, the chords may rupture. All of these factors contribute to or result in insufficiency of the valve.[67]

Mitral valve insufficiency secondary to non-primary valvular abnormalities

One of the more common causes (or indeed, the most common cause) of mitral valve insufficiency is actually not related to a structural problem with the valve itself, but rather is due to dilatation of the mitral valve annulus from other causes. Of the other possible causes, ischemic heart disease is by far the most common. Ischemic heart disease may cause annular dilation by regional wall dysfunction, papillary muscle dysfunction, or global left ventricular dysfunction. Other non-primary valve disorders causing mitral valve insufficiency include dilated cardiomyopathy, hypertrophic cardiomyopathy, and possibly restrictive cardiomyopathy, including amyloidosis.[51,55]

Systemic diseases such as Marfan syndrome, Ehlers–Danlos syndrome, osteogenesis imperfecta, and SLE may cause mitral valve insufficiency and have already been described. Rheumatoid arthritis, hypereosinophilic syndrome, and possibly scleroderma are other systemic diseases that may be associated with mitral valve insufficiency.

External factors such as mediastinal irradiation or trauma, including past surgical procedures or percutaneous intervention, may cause mitral valve insufficiency, usually due to fibrosis of the affected leaflet(s) and related chordae.[32]

References

1. Davachi F, Moller JH, Edwards JE. Diseases of the mitral valve in infancy. An anatomic analysis of 55 cases. Circulation 1971; 43: 565–79.
2. Titus JL. Anatomy and pathology of the mitral valve. In: Ellis FH (ed). Surgery for Acquired Mitral Valve Disease. Philadelphia: WB Saunders, 1967: 49–77.
3. Antunes MJ. Functional anatomy of the mitral valve. In: Barlow JB (ed). Perspectives on the Mitral Valve. Philadelphia: FA Davis, 1987: 1–14.
4. Kearney DL, Titus JL. Cardiovascular anatomy. In: Garson A, Bricker JT, Fisher DF, Neish SR (eds). The Science and Practice of Pediatric Cardiology, 2nd edn. Baltimore: Williams & Wilkins, 1998: 127–53.
5. Ranganathan N, Lam JHC, Wigle ED, Silver MD. Morphology of the human mitral valve II. The valve leaflets. Circulation 1970; 41: 459–67.
6. Kouchoukos NT, Blackstone EH, Doty DB, et al. Anatomy, dimensions and terminology. In: Kouchoukos NT, Blackstone EH, Doty DB, et al (eds). Kirklin/Barratt-Boyes Cardiac Surgery, 3rd edn. Philadelphia: Churchill Livingstone, 2003: 3–65.
7. Silver MM, Silver MD. Examination of the heart and cardiovascular specimens in surgical pathology. In: Silver MD, Gotlieb AI, Schoen FJ (eds).

Cardiovascular Pathology, 3rd edn. Philadelphia: Churchill Livingstone, 2001: 1–29.

8. Rusted IE, Scheifley CH, Edwards JE. Studies of the mitral valve I. Anatomic features of the normal mitral valve and associated structures. Circulation 1952; 6: 825–31.

9. Titus JL, Edwards JE. Mitral insufficiency other than rheumatic, ischemic or infective: emphasis on mitral valve prolapse. Semin Thorac Cardiovasc Surg 1989; 1: 118–28.

10. Bloor CM (ed). Cardiac Pathology. Philadelphia: JB Lippincott, 1978.

11. Abdulla R, Blew GA, Holterman MJ. Cardiovascular embryology. Pediatr Cardiol 2004; 25: 191–200.

12. Wenink ACG, Gittenberger-de Groot AC. Embryology of the mitral valve. Int J Cardiol 1986; 11: 75–84.

13. Colvin EV. Cardiac embryology. In: Garson A, Bricker JT, Fisher DJ Neish SR (eds). The Science and Practice of Pediatric Cardiology, 2nd edn. Baltimore: Williams & Wilkins, 1998: 91–126.

14. Layman TE, Edwards JE. Anomalous mitral arcade. A type of congenital mitral insufficiency. Circulation 1967; 35: 389–95.

15. Titus JL. Congenital malformations of the mitral and aortic valves and related structures. Dis Chest 1969; 55: 358–67.

16. Lam JHC, Ranganathan N, Wigle ED, Silver MD. Morphology of the human mitral valve I. Chordae tendinae: a new classification. Circulation 1970; 41: 449–58.

17. Larsen WJ. Human Embryology, 2nd edn. New York: Churchill Livingstone, 1997: 151–88.

18. Shone JK, Sellers RD, Anderson RC, et al. The developmental complex of 'parachute mitral valve', supravalvular ring of left atrium, subaortic stenosis and coarctation of aorta. Am J Cardiol 1963; 11: 714–25.

19. Schiebler GL, Edwards JE, Burchell HB, et al. Congenital corrected transposition of the great vessels. A study of 33 cases. Pediatrics 1961; 27 (Suppl): 851–88.

20. da Silva CL, Edwards JE. Parachute mitral valve in an adult. Arq Bras Cardiol 1973; 26: 149–53.

21. Tandon R, Moller JH, Edwards JE. Anomalies associated with the parachute mitral valve: a pathologic analysis of 52 cases. Can J Cardiol 1986; 2: 278–81.

22. Rogers HM, Waldron BR, Murphey DFH, Edwards JE. Supravalvular stenosing ring of left atrium in association with endocardial sclerosis (endocardial fibroelastosis) and mitral insufficiency. Am Heart J 1955; 50: 777–81.

23. Elliott LP, Anderson RC, Amplatz K, et al. Congenital mitral stenosis. Pediatrics 1962; 30: 552–62.

24. Kouchoukos NT, Blackstone EH, Doty DB, et al. Congenital mitral valve disease. In: Kouchoukos NT, Blackstone EH, Doty DB, et al (eds). Cardiac Surgery, 3rd edn. Philadelphia: Churchill Livingstone, 2003: 1401–14.

25. Edwards JE. Differential diagnosis of mitral stenosis. A clinicopathologic review of simulating conditions. Lab Invest 1954; 3: 89–115.

26. Di Segni E, Edwards JE. Cleft anterior leaflet of the mitral valve with intact septa. A study of 20 cases. Am J Cardiol 1983; 51: 919–26.

27. Berghuis J, Kirklin JW, Edwards JE, Titus JL. The surgical anatomy of isolated congenital mital insufficiency. J Thorac Cardiovasc Surg 1964; 47: 791–8.

28. Levy MJ, Varco RL, Lillehei CW, Edwards JE. Mitral insufficiency in infants, children and adolescents. J Thorac Cardiovasc Surg 1963; 45: 434–50.

29. Olson LJ, Subramanian R, Ackermann DM, et al. Surgical pathology of the mitral valve: a study of 712 cases spanning 21 years. Mayo Clin Proc 1987; 62: 22–34.

30. Schoen FJ, Edwards WD. Valvular heart disease: general principles and stenosis. In: Silver MD, Gotlieb AL, Schoen FJ (eds). Cardiovascular Pathology. Philadelphia: Churchill Livingstone: 2001: 402–42.

31. Edwards JE. Pathologic aspects of mitral stenosis. AJR Am J Roentgenol 1956; 76: 740–2.

32. Lobo FV, Walley VM, Butany JW. Acquired diseases of the valves and endocardium. In: Bloom S, Lie JT, Silver MD (eds). Diagnostic Criteria for Cardiovascular Pathology of Acquired Diseases. Philadelphia: Lippincott-Raven, 1997: 97–145.

33. Fligner CL, Reichenbach DD, Otto CM. Pathology and etiology of valvular heart disease. In: Otto CM (ed). Valvular Heart Disease, 2nd edn. Philadelphia: WB Saunders, 2004: 18–50.

34. Roldan CA, Shively BK, Crawford MH. An echocardiographic study of valvular heart disease associated with systemic lupus erythematosus. N Engl J Med 1996; 335: 1424–30.

35. Rose AG. Mitral stenosis in Whipple's disease. Thorax 1978; 33: 500–3.

36. Keren DF 'Whipple's disease': the causative agent defined. Its pathogenisis remains obscure. Medicine (Baltimore) 1993; 72: 355–8.

37. Dobbins WO III. The diagnosis of Whipple's disease. N Engl J Med 1995; 332: 390–2.

38. Relman DA. The identification of uncultured microbial pathogens. J Infect Dis 1993; 168: 1–8.

39. McAllister HA Jr, Fenoglio JJ Jr. Cardiac involvement in Whipple's disease. Circulation 1975; 52: 152–6.

40. Fligner CL, Reichenbach DD, Otto CM. Mitral valve prolapse. In: Otto CM (ed). Valvular Heart Disease, 2nd edn. Philadelphia: WB Saunders, 2004: 368–87.

41. Strahan NV, Murphy EA, Fortuin NJ, et al.

Inheritance of the mitral valve prolapse syndrome. Discussion of a three-dimensional penetrance model. Am J Med 1983; 74; 967–72.

42. Chen WW, Chan FL, Wong PH, Chow JS. Familial occurrence of mitral valve prolapse: is this related to the straightback syndrome? Br Heart J 1983; 50: 97–100.

43. Devereux RB. Recent developments in the diagnosis and management of mitral valve prolapse. Curr Opin Cardiol 1995; 10: 107–16.

44. Kielty CM, Phillips JE, Child A, et al. Fibrillin secretion and microfibril assembly by Marfan dermal fibroblasts. Matrix Biol 1994; 14: 191–9.

45. Edwards JE. Floppy mitral valve syndrome. Cardiovasc Clin 1987; 18: 249–71.

46. Lucas RV Jr, Edwards JE. The floppy mitral valve. Curr Prob Cardiol 1982; 7: 1–48.

47. Salazar AE, Edwards JE. Friction lesions of ventricular endocardium. Relation to chordae tendinae of mitral valve. Arch Pathol 1970; 90: 364–76.

48. Guthrie RB, Edwards JE. Pathology of the myxomatous mitral valve. Nature, secondary changes and complications. Minn Med 1976; 59: 637–47.

49. Shrivastava S, Guthrie RB, Edwards JE. Prolapse of the mitral valve. Mod Concepts Cardiovasc Dis 1977; 46: 57–61.

50. Jeresaty RM, Edwards JE, Chawla SK. Mitral valve prolapse and ruptured chordae tendinae. Am J Cardiol 1985; 55: 138–42.

51. Edwards JE. Varieties of valvular heart disease: Part 1. Mitral valvular disease. Pract Cardiol 1982; 8: 111–27.

52. Chesler E, Edwards JE. Mitral valve prolapse and sudden death. Prim Cardiol 1984; 10: 75–87.

53. Chesler E, King RA, Edwards JE. The myxomatous mitral valve and sudden death. Circulation 1983; 67: 632–9.

54. Pocock WA, Bosman CK, Chesler E, et al. Sudden death in primary mitral valve prolapse. Am Heart J 1984; 107: 378–82.

55. Vlodaver Z, Edwards JE. Mitral insufficiency in subjects 50 years of age or older. Clinical–pathologic correlations 2. Cardiovasc Clin 1973; 5: 149–67.

56. Kamensky G, Lisy L, Polak E, et al. Mitral annular calcifications and aortic plaques as predictors of increased cardiovascular mortality. J Cardiol 2001; 37(Suppl 1): 21–6.

57. Dincer I, Ozdol C, Dandachi R, et al. Predictive value of mitral annular calcification for the diagnosis of coronary artery disease in patients with dilated cardiomyopathy. Angiology 2001; 52: 515–20.

58. Adler Y, Fink N, Spector D, et al. Mitral annulus calcification – a window to diffuse atherosclerosis of the vascular system. Atherosclerosis 2001; 155: 1–8.

59. Fox CS, Vasan RS, Parise H, et al. Mitral annular calcification predicts cardiovascular morbidity and mortality: the Framingham Heart Study. Circulation 2003; 107: 1492–6.

60. Osterberger LE, Goldstein S, Khaja F, Lakier JB. Functional mitral stenosis in patients with massive mitral annular calcification. Circulation 1981; 64: 472–6.

61. Volmar KE, Hutchins GM. Aortic and mitral fenfluramine-phentermine valvulopathy in 64 patients treated with anorectic agents. Arch Pathol Lab Med 2001; 125: 1555–61.

62. Connolly HM, Crary JL, McGoon MD, et al. Valvular heart disease associated with fenfluramine–phentermine. N Engl J Med 1997; 337: 581–8.

63. Jollis JG, Landolfo CK, Kisslo J, et al. Fenfluramine and phentermine and cardiovascular findings: effect of treatment duration on prevalence of valve abnormalities. Circulation 2000; 101: 2071–7.

64. Graham DJ, Green L. Further cases of valvular heat disease associated with fenfluramine phentermine. N Engl J Med 1997; 337; 635

65. Libman E, Sacks B. A hitherto undescribed form of valvular and mural endocarditis. Arch Intern Med 1924; 33: 701–37.

66. Bulkley BH, Roberts WC. The heart in systemic lupus erythematosus and the changes induced in it by corticosteroid therapy: a study of 36 necropsy patients. Am J Med 1975; 58: 243–64.

67. Edwards JE, Burchell HB. Pathologic anatomy of mitral insufficiency. Mayo Clin Proc 1958; 33: 497–509.

21

Mitral valve disease

Natesa G Pandian, Francesco Fulvio Faletra, Stefano DeCastro,
Ayan R Patel

Introduction

Mitral valve disease is the most common valvular disorder, and can be due to a primary pathology of the mitral valve or secondary to abnormalities of left heart chambers. The mitral valve is better described as the mitral valve apparatus, constituting the mitral annulus, the anterior and posterior leaflets, the chordae tendinae, the papillary muscles, and the left atrium and left ventricle.[1,2] Both congenital defects and acquired diseases can result in dysfunction of the mitral valve apparatus, the essential consequence being obstruction (mitral stenosis), incomplete closure (mitral regurgitation), or a combination. Symptoms reflecting pulmonary venous congestion, systemic venous congestion, and decreased cardiac output are features of advanced mitral valve disease. The primary diagnostic modality to assess the presence and severity of mitral valve disease is echocardiography. In patients who require an intervention, catheter-based balloon valvuloplasty is the primary therapeutic option for mitral stenosis, with surgery as the next option. Surgical repair is the primary option in patients with severe mitral regurgitation who require an intervention, with valve replacement as the second approach. Novel approaches that employ catheter-based devices or catheter-based repair are emerging; if proven successful in the long term, they could become the primary treatment option in the future.[3,4] This chapter will review the anatomy, pathophysiology, clinical presentation, and treatment of mitral valve disorders, with emphasis on features that have a bearing on percutaneous interventions for mitral valve disease.

Anatomy, physiology, and echocardiographic morphology of the normal mitral apparatus

The mitral valve apparatus is a complex, finely coordinated structure that consists of annulus, leaflets, chordae tendinae, papillary muscles, and left atrial and left ventricular walls. Each of these structures is vital to the valve's function (Figure 21.1). Following isovolumic relaxation, the mitral valve leaflets are forced open when the left atrial pressure exceeds the ventricular diastolic pressure. Following early filling, the leaflets tend to close partially as the ventricle fills. As atrial contraction occurs and the atrial pressure exceeds

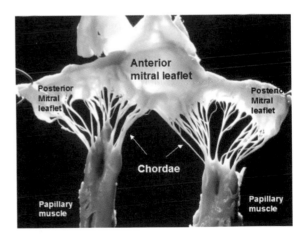

Figure 21.1

Anatomic specimen depicting the various components of the mitral apparatus.

the ventricular pressure again, the leaflets reopen. Besides the filling pressures in the two chambers, flow across the valve influences the degree of valve opening. In the setting of low cardiac output, the extent of the opening excursion of leaflets is decreased even without any intrinsic abnormality of the valve.

Annulus

The mitral annulus is a roughly elliptical structure (with D- or kidney-shaped configuration) (Figure 21.2) whose prominent function is to anchor the leaflets by fusion with their intermediate layer, the 'lamina fibrosa'. In its more elliptical shape (in systole), the ratio of minor to major diameters is approximately 0.75. The longest diameter runs from commissure to commissure, whereas the shortest runs from the middle point of the anterior segment to the middle point of the posterior segment. Both diameters can be measured by two-dimensional (2D) echocardiography in apical two-chamber and parasternal (or apical) long-axis views, respectively (Figure 21.3). Surprisingly, the diameter in the four-chamber apical view has no anatomic reference points for comparison. The mitral annulus can be divided into two portions with a different anatomic consistency: the anterior (the straight line of the 'D') and the posterior portion (the curved line of the 'D') (Figure 21.2).

The anterior annulus

The anterior annulus (also named the mitral–aortic junction, mitral–aortic curtain, or aortic–ventricular membrane) when viewed from an atrial perspective forms a hinge line with the distal margin of the atrial myocardium. However, when seen from its ventricular aspect, the hinge line nearly disappears and a fibrous sheet connects the anterior leaflet to the interleaflet triangle underneath the left and non-coronary aortic cusps (Figure 21.4). The two ends of this region are thickened to form the fibrous trigones (the right trigone is larger and firmer than the left and its fibrous continuity with the membranous septum marks the central fibrous body of the heart).

The posterior annulus

The remainder of the annular circumference continues around the posterior mitral leaflet, where it forms a flexible C-shaped ring in connection with the muscular fibers of both the atrial and the ventricular walls. Externally, the position of the posterior annulus is delineated by the course of the coronary sinus and the left circumflex coronary artery. This portion is histologically rather heterogeneous, with gaps in fibrous continuity, not only among hearts but also within the same heart. Finally, it is 'weaker' than the anterior annulus and most often involved in annular dilatation and calcification.

Echocardiography

Since the annulus is an elliptical subtle structure, when the ultrasound plane of 2D echocardiography transects it perpendicularly (in the long-axis parasternal or apical views) a single dot is imaged

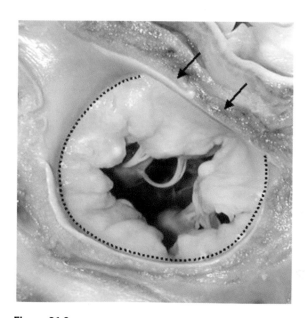

Figure 21.2

The elliptical configuration of the annulus. Arrows point to the anterior annulus (straight line of the D-shaped configuration).

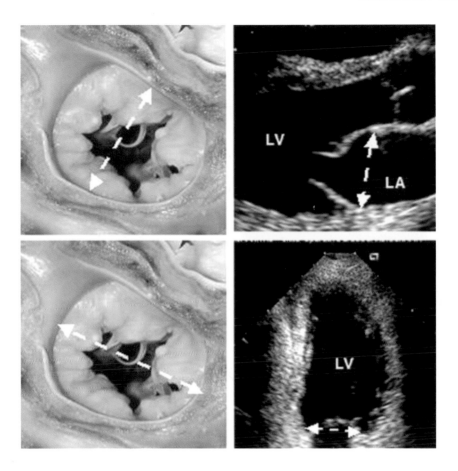

Figure 21.3

The septal–lateral, and commissuro-commissural diameters. On the right, the corresponding echocardiographic cuts are shown. LV, left ventricle; LA, left atrium.

(the hinge point between mitral leaflets and atrial wall) (Figure 21.5A). When short-axis views are used, the translation of the annulus into and out of the echocardiographic plane makes it difficult to image the entire annular circumference in a single image. Conversely, by using 3D echocardiography from an atrial (Figure 21.5B) or ventricular (Figure 21.6) perspective, both the anterior and the posterior annulus can be consistently visualized and the position of fibrous trigones imaged.

Annulus dynamics

The normal mitral annulus is a dynamic structure, which undergoes substantial area changes throughout the cardiac cycle, reaching a maximum in diastole and minimum in systole.[5–7] The maximal area reduction occurs in systole. Reduction of annular area has been attributed mainly to its posterior flexible portion, whereas the anterior annulus has been thought to be relatively fixed during the cardiac cycle. This belief

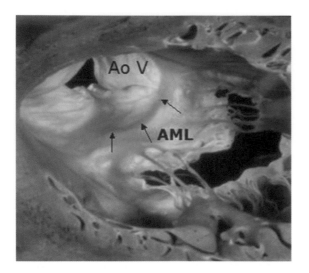

Figure 21.4

Anatomic specimen viewed from above. Arrows point to the connection between the mitral leaflet and the intercuspal triangle. The hinge line is quite evanescent (see text for further details). Ao V, aortic valve; AML, anterior mitral leaflet.

has influenced the development of annuloplasty ring design. Some variability in the anterior annulus extension during the cardiac cycle has been demonstrated.[8] A more 'holistic' approach may give new insights into the annular dynamics. In spite of their close anatomic proximity, the aortic

and mitral valves have been considered, both functionally and surgically, to be separate entities, as if their functions were independent from each other. However, sharing a common pump and a portion of the annulus, the aortic and mitral valves may be considered as a single anatomic and functional unit, like a 'roof' on the ventricular 'house', with an entry way and an exit. Because of such strict continuity, a certain degree of valve interdependence may intuitively be expected. Some studies performed in normal adult sheep using radio-opaque marker technology have shown that the valves not only work in synchrony but also contribute to each other's geometric annular changes. (Figure 21.7). During isovolumic contraction and early systole, the expansion of aortic orifice causes a posterior displacement of the anterior annulus, contributing (together with the posterior annular contraction) to septal–lateral diameter reduction and leaflet coaptation. During isovolumic relaxation and early diastole, the annular enlargement is caused by the expansion of the posterior annulus and by the displacement of the anterior annulus towards the aortic orifice. In other words, the anterior annulus seems to act like a piston, facilitating mitral valve closure in systole and atrial filling in diastole. It is interesting to note that both aortic root and mitral annulus expansion anticipate the hemodynamic events. Using 2D echocardiography, the piston-like movement of the anterior annulus may not

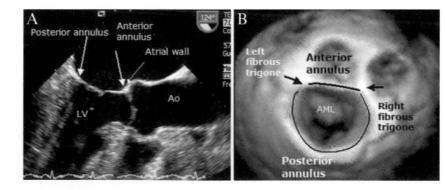

Figure 21.5

Two- and three-dimensional images of the mitral annulus. (A) With 2D echocardiography, the annulus is imaged as a single point (hinge point) connecting the anterior and posterior leaflets with the atrial wall. (B) With 3D transesophageal echocardiography from the atrial perspective, the anterior annulus (black line), the posterior annulus (red line), and the location of fibrous trigones (arrows) can be imaged. LV, left ventricle; Ao, aorta; AML, anterior mitral leaflet.

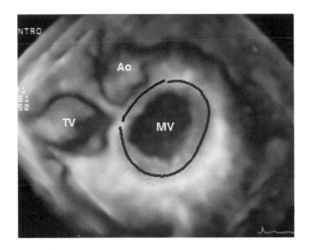

Figure 21.6

Three-dimensional image of the mitral annulus. With 3D transthoracic echocardiography from the ventricle, the posterior annulus (red line) and the anterior annulus (black line) can easily be imaged. MV, mitral valve; TV, tricuspid valve; Ao, aorta.

easily be noted. Conversely, with 3D echocardiography, it can be appreciated, even in still frame images. Moreover, expansion and reduction of the entire annular area can be imaged (Figure 21.7). The annulus is not lying in a plane but rather has a 3D 'saddle-shaped' configuration.[9] 'Peaks' are located in the middle points of the anterior and posterior segments, whereas 'valleys' lie near the commissures. Although many studies have confirmed this configuration, the reason why the mitral valve annulus has such a complex 3D shape is not clear. In theory, since the leaflets are anchored to the annulus, the reduction of annular perimeter during annular contraction should compromise the geometry of leaflet insertion, making valve tissue redundant so that posterior scallops, for instance, might superimpose on each other and bulge. The saddle-shaped configuration mitigates this potential limiting factor of annular contraction; by increasing the height and eccentricity of annular configuration during contraction, the annular area will decrease without a corresponding reduction in the annular perimeter, so that leaflet–annular geometric relationships remain constant. Moreover, the increase of annulus eccentricity during contraction makes the leaflet curvature more pronounced, thus reducing stress against leaflets. By Laplace's law, curvature of leaflets minimizes stress forces. The saddle shape of the annulus may contribute to reductions in leaflet stress (in addition to leaflet billowing: see later) by enhancing leaflet curvature.

Leaflets

Unequivocally, the most important components of the valve are the leaflets. Two main indentations separate the valve tissue into anterior (or aortic) and posterior (or mural) leaflets. (Figure 21.8). These indentations do not reach the annulus, but end about 5 mm short. Thus, from a strictly anatomic point of view, being anchored along the entire annulus circumference, the mitral valve can be considered as a single veil. The anterior leaflet has a roughly triangular free edge and occupies one third of the annular circumference (nearly 3 cm). However, it is deeper than the posterior leaflet (1.5–2.5 cm vs 0.8–1 cm); thus, the overall orifice areas covered by each leaflet are equivalent. The posterior leaflet is long and narrow, attached to the remaining two-thirds of the annular circumference. Small indentations divide the mural leaflet into three or more scallops. Using the surgeon's language these scallops are denominated from lateral to medial P1, P2, and P3 (P stands for 'posterior'), with the middle scallop (P2) usually being larger than the other two. The corresponding areas of the anterior leaflet are denominated A1, A2, and A3 (although no anatomic subdivision can be seen). In both leaflets, two different zones of lines of coaptation can be distinguished: a clear and a rough zone. This distinction is more evident in the anterior leaflet. The chordal apparatus inserts to the ventricular side of the rough zone, making it irregular and thick. Conversely, the clear zone is thin and translucent. In systole, the clear zone of the anterior leaflet bulges towards the left atrial cavity. Far from being a pathologic feature, this curvature reduces the stress against the leaflets. In systole, the ventricular sides of the rough zones of both leaflets meet each other to assure valve competence. From a left atrial perspective, the leaflet apposition forms a cavo-convex zone 5–8 mm deep, which prevents valve incompetence when a moderate

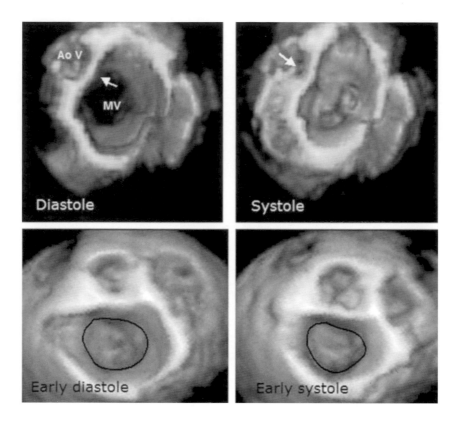

Figure 21.7

Three-dimensional images of the mitral annulus at diastole and systole. Displacement of the mitral–aortic junction can be appreciated (arrows). The entire annular circumference and its variation through the cardiac cycle can be imaged (black line). MV, mitral valve; Ao V, aortic valve.

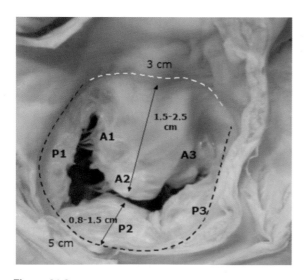

Figure 21.8

Anatomic specimen of mitral valve leaflets.

degree of annular dilation occurs (valve reserve). The line or surface of contact between two structures is called a commissure. Thus, literally speaking, the mitral valve has a single commissure. However, by convention, each end of the closure line is considered one commissure, so that the current literature designates the mitral valve as having two commissures (anterolateral and posteromedial). Such commissures are the first to be involved in the scar process following rheumatic fever and their fusion is responsible for valve area reduction in mitral stenosis. M-mode echocardiography could easily distinguish the anterior from the posterior leaflet. However, only a single point of the valve can be imaged. 2D echocardiography shows the finer anatomic details of the leaflets, and the scallops of the posterior leaflet can be identified (Figures 21.9 and 21.10). However, it must be kept in mind that

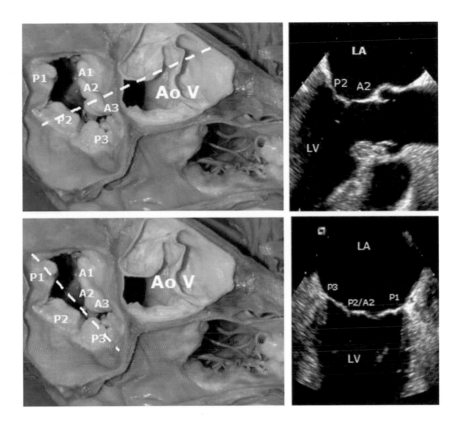

Figure 21.9

Two-dimensional transesophageal echocardiographic images of the posterior scallops. The dashed lines on the anatomic specimen mark the echocardiographic cuts. LA, left atrium; LV, left ventricle.

these images are *not* the anterior or posterior leaflets, but they rather represent a thin (1–2 mm thick, depending on resolution) slice of mitral leaflets. Only with 3D echocardiography can the entire surface of the leaflets be seen 'en face' from both the atrial and the ventricular perspectives. Using 3D echocardiography, leaflet area rather than leaflet length can be measured and deficiency of leaflet tissue (as occurs in functional mitral regurgitation) can be better appreciated.

Chordae tendinae and papillary muscles

Chordae tendinae are string-like structures that connect the rough zone and free edge of the leaflets to the papillary muscles. Since chordae usually branch distal to their muscular origins, there are four or five times more chordae attached to the leaflets than to the papillary muscles. There are numerous classifications of chordae tendinae arrangement. There is a wide variability from heart to heart, and only a rough organization can be recognized. One of the most commonly used classifications is one that distinguishes chordae tendinae as first-, second-, or third-order chordae according to their insertion on the leaflet's margin, rough zone, or basal area, respectively. The first-order chordae are thought to prevent valve incompetence; the second-order chordae (among which are the thickest chordae, called 'strut chord') are thought to maintain 'mitral–papillary muscle–ventricle wall continuity', thus supporting longitudinal shortening of

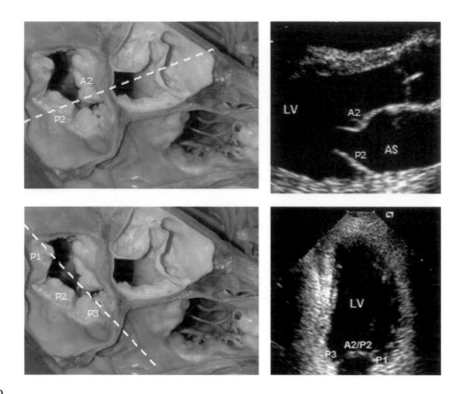

Figure 21.10

Two-dimensional transthoracic echocardiographic images of the posterior scallops. The dashed lines on the anatomic specimen mark the echocardiographic cuts. LA, left atrium; LV, left ventricle.

the left ventricle. The role of the basal chordae (small chordae connecting the basal area of the posterior leaflet to the ventricular wall) is unknown. The two papillary muscles, the antero-lateral and posteromedial units, are the anchors from which chordae tendinae emerge. The integrity and function of the myocardium subja-cent to the papillary muscles are more important than the 'function' of the papillary muscles them-selves. Isolated destruction of papillary muscles alone may not cause mitral regurgitation, but when associated with distortion or dysfunction of the subjacent myocardium, incomplete mitral valve closure and regurgitation can occur. Given their string-like structure, chordae tendinae can-not be easily classified using a tomographic tech-nique such as 2D echocardiography, but ruptured chords can be recognized by 2D and 3D echocar-diography, and particularly by transesophageal

echocardiography. Papillary muscles are well imaged by 2D and 3D echocardiography.

Left ventricle and left atrium

Normal size, shape, proportion, and function of the left heart chambers are essential for optimal closure of the mitral valve. Marked dilatation of the left atrium can distort the mitral annulus. More importantly, the size, geometry, and func-tion of the left ventricle have significant bearings on the function of the mitral valve. Regional or global left ventricular dilatation or dysfunction interferes with the synchrony and integrity needed for mitral valve closure and are common mechanisms of mitral regurgitation. 2D echocar-diography has been the mainstay in the evaluation of the left heart chambers, while 3D echocardiography provides more accurate estimates of left ventricular and atrial volumes and function.

Mitral stenosis

Etiology and pathology

The most common etiology of mitral stenosis is chronic scarring caused by rheumatic heart disease. The leaflets become thick because of fibrosis, and commissures become fused. As a result, the opening orifice is reduced. When the degenerative process involves primarily the tips of the leaflets, the belly of the leaflets exhibit doming during diastole. In severe cases, degeneration and calcification involve the whole span of leaflets, including the annulus. The fibrotic fusion may extend to the submitral structures as well. Less common causes of mitral stenosis include severe fibrodegenerative calcification of the mitral annulus and the base of the leaflets (particularly in the elderly), drug-induced valvulopathy, carcinoid heart involvement, and systemic lupus erythematosus.

Pathophysiology and clinical features

The mechanical obstruction at the mitral valve level elevates left atrial pressure and increases the pressure gradient between the left atrium and left ventricle. For a given flow rate, a smaller orifice is associated with a higher transmitral gradient. For a given orifice size, increased or decreased flow rate results in similar changes in the gradient. Elevated left atrial pressures lead to pulmonary venous hypertension and eventually to pulmonary arterial hypertension and pressure overload to the right heart chambers. Increased heart rate associated with a tachyarrhythmia or physical effort increases the transmitral gradient, left atrial pressure, and pulmonary artery pressures and results in a decrease in forward output. The normal mitral valve area ranges from 4 to 6 cm^2. Generally, mitral valve narrowing not associated with any significant transmitral gradient, even when the valve area is decreased to 2 cm^2.

As the valve area decreases further, symptoms may be exhibited first with effort and later at rest. A valve area of 1–1.5 cm^2 is considered to reflect moderate mitral stenosis and area of 1 cm^2 or less is considered as severe mitral stenosis, warranting mechanical intervention.

Elevation of left atrial pressure causes left atrial enlargement. Marked dilatation of the left atrium can compress adjacent structures such as the esophagus, left main bronchus, and left recurrent laryngeal nerve, and may cause symptoms related to such compression. High left atrial pressure also causes impediment to inflow into the left atrium and subsequent blood swirling and stasis. This is compounded by atrial fibrillation. Slow blood flow patterns and blood stasis in the body of the atrial chamber and even more prominently in the left atrial appendage are the common mechanisms for formation of left atrial clots and the risk of systemic embolism.

As mitral stenosis becomes severe, patients exhibit symptoms of decreased cardiac output and pulmonary venous congestion. Easy fatigueability and exertional dyspnea are common symptoms. As the disease progresses, patients may experience dyspnea at rest, orthopnea, paroxysmal nocturnal dyspnea, and pulmonary edema. Advanced cases with pulmonary hypertension will exhibit features of systemic venous congestion. Severe pulmonary hypertension may be associated with hemoptysis. Symptoms caused by compression of the left atrium include dysphagia and hoarseness of the voice. Mitral stenosis is a slowly progressive disease and many patients slow their activity even without being aware of it. Exercise evaluation will help unmask the symptoms in such patients.

Patients with severely advanced mitral stenosis may have peripheral and facial cyanosis. In those with severe pulmonary hypertension and elevated right atrial pressure, jugular venous distention and elevated venous pressure are present and the pulmonic component of the second heart sound may be loud. The characteristic auscultatory findings in mitral stenosis include a loud first heart sound, an opening snap, and a rumbling mid–late-diastolic murmur with late-diastolic accentuation. The murmur is often localized to the cardiac apex and better appreciated with the patient in the left lateral position. In the presence of atrial fibrillation, the late-diastolic accentuation of the murmur is absent. Opening snap generally indicates pliable valve leaflets and may be absent in patients with severely calcified leaflets.

Diagnostic evaluation

The electrocardiogram may show features of left atrial enlargement and, in some cases, right ventricular hypertrophy. Chest radiography may reveal evidence of left atrial enlargement and pulmonary venous congestion. Cardiac catheteriza-tion used to be the diagnostic method. Employing left and right heart catheterization, transmitral pressure gradient and cardiac output data were recorded, from which mitral valve area was cal-culated with the use of the Gorlin formula. During the last two decades, echocardiography has replaced cardiac catheterization methods for the assessment of mitral stenosis. Today, invasive hemodynamic recordings are performed only during an interventional procedure or to calculate pulmonary vascular resistance in a few patients in whom such information is necessary.

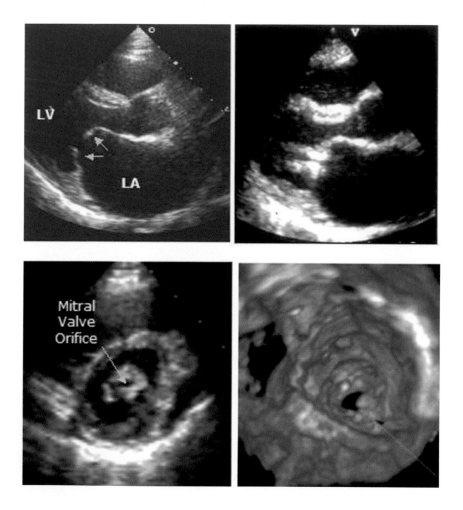

Figure 21.11

Two- and three-dimensional images of the mitral valve in mitral stenosis. The top panels depict long-axis views of the mitral valve in two patients with mitral stenosis. In the left-hand example, the mitral valve leaflets appear mildly thickened with diastolic doming with restricted opening, while more severe thickening is noted in the right-hand example. The bottom images, from two other patients, depict the narrowed mitral valve orifice in the short-axis 2D view (left) and in the 3D view from the ventricle (right). LA, left atrium; LV, left ventricle.

The different modalities of echocardiography provide comprehensive information regarding the morphologic abnormalities of the mitral apparatus, and the size and function of the cardiac chambers, as well as hemodynamic derangements.[10–15] With 2D and 3D echocardiography, the degree of valve thickening, commissural fusion, and valve area by planimetry are ascertained (Figure 21.11). With pulsed and continuous-wave Doppler echocardiography, the transmitral pressure gradient and cardiac output are calculated (Figure 21.12). Doppler echocardiography provides other methods of obtaining valve area by the pressure half-time method and the continuity equation method. In addition, the pulmonary artery pressure can be derived from the tricuspid regurgitation velocity and the estimated right atrial pressure. Doppler methods, particularly color Doppler, allow for assessment of mitral regurgitation if present. The size and function of the left atrium, left ventricle, and right ventricle are easily assessed with 2D echocardiography. 3D echocardiography is ideally suited to assess the mitral apparatus.

Currently, the most accurate method for determining mitral valve area remains the planimetric area by 2D echocardiography (Figure 21.11). Given a funnel-shaped configuration of mitral stenosis, the valve area perimeter must be drawn in its narrowest and deepest orifice. The major limitation of 2D planimetry in mitral stenosis is that there is no controlled sectioning of mitral valve orifice. Sometimes, due to distortion of the leaflets, the contour of the valve area cannot be drawn accurately in a single plane. In some cases, the echocardiographic plane in the parasternal short-axis view cannot be properly oriented perpendicular to the narrowest orifice; of course, oblique cuts of valve area overestimate the degree of obstruction. Such technical problems are overcome by 3D echocardiography. With this, the narrowest area is always imaged, irrespective of orientation; moreover, the area can be traced using novel approaches such as the apical view. This improves accuracy and interobserver variability. The extent of commissural fusion cannot be appreciated fully by 2D echocardiography. However, with 3D echocardiography, this evaluation will be possible and it is likely that such information will be relevant before surgical commissurotomy (Figure 21.13). Whether commissural fusion is 'symmetrical' or 'asymmetrical' (i.e. whether it is more pronounced in one commissure than in the other, or, conversely, both commissures are equally affected) may be important before balloon mitral valvuloplasty; the procedure may, for instance, be more technically complicated in a case of asymmetrical fusion and the results less consistent. Moreover, after the procedure, imaging obtained by 3D echocardiography may better elucidate results (if, for instance, one or both commissures have been split). Furthermore, novel 3D projections provide new visualization perspectives. After balloon valvuloplasty, for example, the split of the commissure extending from the narrow orifice to the annulus should produce an optimal result. Such information can be given by 3D echocardiography,

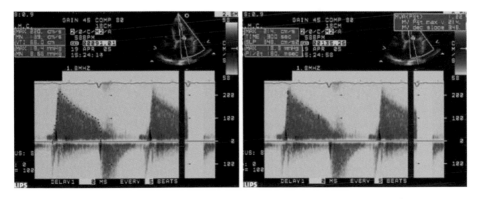

Figure 21.12

Continuous-wave Doppler recordings of transmitral flow from a patient with mitral stenosis. From the velocity profile, the transmitral mean gradient (left) and the mitral valve area (right) are obtained.

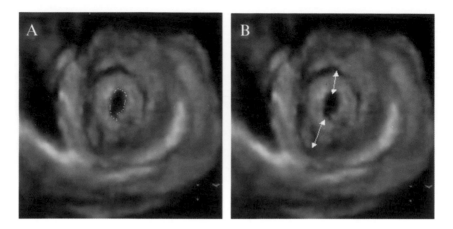

Figure 21.13

Three-dimensional transthoracic echocardiographic section of the mitral valve, viewed from the ventricular perspective, from a patient with mitral stenosis. The extent of commissural fusion (arrows) is easily assessed.

by cropping the set of volumetric data in a proper way.

In patients with severe mitral stenosis in whom an intervention is contemplated, echocardiography yields all the necessary information. The degree of morphologic abnormalities of the mitral apparatus influences the decision regarding mechanical interventions. Catheter-based balloon mitral valvuloplasty is the preferred method of relieving mitral obstruction in the modern era. Patients with pliable mitral leaflets with only moderate mitral valve thickening, minimal or no subvalvular abnormalities, minimal or no calcification in the valve apparatus, and mild or no mitral regurgitation are optimal candidates for balloon valvuloplasty. On the other hand, in patients with severe valve thickening and calcification, non-pliable valves, thickening and shortening of submitral structures, and/or significant mitral regurgitation, balloon valvuloplasty is unlikely to yield a good result and is more likely to be associated with complications such as tearing of the valve leaflets, injury to submitral structures, and/or severe mitral regurgitation. Information regarding all these issues is easily obtained by echocardiography. Transesophageal echocardiography is indicated to exclude the presence of left atrial thrombi and to assess the mitral apparatus in patients in whom

transthoracic imaging is unable to provide the needed information. Transesophageal echocardiography is also frequently used to guide the trans-septal catheterization and balloon valvuloplasty procedures (Figure 21.14).[16] In addition, echocardiography is useful in assessing the effects and complications of the procedure as well as in the follow-up of patients (Figure 21.15).

Management

The primary treatment for a mechanical problem such as mitral stenosis is mechanical relief. Medical therapy consists of serial clinical evaluation of the patient, antibiotic prophylaxis to prevent endocarditis, correction or control of atrial fibrillation, anticoagulation in patients with severe mitral stenosis and/or atrial fibrillation, treatment of heart failure symptoms, and evaluating the patient for the optimal procedure and timing of intervention. In patients with symptomatic and/or severe mitral stenosis, balloon valvuloplasty is the preferred procedure when mitral valve morphology deems those patients optimal for such a procedure.[17–21] In others, surgical commissurotomy or valve replacement is performed.

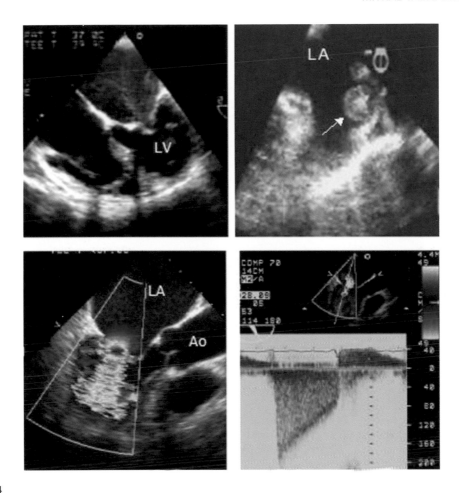

Figure 21.14

Transesophageal images from patients with mitral stenosis displaying a stenotic mitral valve (top left), a clot in the left atrial appendage (top right), high-velocity flow across the mitral valve (bottom left), and the velocity profile of the transmitral flow (bottom right). Ao, aorta; LA, left atrium; LV, left ventricle.

Mitral regurgitation

Etiology and pathology

All components of the mitral apparatus should work in synchrony and in proportion for optimal mitral valve closure. Intrinsic abnormalities in valve leaflets, mitral annulus, chordae tendinae, or papillary muscles can cause mitral regurgitation, referred to as primary mitral regurgitation. Incomplete coaptation of the leaflets caused by regional or global left ventricular dilatation or dysfunction results in secondary mitral regurgitation, also called functional mitral regurgitation.[22,23]

Leaflet abnormalities that are associated with mitral regurgitation include excessive leaflet tissue, deficient leaflet tissue, or restricted leaflet mobility. The most common pathology in primary mitral regurgitation is myxomatous degeneration of the mitral valve, resulting in prolapse. This condition can also result in flail leaflet, caused by ruptured chordae tendinae. Mitral valve prolapse can involve one or more segments of the mitral leaflet and one or both of the mitral leaflets. Other etiologies of leaflet disorders include endocarditis, congenital defects, rheumatic valve disease, and drug-induced pathology. Secondary or functional mitral regurgitation is caused by regional

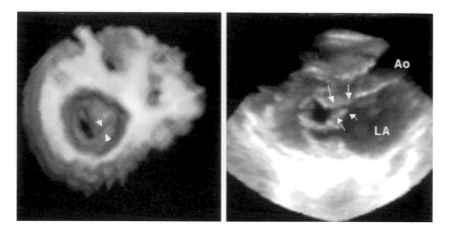

Figure 21.15

Three-dimensional echocardiographic images in patient with mitral stenosis, after balloon valvuloplasty. Only one commissure has been split (arrows) in one patient (left panel), and the split of the commissure extends from the narrowest orifice to the annulus in the second patient (right panel). LA, left atrium; Ao, aorta.

or global left ventricular dilatation in ischemic heart disease and by global left ventricular dilatation and dysfunction in non-ischemic dilated cardiomyopathy. Regurgitation noted in patients with acute or chronic ischemic heart disease is also referred to as ischemic mitral regurgitation, although it is preferable to avoid this term. Partial or complete papillary muscle rupture or chordal rupture in the setting of acute myocardial infarction causes acute mitral regurgitation. Mitral regurgitation during ischemia or infarction without papillary muscle rupture has been termed papillary muscle dysfunction. It is now recognized that it is the dysfunction of the subjacent myocardium that plays a bigger role than dysfunction of the papillary muscle itself. In hypertrophic obstructive cardiomyopathy, mitral regurgitation occurs because of systolic deformation of the mitral leaflets during systole (systolic anterior motion). In addition, some patients with hypertrophic cardiomyopathy have primary abnormalities of papillary muscle origin and/or size causing mitral regurgitation.

Pathophysiology and clinical features

The left ventricle is subjected to volume overload because of mitral regurgitation.

The left ventricle has to contract to a greater degree to maintain adequate forward output. In patients with acute severe mitral regurgitation, the acute volume overload causes acute severe elevation of left ventricular filling pressure and decreases forward stroke volume. These patients present with severe left heart failure and hypotension. In patients with chronic mitral regurgitation, the left ventricle enlarges secondary to the volume overload.

Left ventricular enlargement, eccentric hypertrophy, normal wall stress, and normal or mildly increased ejection fraction are markers of the compensatory phase in those with chronic mitral regurgitation. These patients may remain asymptomatic for many years. Eventually, however, the wall stress increases, further left ventricular dilatation occurs, and systolic dysfunction sets in. A decrease in ejection fraction indicates that significant systolic dysfunction has occurred. Subtle degrees of left ventricular dysfunction may go undetected because the ejection fraction may remain within normal limits owing to unloading of blood into the left atrium as well as increased left ventricular preload. Left atrial enlargement reflects the chronicity of mitral regurgitation, and increased left atrial compliance may be associated with a very large left atrium. At a certain stage, ventricular decompensation occurs and left ventricular filling pressure increases further, leading to symptoms of pulmonary congestion and left heart failure. Chronic elevation of left-sided filling pressures and pulmonary venous hypertension result in pulmonary arterial hypertension and in right heart failure. In patients with left ventricular dilatation and dysfunction, development of mitral regurgitation exacerbates the symptoms of heart failure and is associated with worsening prognosis.

Physical examination in patients with chronic mitral regurgitation may reveal a brisk pulse. The first heart sound may be normal or muffled. The pulmonic component of the second heart sound may be accentuated if pulmonary hypertension is present. One or more systolic clicks may be audible in patients with mitral valve prolapse. Absence of a click does not exclude mitral valve prolapse. While the classic description of mitral regurgitation murmur is that of a soft blowing holosystolic murmur audible at the apex with radiation to the axilla, it should be noted that the mechanism and severity of mitral regurgitation determine the characteristics of the murmur. Some patients with mitral valve prolapse may have only a late-systolic murmur. The direction of the mitral regurgitation jet may influence the direction of radiation. If the jet is directed anteriorly, the murmur may radiate to the parasternal region. Likewise, some patients, particularly those with acute severe mitral regurgitation, may have an ejection type of systolic murmur. In the setting of low-output state, the murmur may be soft or even inaudible. In some patients, the murmur may be heard only with an afterload-increasing maneuver such as hand-grip exercise.

Diagnostic evaluation

The electrocardiogram may show features of left ventricular hypertrophy and left atrial enlargement and generally is non-specific. Chest radiography may reveal left atrial enlargement, left ventricular enlargement, and, in severe cases, pulmonary congestion. Echocardiography provides comprehensive information on the morphologic and functional abnormalities responsible for mitral regurgitation, the severity of mitral regurgitation, and its impact on left ventricular size and function as well as left atrial size. Cardiac catheterization is not necessary for the assessment of mitral regurgitation. If performed, left atrial or pulmonary capillary wedge pressure may show augmented v-wave and increased pressure, and, in advanced cases, evidence of pulmonary hypertension. Left ventricular angiography yields a semi-quantitative estimate of mitral regurgitation severity on a scale of 1–4 or 1–3.

All modalities of echocardiography are useful in the evaluation of mitral regurgitation (Figures 21.16–21.20).[11 27] 2D and 3D echocardiography

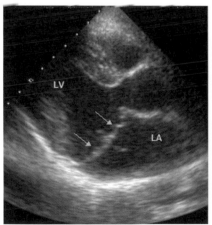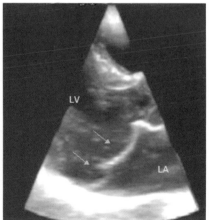

Figure 21.16

Two-dimensional (left) and three-dimensional (right) images from a patient with bileaflet mitral valve prolapse. LA, left atrium; LV, left ventricle.

depict the morphologic abnormalities responsible for mitral regurgitation (Figures 21.16 and 21.18). In patients with suboptimal surface windows, transesophageal echocardiography yields higher-resolution images of the mitral leaflets, chordae tendinae, and papillary muscles. With 3D echocardiography, it is possible to precisely define topography and size of prolapsed tissue; in addition, the ratio of prolapsed to non-prolapsed tissue, the extension of prolapsed tissue measured at its annular insertion, or the size of the prolapsed area can be measured (Figure 21.19). Direct imaging of regurgitant orifices is also possible. Such orifices are often irregularly shaped and can be multiple. Novel orientations with 3D echocardiography may allow better images of chordae tendinae and papillary muscles (Figure 21.21). In patients with secondary or functional mitral regurgitation, 2D and 3D examination dis-

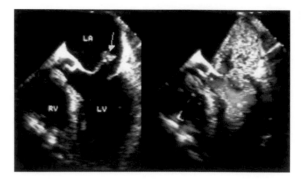

Figure 21.18

Transesophageal images from a patient with a ruptured papillary muscle (arrow) and severe mitral regurgitation. LA, left atrium; LV, left ventricle; RV, right ventricle.

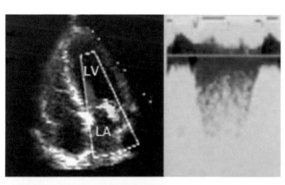

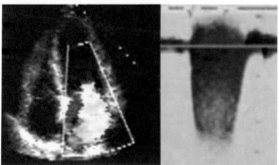

Figure 21.17

Color Doppler and continuous-wave Doppler recordings in patients with mild (top panels) and severe (bottom panels) mitral regurgitation. The top example, from a patient with mild regurgitation, shows a small mitral regurgitation jet in color Doppler with light intensity in continuous-wave Doppler; the bottom example displays a large jet with intense signals. LA, left atrium; LV, left ventricle.

play underlying left ventricular and left atrial abnormalities, such as regional dilatation and dysfunction, global dilatation and dysfunction, the degree of apical displacement of leaflet coaptation, the distorted geometry of the papillary muscle(s), mitral annular dilatation, and/or left atrial enlargement.

Color Doppler examination displays the presence, size, and direction of the mitral regurgitation jet (Figure 21.17). The presence of mitral regurgitation and the antegrade diastolic mitral velocity are recognized by pulsed Doppler examination. In the absence of mitral stenosis, the early diastolic E-wave velocity increases as mitral regurgitation severity increases. Pulsed Doppler examination of the pulmonary venous flow may show attenuation or reversal of the systolic wave in severe cases, if the left atrial compliance is decreased and the pressure is high. Absence of systolic reversal or attenuation, however, does not exclude severe mitral regurgitation, since the left atrium could be compliant and have normal pressures in the setting of severe chronic mitral regurgitation. Continuous-wave Doppler reveals the mitral regurgitation velocity profile and the pressure gradient between the left ventricle and left atrium. The intensity of the mitral regurgitation velocity profile reflects the severity of mitral regurgitation – more intense in severe cases and of light intensity in mild cases (Figure 21.17). Color Doppler has become the initial mode in the assessment of mitral regurgitation jets. A trace amount of mitral regurgitation can be present even in normal individuals, and such a presence

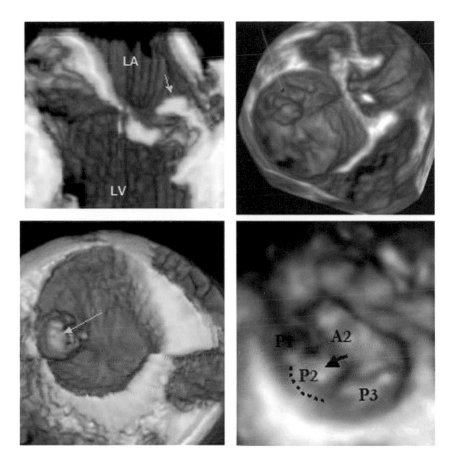

Figure 21.19

Three-dimensional echocardiographic views (longitudinal section, top left, and views from the left atrium, other images) of mitral valve prolapse depicting the location and number of the abnormal segments (arrows). LA, left atrium; LV, left ventricle.

does not necessarily connote any pathology. Besides showing the presence of mitral regurgitation, color Doppler displays the origin of the jet, the size of the jet proximal to, at, and distal to the valve, as well as the direction of the jet. Some patients may have more than one jet identified by color Doppler. The jet area within the left atrium or the ratio of the jet area to the left atrial area have been reported to correlate with mitral regurgitation severity, but caution needs to be exercised in using such an approach; such measurements in one frame in systole may not reflect the true severity, and eccentric jets could be misjudged. The flow convergence of the jet proximal to the regurgitant orifice (proximal flow convergence) is useful in pointing out the location of the jet orifice(s), and the size of the flow convergence correlates with the severity of mitral regurgita-

tion. Adjusting the scale calibration of color Doppler can help bring out the flow convergence zone better. The narrow portion of the jet immediately distal to the regurgitant orifice is known as the vena contracta, and its size also correlates with the mitral regurgitation severity. The overall severity of mitral regurgitation can be gauged on a semiquantitative scale of mild, moderate, or severe, or a scale of 1 to 4+ by examining the jet in different views and using a multiparametric approach of pulsed Doppler E-wave, continuous Doppler intensity, and color Doppler evaluation of the different facets of the jet.

There are several approaches to quantify the regurgitant volume and regurgitant fraction. The left ventricular filling volume can be calculated by measuring the time–velocity integral of mitral flow (pulsed Doppler) and mitral annular

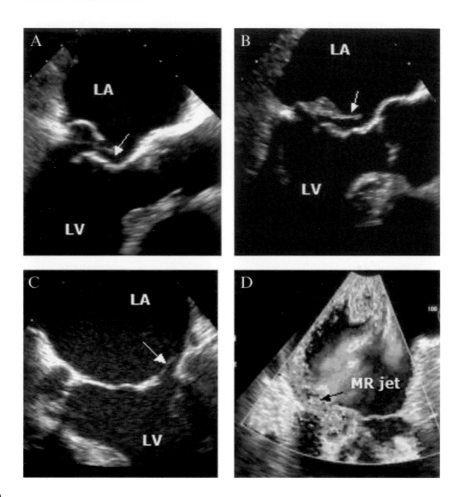

Figure 21.20

(A–D) Transesophageal echocardiographic images of flail mitral leaflets and ruptured chordae tendinae and severe mitral regurgitation (MR). LA, left atrium; LV, left ventricle.

dimension from 2D images. From the dimension, the mitral annular area is calculated assuming that it is circular. The time–velocity integral of mitral flow (sampled at the annular level) is multiplied by the annular cross-sectional area to yield the total left ventricular filling volume. Using the left ventricular outflow dimension and the time–velocity integral of forward flow (sampled at the outflow tract) yields the forward stroke volume. The total filling volume minus the forward stroke volume is the regurgitant volume. The regurgitant fraction is the ratio of the regurgitant volume to the total filling volume. Another approach is to calculate the total stroke volume of the left ventricle (which includes both the regur-

gitant volume and the forward stroke volume) by 2D echocardiography using a modified Simpson equation, and subtracting the forward stroke volume derived at the left ventricular outflow. Color Doppler allows two other approaches. One is to measure the radius of the proximal flow convergence zone, calculate the surface area of this zone $(2\pi r^2)$, and multiply it by the velocity of the flow convergence zone. The regurgitant orifice area is then calculated by dividing the regurgitant flow by the velocity of the mitral regurgitant jet recorded by continuous-wave Doppler. Another color Doppler method to calculate the regurgitant flow is to derive the cross-sectional area of the vena contracta of the jet from its radius, and mul-

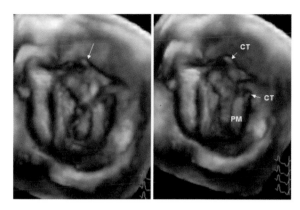

Figure 21.21

Three-dimensional echocardiographic view of the mitral apparatus viewed from above in a patient with ruptured chordae tendinae (CT). The two heads of the ruptured chordae tendinae – one attached at the papillary muscle, the other at the anterior leaflet – can be seen (arrows). PM, papillary muscle.

tiply it by the mitral regurgitant velocity recorded by continuous-wave Doppler. The color Doppler methods, while apparently simple, are fraught with some flaws because of the assumptions involved. The assumptions that the proximal flow convergence zone is a perfect hemisphere, that the vena contracta is circular, and that measurement in one frame during systole reflects the overall regurgitant flow are often incorrect. Furthermore, these methods are not applicable when there is more than one regurgitant orifice. The quantitative approach using 2D and pulsed Doppler is more reliable than the color Doppler methods of flow quantitation. 3D echocardiography offers another approach to quantitation of mitral regurgitation without undue assumptions, as long as mitral regurgitation is the only regurgitant lesion. The total stroke volumes of left and right ventricles can be derived using the unmodified Simpson equation in 3D imaging. The left ventricular stroke volume minus the right ventricular stroke volume yields the mitral regurgitant volume.

Besides the definition of functional pathology and severity of mitral regurgitation, echocardiography also allows for evaluation of the hemodynamic state and left heart chambers. An accentuated E-wave with rapid deceleration in the mitral flow and attenuated or reversed systolic

wave in the pulmonary venous flow are markers of elevated filling pressures in the left heart chambers. A steep decline in the mitral regurgitation velocity profile in late systole indicates elevated left atrial pressure and is often noted in acute severe mitral regurgitation. Using the tricuspid regurgitation velocity and the estimated right atrial pressure, the presence and severity of pulmonary hypertension can be assessed. The left ventricular volume, mass, and radius-to-wall thickness ratio, which are useful indices in clinical decision-making, can be estimated by 2D or 3D echocardiography.

Transesophageal echocardiography is frequently employed preoperatively and in the operating room to guide the surgeon in planning the type of valve repair.[27] Intraoperative echocardiography also aids in assessment of the success of surgical repair and in the detection of complications, if any, related to surgery. Transesophageal echocardiographic imaging is a necessity in patients undergoing catheter-based mitral valve repair procedures, currently under investigation.

Exercise testing is useful in the assessment of effort tolerance in patients with asymptomatic severe mitral regurgitation and in those where there is discordance between symptoms and the severity of mitral regurgitation at rest. Coupling echocardiographic imaging with exercise adds an advantage. Worsening of mitral regurgitation could be an indicator of the dynamic nature of mitral regurgitation and may explain the symptoms in some patients, particularly those with functional mitral regurgitation. Exercise-induced changes in left ventricular volumes and function may provide prognostic information as well.

Cardiac catheterization is necessary only in patients in whom the coronary anatomy needs to be defined. The roles of other imaging techniques such as magnetic resonance imaging and computed tomography in patients with mitral regurgitation are discussed elsewhere in this book.

Management

Acute severe mitral regurgitation caused by papillary muscle rupture or endocarditis often warrants surgery. Unloading agents and intra-aortic balloon pump support are useful as interim measures and in those not suitable for surgery.

Treatment of the underlying coronary artery disease, endocarditis, or trauma is indicated.

Medical therapy for asymptomatic patients with mitral regurgitation includes antibiotic prophylaxis against endocarditis. Vasodilators and angiotensin-converting enzyme inhibitors are often used, but there is no clear evidence that medical therapy will prevent the progression of mitral regurgitation, delay the development of left ventricular dysfunction, or postpone the timing of surgery in patients with moderate mitral regurgitation. Patients with dilated ventricles associated with cardiomyopathy and functional mitral regurgitation are likely to benefit from medical measures, but the definitive means of correcting mitral regurgitation remains surgical intervention.

Patients with mitral regurgitation due to primary valvular disease do well for many years without symptoms. Those with symptoms, pulmonary hypertension, or atrial fibrillation are candidates for repair or replacement of the mitral valve. Valve repair is preferable to valve replacement. In the present era, atrial maze procedure is combined with mitral valve surgery in those patients with mitral regurgitation and chronic atrial fibrillation.

The timing of intervention in patients with asymptomatic severe primary mitral regurgitation remains controversial.[21,28] Ideally, such patients should have surgery before left ventricular dysfunction develops and before valve degeneration progresses to an unrepairable stage. Some reports suggest that valve repair is indicated even in asymptomatic patients with flail mitral valve because of the fear of sudden death or poor outcome with medical therapy. While the issue has not been resolved, the general approach is to delay surgery and follow the patient when mitral regurgitation is not associated with any symptoms, and when left ventricular size (end-systolic dimension <45 mm) and function (ejection fraction >60%) are normal, unless one is absolutely certain that the valve could be repaired successfully. If there is left ventricular enlargement or dysfunction (end-systolic dimension ≥45 mm, ejection fraction ≤60%), or there is even a trend towards such a change, valve repair or replacement should be performed.

Symptomatic patients with marked left ventricular dysfunction (ejection fraction <30%) are preferably treated medically because of the high risk associated with surgery.

The issue of secondary or functional mitral regurgitation in patients with ischemic or non-ischemic dilated cardiomyopathy is under intense study. The presence of mitral regurgitation is an independent predictor of decreased survival. If myocardial revascularization surgery is planned in a patient with ischemic left ventricular dysfunction and severe mitral regurgitation, then concurrent mitral annuloplasty or repair is generally performed. Decision-making in cases of only moderate mitral regurgitation in such a patient remains difficult. If the ventricle is dilated, the mitral annulus is enlarged and the leaflet coaptation is distorted, it is preferable to correct mitral regurgitation even if it is only moderate. On the other hand, if the primary problem is coronary artery disease in a patient with only mild or moderate mitral regurgitation and normal left ventricular size and function, then there may not be a need to perform mitral valve surgery.

Secondary mitral regurgitation associated with marked left ventricular dilatation and dysfunction due to advanced ischemic or non-ischemic dilated cardiomyopathy is becoming a common problem. Even though some experience suggests that mitral annuloplasty could be performed in such patients with a relatively low mortality,[29] these patients are generally not considered for open-heart surgery because of the high risk. Many approaches that are directed towards favorably improving left ventricular remodeling, such as biventricular pacing or placement of cardiac support devices, may decrease mitral regurgitation as well, but they are still under investigation. Intense effort is also afoot in developing catheter-based techniques to decrease the mitral annular size or improve mitral valve coaptation (see elsewhere in this book). The initial results in experimental and clinical trials are encouraging, and it is highly likely that the future will see one or more of these percutaneous techniques as a preferred treatment option in secondary mitral regurgitation or even in primary mitral regurgitation (Figure 21.22).

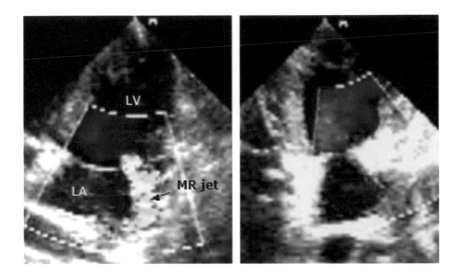

Figure 21.22

Two-dimensional images depicting mitral regurgitation (MR) in an animal model of ischemic mitral regurgitation (left) and the abolition of mitral regurgitation after pervenous catheter-based mitral annuloplasty. LA, left atrium; LV, left ventricle.

Conclusion

New insights have been gained into the pathophysiology of mitral regurgitation during the last few decades. Echocardiography has revolutionized the diagnostic evaluation of stenotic and regurgitant mitral valve lesions and has led to a better appreciation of the importance of the functional morphology of the mitral apparatus. Novel surgical approaches to valve repair and innovative percutaneous techniques to correct mitral valve disease have been developed, providing an impetus for early intervention in patients with mitral valve disease.

References

1. Perloff JK, Roberts WC. The mitral apparatus. Functional anatomy and mitral regurgitation. Circulation 1972; 46: 227–39.
2. Kanani M, Anderson RH. The anatomy of the mitral valve: a retrospective analysis of yesterday's future. J Heart Valve Dis 2003; 12: 180–5.
3. Liddicoat JR, MacNeill BD, Gillinov AM, et al. Percutaneous mitral valve repair: a feasibility study in an ovine model of acute ischemic mitral regurgitation. Catheter Cardiovasc Interv 2003; 60: 410–16.
4. Rodriquez LL, Acquatella H, Wiegers S, et al. Percutaneous edge-to-edge repair for mitral regurgitation guided by transesophageal and transthoracic echocardiography. J Am Coll Cardiol 2004; 43: 25A.
5. Tsakiris AG, von Bernuth G, Rastelli GS, et al. Size and motion of the mitral valve annulus in anesthesized intact dogs. J Appl Physiol 1971; 30: 611–18.
6. Ormiston JA, Shah PM, Tei C, Wong M. Size and motion of the mitral valve annulus in man. I. A two-dimensional echocardiographic method and findings in normal subjects. Circulation 1981; 64: 113–20.
7. De Casto S, Saladin V, Cartoni D, et al. Qualitative and quantitative evaluation of mitral valve morphology by intraoperative volume-rendered three-dimensional echocardiography. J Heart Valve Dis 2002; 11: 2: 173–80.
8. Timek TA, Miller DC. Experimental and clinical assessment of mitral annular area and dynamics: What are we actually measuring? Ann Thorac Surg 2001; 72: 966–74.
9. Levine RA, Handschumacher MD, Sanfilippo AJ, et al. Three-dimensional echocardiographic reconstruction of the mitral valve, with implications for the diagnosis of mitral valve prolapse. Circulation 1989; 80: 589–98.
10. Wann LS, Weyman AE, Feigenbaum H, et al. Determination of mitral valve area by cross-sectional echocardiography. Ann Intern Med 1978; 88: 337–41.
11. Hatle L, Brubakk A, Tromsdal A, Angelsen B. Noninvasive assessment of pressure drop in mitral

stenosis by Doppler ultrasound. Br Heart J 1978; 40: 131–40.

12. Cheitlin MD, Armstrong WF, Aurigemma GP, et al. ACC/AHA/ASE 2003 Guideline Update for the Clinical Application of Echocardiography: summary article: a report of the American College of Cardiology/American Heart Association Task Force on Practice Guidelines (ACC/AHA/ASE Committee to Update the 1997 Guidelines for the Clinical Application of Echocardiography). Circulation 2003; 108: 1146.

13. Faletra F, Pezzano JA, Fusco, R et al. Measurement of mitral valve area in mitral stenosis: four echocardiographic methods compared with direct measurement of anatomic orifices. J Am Coll Cardiol 1996; 28: 1190–7.

14. Mohan JC, Mukherjee S, Kumar A, et al. Does chronic mitral regurgitation influence Doppler pressure half-time-derived calculation of mitral valve area in patients with mitral stenosis? Am Heart J 2004: 148: 703–9.

15. Zamorano J, Cordeiro P, Sugeng L, et al. Real-time three-dimensional echocardiography for rheumatic mitral valve stenosis evaluation: an accurate and novel approach. J Am Coll Cardiol 2004; 43: 2091–6.

16. Kronzon I, Tunick PA, Schwinger ME, et al. Transesophageal echocardiography during mitral valvuloplasty. J Am Soc Echocardiogr 1989; 2: 380–5.

17. Lock JE, Khalilullah M, Shrivastava S, et al. Percutaneous catheter commissurotomy in rheumatic mitral stenosis. N Engl J Med 1985; 313: 1515–18.

18. Carroll JD, Feldman T. Percutaneous mitral balloon valvotomy and the new demographics of mitral stenosis. JAMA 1993; 270: 1731–6.

19. Reyes VP, Raju BS, Wynne J, et al. Percutaneous balloon valvuloplasty compared with open surgical commissurotomy for mitral stenosis. N Engl J Med 1994; 331: 961–7.

20. Ben Farhat M, Ayari M, Maatouk F, et al. Percutaneous balloon versus surgical closed and open mitral commissurotomy: seven-year follow-up results of a randomized trial. Circulation. 1998; 97: 245–50.

21. Bonow RO, Carabello B, de Leon AC Jr, et al. Guidelines for the Management of Patients with Valvular Heart Disease. A report of the American College of Cardiology/American Heart Association. Task Force on Practice Guidelines. J Am Coll Cardiol 1998; 32: 1486–588.

22. Carabello, BA. Mitral valve disease. Curr Prob Cardiol 1993; 18: 423–78.

23. Enriquez-Sarano M, Freeman WK, Tribouilloy CM, et al. Functional anatomy of mitral regurgitation. J Am Coll Cardiol 1999; 34: 1129–36.

24. Patel A, Mochizuki Y, Yao J, Pandian NG. Mitral regurgitation: comprehensive assessment by echocardiogram. Echocardiography 2000; 17: 275–83.

25. Yao J, Masani ND, Cao QL, Nikuta P, Pandian NG. Clinical application of transthoracic volume-rendered three-dimensional echocardiography in the assessment of mitral regurgitation. Am J Cardiol 1998; 82: 189–96.

26. Kwan J, Shiota T, Agler DA, et al. Geometric differences of the mitral apparatus between ischemic and dilated cardiomyopathy with significant mitral regurgitation: real-time three-dimensional echocardiography study. Circulation 2003; 107: 1135–40.

27. Matsunaga A, Shah PM, Raney AA. Impact of intraoperative echocardiography/surgery on successful mitral valve repair: a community hospital experience. J Heart Valve Dis 2005; 14: 1–7

28. Enriquez-Sarano M. Timing of mitral valve surgery. Heart 2002; 87: 79–85.

29. Bolling SF, Pagani FD, Deeb GM, Bach DS. Intermediate-term outcome of mitral reconstruction in cardiomyopathy. J Thorac Cardiovasc Surg 1998; 115: 381–6.

22

Cardiovascular magnetic resonance imaging in the evaluation of mitral regurgitation

Susan M Sallach, Ronald M Peshock

Introduction

The evaluation of patients with mitral regurgitation for valve repair is complex. The cardiologist must know the details of valve structure and function and the effects of chronic loading on ventricular size and function. In addition, it is important to know if other valvular or myocardial disease is present. At present, transthoracic and transesophageal echocardiography are the primary tools for the evaluation of mitral valve disease.

Recently, cardiovascular magnetic resonance (CVMR) imaging has emerged as an effective tool for the evaluation of patients with valvular heart disease.[1] CVMR can evaluate valve morphology, assess valve motion and function, and accurately quantify ventricular volumes and function. It can also provide important information on the extent of myocardial scarring due to infarction and detect the presence of non-ischemic myopathic processes.[2,3] Importantly, it can obtain this information non-invasively without ionizing radiation and without the limitations of acoustic window.

This chapter will (1) describe the CVMR approach to the patient with mitral regurgitation, (2) examine its use in the assessment of the patient with mitral regurgitation prior to and after mitral valve repair, (3) briefly discuss the issue of CVMR and implants and devices, and (4) consider potential future applications.

CVMR approach to the patient with mitral regurgitation

A standard CVMR examination is now widely used, and consists of bright-blood imaging (cine gradient echo or steady-state free precession) to assess structure and function, dark-blood imaging (typically a form of double inversion recovery spin echo) for tissue characterization and detailed structure, and cine phase contrast imaging for quantification of flow.[4] Similar to echocardiography, standard two-chamber, four-chamber, short-axis, and three-chamber cine MR views are the absolute minimum set of images that can provide useful information about the mitral valve (Figure 22.1).

In the standard examination, 8–10 short-axis images are routinely acquired from the ventricular apex to the base of the heart so that accurate quantification of right and left ventricular volumes can be performed (Figure 22.2A). In addition, this provides additional images to evaluate right and left ventricular segmental function. At present each set of CVMR images is generally acquired using electrocardiographic (ECG) gating during a 10–15 s breath-hold. At a magnetic field of 1.5 T, typically images have a slice thickness of 6–8 mm, an in-plane resolution of 1.5 mm or less, and a temporal resolution of 40 ms or less.

Cine phase contrast images are used for quantification of flow in the aorta and pulmonary artery (Figure 22.2B). Similar to Doppler echocardiography, the imaging can be adjusted to prevent aliasing of velocities. Generally, flow through the CVMR imaging plane is measured, although it is possible to measure in-plane velocities (similar to Doppler echocardiography) or along all axes to determine the flow vector at each point in the image.[5] CVMR is not restricted by acoustic window or attenuation and thus can obtain images in any plane. It can be used to directly image the mitral valve in cross-section to

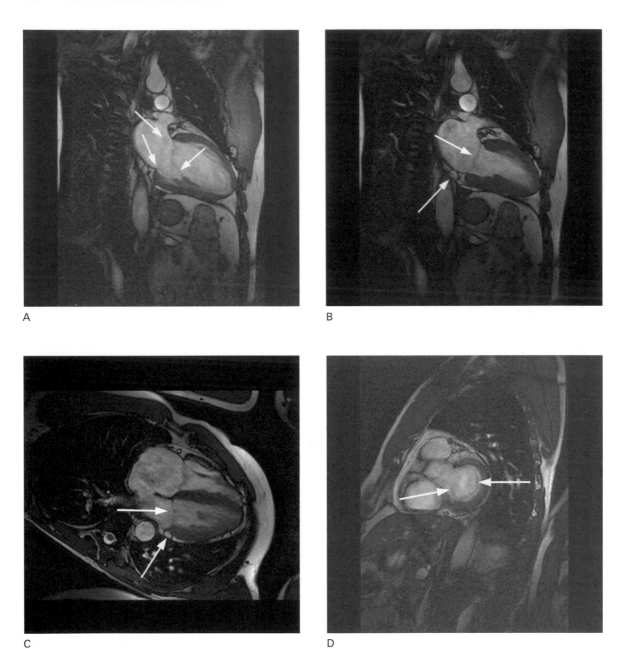

Figure 22.1

Normal mitral valve by CVMR. (A) White-blood, two-chamber mid-diastolic image. The anterior mitral valve leaflet, posterior mitral valve leaflet, chordae, and papillary muscle are well visualized (arrows). (B) White-blood, two-chamber systolic image. The mitral valve leaflets are again well visualized (arrow). Note the location of the coronary sinus in this view (yellow arrow). (C) White-blood, four-chamber systolic image. The mitral valve leaflets (arrow) and the coronary sinus are again indicated (yellow arrow). (D) White-blood, short-axis image through the mitral valve leaflets during diastole. The posterior leaflet is seen, as well as a portion of the anterior leaflet (arrows). (E) White-blood, three-chamber early diastolic image. This image could be used to measure anterior leaflet length, posterior leaflet length, and distance from the coaptation point to the septum, comparable to measurements made using echocardiography. (F) Black-blood, four-chamber image obtained in diastole. The change in contrast is obtained by varying the imaging sequence without the use of any contrast agent.

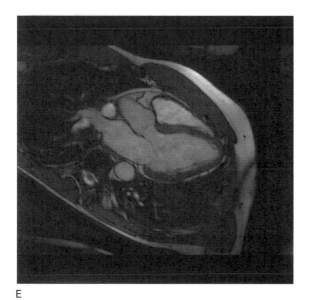

E

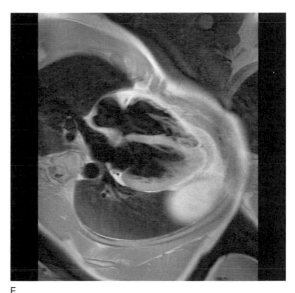

F

Figure 22.1 *contd*

measure stenotic or regurgitant orifice flow (Figure 22.2E–H). As in echocardiography, this approach is complicated by the motion of the base of the heart towards the apex with systole, so that the valve moves through the imaging plane, resulting in differing cross-section due to translation of the valve. Although it is technically feasible, color flow MRI is not presently available as a standard tool on any commercial MRI system.[6]

A recent important addition to the standard CVMR examination is delayed imaging after gadolinium contrast. This method is now used routinely to identify the extent of myocardial scaring following infarction and can be used to help identify regions that are viable and will respond to revascularization.[7] It is also of increasing importance in the evaluation of non-ischemic cardiomyopathies and acute myocarditis.

CVMR assessment of the patient prior to and following mitral valve repair

From extensive studies using transesophageal echocardiography prior to mitral valve repair, it is known that several questions must be addressed:[8,9] How severe is the mitral regurgitation and is mitral stenosis present? What are the

specific locations of prolapsing or flail leaflets, areas of tethering and restriction, and areas of normal leaflet function? Are the leaflets perforated, calcified, excessively long, thickened, or immobile? Is there superior displacement of the valve? Is mitral annular calcification present? Are the chordae thickened? What is the status of the papillary muscle and ventricular wall? Finally, what is the status of overall ventricular function?

To utilize CVMR effectively in the evaluation of mitral regurgitation, it is important to understand several features of MRI that influence the appearance of valves. Virtually all images acquired using CVMR are not obtained in real time. As mentioned above, they are typically obtained during a breath-hold (10–15 s) using ECG gating. Thus, they represent valve motion 'averaged' over the 10–20 cardiac cycles that occur during the breath-hold. In some ways, it is actually surprising that valve motion is so highly reproducible over 10–20 cardiac cycles to permit imaging of valvular structures down to a millimeter in size. Abnormal valve motion, such as that seen with mitral valve prolapse (Figure 22.3) is readily detected on bright-blood cine studies. It is also apparent that measures of mitral annular circumference, anterior leaflet length, posterior leaflet length, and the distance from the septum to the coaptation point can be obtained. Finally,

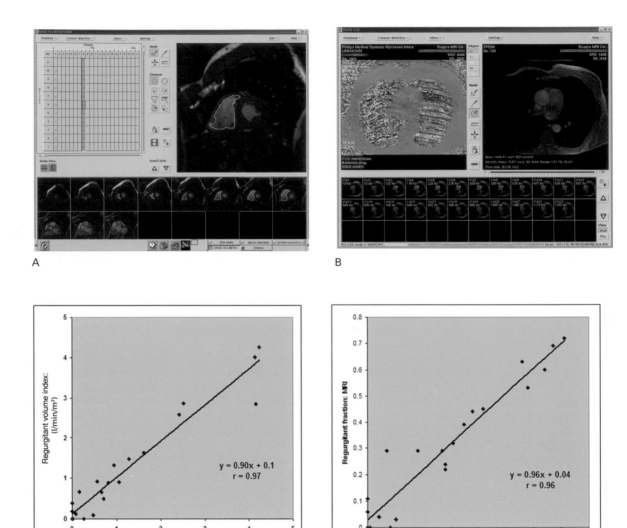

Figure 22.2

Quantitative assessment of function and regurgitation. (A) Typical short-axis images used for the calculation of left and right ventricular volumes and stroke volumes. The left (red) and right (yellow) endocardial contours at end-systole are shown. (B) Axial images obtained for measurement of flow in the ascending aorta. The quantitative flow map is in the left panel, with the magnitude image on the right. (C) Comparison of CVMR with invasive catheterization in the measurement of regurgitant volume. (D) Comparison of CVMR with invasive catheterization in the measurement of regurgitant fraction. (E) Short-axis image obtained through the mitral orifice during diastole. The three posterior leaflet segments are visualized (arrows), as well as the anterior leaflet. (F) Short-axis flow image obtained through the mitral orifice during diastole. Flow from the left atrium into the left ventricle is white relative to the relatively stationary tissue of the heart and chest wall. (G) Short-axis image obtained through the left atrium just distal to the mitral orifice during systole. There is now signal loss in the region of the regurgitant jet (yellow arrow). (H) Short-axis flow image obtained through the left atrium just distal to the mitral orifice during systole. The flow is now from the left ventricle into the left atrium and is shown as dark relative to heart and other structures (yellow arrow). (Parts C and D are reproduced from Hundley et al. Circulation 1995; 92: 1151–8.[16])

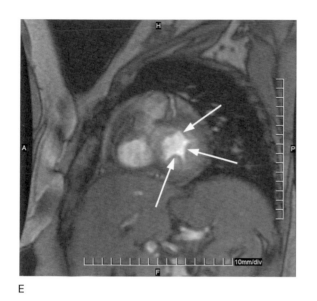

E

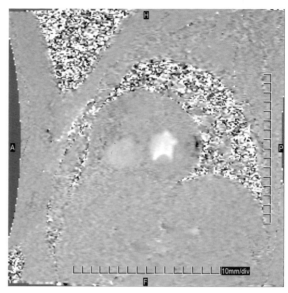

F

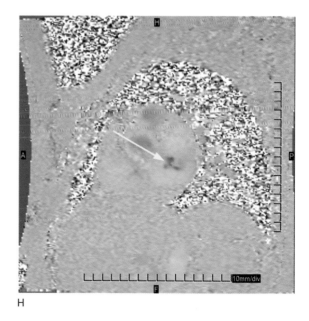

G

H

Figure 22.2 *contd*

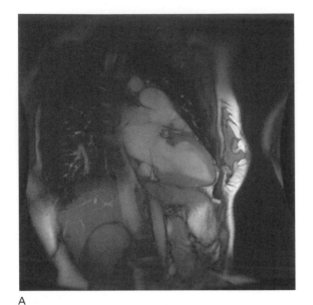

A

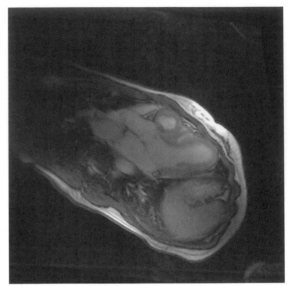

B

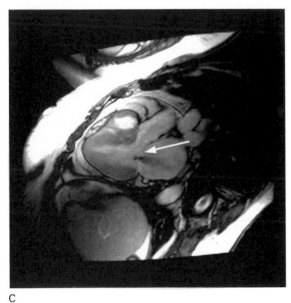

C

Figure 22.3

Mitral valve prolapse. (A) Bright-blood, two-chamber systolic image in a patient in mitral valve prolapse without regurgitation. (B) Bright-blood, three-chamber, systolic image in the same patient demonstrating anterior mitral valve leaflet prolapse. (C) Bright-blood, three-chamber late-systolic image in a different patient with prolapse of the anterior mitral valve leaflet (arrow) with moderate mitral regurgitation.

CVMR can be particularly helpful in determining papillary muscle orientation and in cases of unusual ventricular geometry.

However, the need to acquire the data over a number of cardiac cycles has several implications. First, chaotic motion that is not reproducible from cycle to cycle will result in 'blurring' of the image and loss of that detail. This makes it difficult, if not impossible, to detect small vegetations using CVMR, due to their non-reproducible motion. Similarly, it may make detection of chordal rupture difficult. Second, the quality of CVMR images of valves is dependent upon the consistency of the heart rate and the ability of the patient to maintain a breath-hold. Thus, it is critical to obtain a good ECG for gating during the examination. Interestingly, it is possible to obtain good images for evaluation of ventricular function in patients in atrial fibrillation if the rate is relatively well controlled.[10] However, the precise effects of atrial fibrillation on valve imaging have not been investigated. An alternative to breath-hold is the use of a 'navigator-echo' approach, which essentially gates the image to the respiratory cycle. This approach has been used extensively in coronary artery imaging using CVMR.[11] Although this has not been extensively evaluated, anecdotal evidence suggests that one can obtain excellent images of the valves using this technique. Unfortunately, this form of respiratory gating significantly increases scan time, which may limit its applicability in patients with valvular disease.

Another important feature of CVMR is that there are multiple mechanisms that play a role in image contrast. A complete discussion of these factors is beyond the scope of this chapter, but there are several points that are relevant to the assessment of structural abnormalities of the mitral valve. The CVMR signal arises from hydrogen nuclei in water and fat. Signal intensity in a given tissue is then influenced by a large number of factors, including the number of hydrogen nuclei present, the characteristic relation times of the tissues (T1 and T2), and the presence of materials that alter the local magnetic field in the tissue (such as the presence of a prosthetic valve). Thus, signal intensity in CVMR images is dependent on the composition of the tissue being imaged, and the imaging approach can then be designed to accentuate difference in tissues. By simply changing the settings on the MR imaging

device, one can obtain black-blood or white-blood images of the heart without the use of contrast agents. These differences lead to the contrast between valve apparatus and blood pool to identify thickening and other structural abnormalities (Figure 22.4) and mitral annular calcification (Figure 22.5).

Qualitative assessment of mitral regurgitation

A second important point is that CVMR is intrinsically sensitive to motion. Signal loss occurs in regions of turbulent or disordered blood flow due to dephasing. This is the basis for the ability to visually detect the regurgitant jet using CVMR (Figure 22.3C). Interestingly, it is quite effective in identifying multiple jets (Figure 22.6) and regions of proximal flow acceleration on the ventricular side of the valve (Figure 22.4D). However, if there is disordered flow near a valve leaflet, this can result in signal loss, with a false increase in the apparent valve 'thickness' on CVMR. This artifact can be distinguished by its changes over the cardiac cycle. However, it is important that the person interpreting CVMR studies of the mitral valve have sufficient experience to recognize this potential artifact.

Qualitative assessment of the severity of regurgitation is dependent upon identifying signal loss in regions of turbulent or otherwise-disordered blood flow. Determination of the location and direction of the regurgitant jet is very similar to that used in echocardiography. The major difference is the absence of color flow for CVMR. Visual assessment of mild, moderate, and severe lesions correlates with echocardiographic or angiographic grading and demonstrates good interobserver variability.[12]

Quantitative assessment of ventricular volumes and function and the presence of myocardial scar

CVMR is essentially the 'gold standard' for the accurate and reproducible measurement of

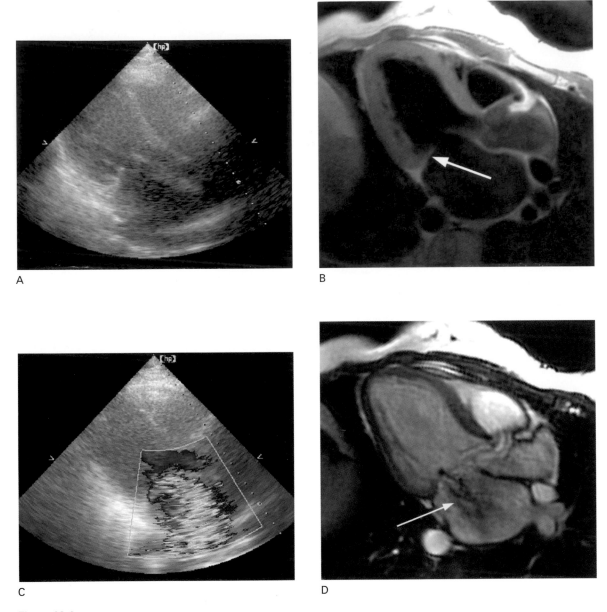

Figure 22.4

Rheumatic mitral valve disease. (A) Transthoracic echocardiogram in a patient with rheumatic mitral valve disease with thickening of the mitral valve leaflets. (B) CVMR, black-blood image obtained in the same patient demonstrates thickening of the posterior mitral valve leaflet (arrow). (C) Three-chamber color flow image demonstrating mitral regurgitation. (D) CVMR, bright-blood, three-chamber systolic image demonstrating loss of signal in the left atrium due to mitral regurgitation (yellow arrow).

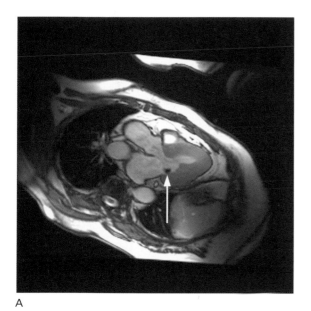
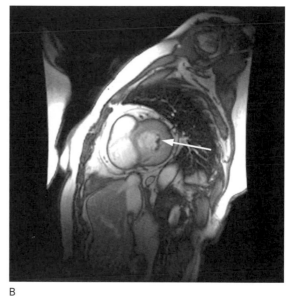

A   B

Figure 22.5

Mitral annular calcification. (A) Bright-blood, three-chamber systolic image in a patient with severe mitral annular calcification (arrow) that involves the posterior mitral valve leaflet. (B) Bright-blood, short-axis, early diastolic image at the level of the mitral annulus, again demonstrating severe mitral annular calcification posteriorly (arrow).

ventricular volumes and function.[13,14] Thus, it is an effective means for determining and following ventricular size and function. With the advent of delayed-enhancement imaging, it is now possible to reliably identify those patients with significant regions of myocardial scarring due to ischemic disease (Figure 22.6). It has been shown that segments that demonstrate less than 50% of the wall involved by scar contain viable myocardium, which will improve with revascularization.[7]

Quantitative assessment of regurgitation

A major role for CVMR is in the quantification of regurgitation.[15] In the absence of additional valvular disease, one can directly compare right and left ventricular stroke volumes to quantify the amount of regurgitation present. Right and left ventricular stroke volumes typically differ by less than 10%, permitting detection of regurgitation of clinical importance.

In the case of multiple regurgitant valves, it is necessary to compare the left ventricular stroke volume with an independent measure of forward cardiac output obtained using quantitative flow. In a patient with both mitral and aortic regurgitation, the quantitative flow sequence could be used to directly measure forward cardiac output and regurgitant flow across the aortic valve. This regurgitant flow would be subtracted from the total left ventricular stroke volume to yield the mitral regurgitant flow. Alternatively, one could directly measure the regurgitant flow across the mitral valve. In complex cases, it may be advisable to obtain both measures to compare the results obtained with each approach.

The assessment of regurgitant volume and regurgitant fraction has been directly compared with invasive measures in patients with mitral regurgitation.[16] These studies demonstrated an excellent correlation over a wide range of regurgitant volumes (Figure 22.2C, D). There are also studies demonstrating a good correlation between quantitative measurements by echocardiography and CVMR.[17] Quantitative flow images acquired

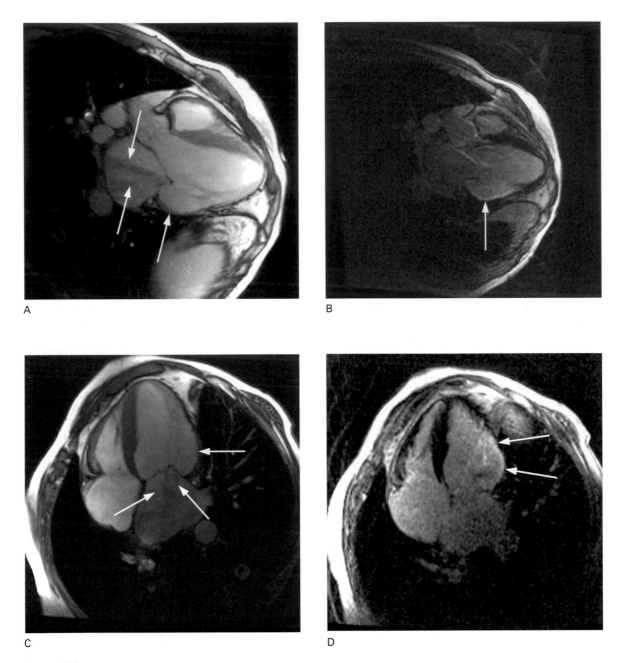

Figure 22.6

Ischemic mitral regurgitation. (A) Bright-blood, three-chamber systolic image in a patient with ischemic heart disease and mitral regurgitation. Two jets are seen in the left atrium (arrows). There is thinning of the basal posterior left ventricular wall (yellow arrow). (B) Delayed-enhancement, three-chamber image obtained after gadolinium contrast. There is evidence of extensive subendocardial scar posteriorly (yellow arrow). (C) Bright-blood, four-chamber systolic image in the same patient. The mitral regurgitant jets (arrows) are again seen and there is thinning of the lateral wall yellow arrow). (D) Delayed-enhancement, four-chamber image obtained after gadolinium contrast. There is evidence of scar in the basal and midlateral walls to the base of the papillary muscle (arrows).

in the short axis at the level of the mitral annulus (Figure 22.2) can also be compared with velocity-encoded assessment of ascending aortic flow volume to calculate regurgitant fraction and volume in patients with isolated mitral regurgitation, with good correlation with echocardiographic severity ($r = 0.87$).[18] Direct measurement of the flow across the mitral valve is possible using CVMR and has recently been used in patients selected for mitral valve repair.[19] Recently, the utility of measurement of regurgitant orifice area has been emphasized in echocardiography.[20] All of these methods can be used to assess the severity of mitral regurgitation by CVMR.

CVMR and implants and devices

Given that MRI uses magnetic fields and radio-frequency waves to image the heart, there has been extensive investigation of the effects of these fields on metallic implants, including prosthetic valves.[21,22] The force exerted on a prosthetic valve by the main magnetic field has been shown to be low at both 1.5 T and more recently at 3.0 T. Tissue heating has also been shown to be negligible at 1.5 T. However, the metal artifact produced by the valve can be significant and will depend upon details of the pulse sequence (Figure 22.7). The artifact complicates evaluation of prosthetic valve motion with CVMR, suggesting that some other imaging technique may be preferable when the primary question is prosthetic valve motion. CVMR can be particularly useful in the evaluation of perivalvular abscess in the setting of prosthetic valve endocarditis, where shadowing of the ultrasound beam due to the prosthetic valve apparatus can be significant.

With the rapid development of new devices, there is now an annually revised manual dealing with the safety of implants and devices in patients sent for CVMR and a regularly updated website (www.mrisafety.com).[23] Certain materials have been shown to be MR-compatible and to result in minimal artifact. In a study of materials used in stents,[24] signal loss was lowest for nitinol stents, with increasing loss for platinum and cobalt alloy stents. Stainless steel stents were associated with the greatest signal loss. In the design of future leaflet clips and coronary sinus annuloplasty devices, it would be highly desirable to construct them of materials that are MR-compatible, with minimal artifact if possible.

Potential future applications

Clearly, a major limitation of CVMR at present is the inability to use it for intraoperative monitoring of mitral valve repair. However, an area of active investigation at the present time is the use of CVMR in interventional procedures.[25] This poses a number of challenges: (1) the design of magnets that provide reasonable access of the physician to the patient, (2) the development of MR-compatible interventional devices, (3) tracking the position of devices in the magnet, and (4) monitoring of the patient in the MR environment. A number of groups have made substantial progress in addressing these challenges.[26] Specifically, innovative magnet designs have been developed (Figure 22.8A) that combine the capability of CVMR and conventional X-ray angiography. There has also been significant investigation of tracking of the position of catheters on the basis of artifact associated with them or with the use of specially designed catheters that actively report the position in the magnet, similar to techniques used for catheter tracing in electrophysiology (Figure 22.8B).

Interventional CVMR has been used successfully in the pediatric population to monitor the position of atrial septum occlusion devices.[25] More recently, investigators have described the intravascular placement of prosthetic pulmonary valves under CVMR guidance[27] in animal models.

Conclusion

Clinicians will increasingly require approaches to assess the severity of mitral valve disease in an increasing elderly population with important comorbidities such as coronary artery disease and cardiac dysfunction. New catheter-based therapeutic techniques substantially increase the range of patients who are candidates for intervention. This suggests that the assessment of patients with mitral valve disease will require highly accurate and quantitative methods to assess the extent and nature of the underlying pathology and the response to therapy. CVMR

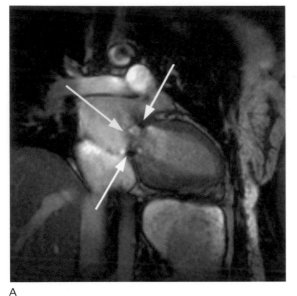

A

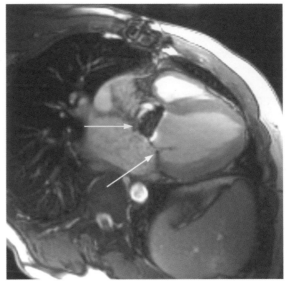

B

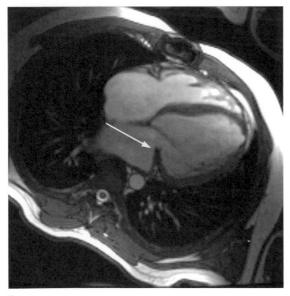

C

Figure 22.7

Mitral annuloplasty. (A) Bright-blood, two-chamber systolic image in a patient with a mitral annuloplasty ring. There is an artifact from the metallic ring (arrows) and evidence of continued mitral regurgitation (yellow arrow). (B) Bright-blood, three-chamber systolic image in a patient with a #32 Cosgrove ring annuloplasty and P2 to A2 chordal transfer. Artifact from the ring is seen posteriorly (arrow). There is also artifact from a prosthetic aortic valve (yellow arrow). (C) Bright-blood, four-chamber diastolic image in the same patient, demonstrating the alteration in the shape of the lateral mitral annulus (arrow).

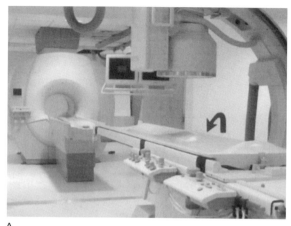
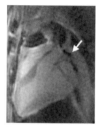
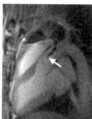
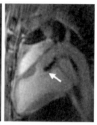

A   B

Figure 22.8

Interventional CVMR. (A) Interventional CVMR and angiography suite in which the two adjoining units are connnected by a sliding table (arrow). (Reproduced from Kuehne et al. Radiology 2003; 226: 475–81[27] with permission from the Radiological Society of North America). (B) CVMR images obtained in an animal model demonstrating catheter positioning (arrow) under CVMR guidance. (Reproduced from Buecker et al. Invest Radiol 2004; 39: 656–60.[28])

offers important advantages in the assessment of cardiac structure and function, and will play an increasing role in the evaluation of patients with mitral regurgitation.

References

1. Fogli M, Reimold S, Peshock RM. Valvular heart disease. In: Edelman RR, Hesselink JR, Zlatkin MI (eds). Clinical Magnetic Resonance Imaging, 3rd edn. Amsterdam: Elsevier, 2005.
2. Rutherford JD, Yeung AC, Reimold SC, et al. Coronary heart disease – acute coronary syndromes. In: Sutton MG, Rutherford JD (eds). Clinical Cardiovascular Imaging. A Companion to Braunwald's Heart Disease. Philadelphia: WB Saunders, 2004.
3. McCrohon JA, Moon JCC, Prasad SK, et al. Differentiation of heart failure related to dilated cardiomyopathy and coronary artery disease using gadolinium-enhanced cardiovascular magnetic resonance. Circulation 2003; 108: 54–9.
4. Peshock R, et al. Normal cardiac anatomy, orientation and function. In: Manning WJ, Pennell DJ (eds). Cardiovascular Magnetic Resonance. New York: Churchill Livingstone, 2002.
5. Kilner PJ, Yang GZ, Wilkes AJ, et al. Asymmetric redirection of flow through the heart. Nature: 2000; 404: 13.
6. Nayak KS, Cunningham CH, Santos JM, et al. Real-time color flow MRI. Magn Reson Med 2000; 43: 251 8.
7. Kim RJ, Wu E, Rafael A, et al. The use of contrast-enhanced magnetic resonance imaging to identify reversible myocardial dysfunction. N Engl J Med 2000; 343: 1445–53.
8. Hirsch KJ, Hirsch GM. Mitral valve repair. In: Perrino AC, Reeves ST (eds). A practical approach to Transesophageal Echocardiography. Philadelphia: Lippincott, Williams and Wilkins, 2003.
9. Shanewise JS, Cheung AT, Aronson S, et al. ASE/SCA Guidelines for Performing a Comprehensive Intraoperative Multiplane Transesophageal Echocardiography Examination: recommendations of the American Society of Echocardiography Council for Intraoperative Echocardiography and the Society of Cardiovascular Anesthesiologists Task Force for Certification in Perioperative Transesophageal Echocardiography. J Am Soc Echocardiogr 1999; 12: 884–900.
10. Hundley WG, Meshack BM, Willett DL, et al. Quantitation of left ventricular volumes, ejection fraction and cardiac output in patients with atrial fibrillation by cine magnetic resonance imaging: a comparison with invasive measurements. Am J Cardiol 1996; 78: 1119–23.

11. Kim WK, Damas PG, Stuber M, et al. Coronary magnetic resonance angiography for the detection of coronary stenosis. N Engl J Med 2001; 345: 1863–9.

12. Wagner S, Anffermann W, Buser P, et al. Diagnostic accuracy and estimation of the severity of valvular regurgitation from the signal void on cine magnetic resonance images. Am Heart J 1989; 118: 760–7.

13. Grothues F, Smith GC, Moon JC, et al. Comparison of interstudy reproducibility of cardiovascular magnetic resonance with two-dimensional echocardiography in normal subjects and in patients with heart failure or left ventricular hypertrophy. Am J Cardiol 2002; 90: 29–34.

14. Boxt LM, Katz J, Kolb T, et al. Direct quantitation of right and left ventricular volumes with nuclear magnetic resonance imaging in patients with primary pulmonary hypertension. J Am Coll Cardiol 1992; 19: 1508.

15. Zoghbi WA, Enriquez-Sarano M, Foster E, et al. Recommendations for evaluation of the severity of native valvular regurgitation with two-dimensional and Doppler echocardiography. J Am Soc Echocardiogr 2003; 16: 777–802.

16. Hundley WG, Li HF, Willard JE, et al. Magnetic resonance imaging assessment of the severity of mitral regurgitation: a comparison with invasive techniques. Circulation 1995; 92: 1151–8.

17. Kizilbash AM, Hundley WG, Willett DL, et al. Comparison of quantitative Doppler with magnetic resonance imaging for assessment of the severity of mitral regurgitation. Am J Cardiol 1998; 81: 792–5.

18. Fujita N, Chazouilleres AF, Hartiala JJ, et al. Quantification of mitral regurgitation by velocity-encoded cine nuclear magnetic resonance imaging. J Am Coll Cardiol 1994; 23: 951–8.

19. Westenberg JJ, Doornbos J, Versteegh MI, et al. Accurate quantitation of regurgitant volume with MRI in patients selected for mitral valve repair. Eur J Cardiothorac Surg 2005; 27: 462–6.

20. Enriquez-Sarano M, Avierinos J-F, Messika-Zeitoun D, et al. Quantitative determinants of the outcome of asymptomatic mitral regurgitation. N Engl J Med 2005; 352: 875–83.

21. Shellock FG. Prosthetic heart valves and annuloplasty rings: assessment of magnetic field interactions, heating, and artifacts at 1.5 Tesla. J Cardiovascr Magn Reson 2001; 3: 317–24.

22. Shellock FG. Biomedical implants and devices: assessment of magnetic field interactions with a 3.0-Tesla MR system. J Magn Reson Imaging 2002; 16: 721–32.

23. Reference Manual for Magnetic Resonance Safety, Implants and Devices. Los Angeles: Biomedical Research Publishing Group, 2005.

24. Wang Y, Truong TN, Yen C, et al. Quantitative evaluation of susceptibility and shielding effects of nitinol, platinum, cobalt-alloy, and stainless steel stents. Magn Reson Med 2003; 49: 972–6.

25. Razavi R, Hill DL, Keevil SF, et al. Cardiac catheterisation guided by MRI in children and adults with congenital heart disease. Lancet 2003; 362: 1877–82.

26. Barbash IM, Leor J, Feinberg MS, et al. Interventional magnetic resonance imaging for guiding gene and cell transfer in the heart. Heart 2004; 90: 87–91.

27. Kuehne T, Saeed M, Higgins CB, et al. Endovascular stents in pulmonary valve and artery in swine: feasibility study of MR imaging-guided deployment and postinterventional assessment. Radiology 2003; 226: 475–81.

28. Buecker A, Spuentrup E, Schmitz-Rode T et al. Use of a nonmetallic guide wire for magnetic resonance-guided coronary artery catheterization. Invest Radiol 2004; 39: 656–60.

23

Invasive hemodynamics for the assessment of the mitral valve

Michael J Lim, Jack L Collier, Morton J Kern

Introduction

Although echocardiography (transthoracic and transesophageal) has become the diagnostic testing modality of choice in the evaluation of the patient with mitral valve disease, direct hemodynamic assessments of valvular dysfunction in the catheterization laboratory with fluid-filled catheters remains a vital and necessary tool in the complete evaluation of many patients. Furthermore, invasive hemodynamics remains the guide for the monitoring of the effectiveness of currently available catheter-based treatment of mitral stenosis (i.e. balloon valvuloplasty), as well as forthcoming percutaneous approaches to the regurgitant valve. Because of operator and laboratory variability of some echocardiographic findings, many physicians still consider invasive hemodynamic data as among the most reliable diagnostic approach when considering the need for surgical correction. Furthermore, intraprocedural hemodynamic data are often critical to interim decisions for proceeding or terminating an intervention.

Normal mitral valve hemodynamics

Hemodynamically, mitral valve function is assessed by comparing the pressure waveforms of the left atrium (LA) and left ventricle (LV) throughout the cardiac cycle. A true LA pressure is the most reliable pressure, but for nearly all clinical measurements, the pulmonary capillary wedge pressure (PCWP) is commonly substituted for LA pressure (Figure 23.1).[1]

In normal subjects during sinus rhythm, atrial contraction produces a systolic wave (a-wave), followed by an x-descent. During atrial filling, a v-wave is produced, with its characteristic y-descent. These four typical and distinct waveforms are easily identified on the right atrial (RA), PCW, and LA hemodynamic tracings, and can be distinguished by timing the occurrence of the peak wave with the corresponding wave on the electrocardiogram (ECG) tracing (Figure 23.2). The a-wave is generally larger on the right heart tracing and the v-wave is larger on the PCW/LA tracing. When matched up against a simultaneous ECG, the a-wave, a late-diastolic event, occurs about 40 ms after the p-wave. In some tracings the x-descent will be interrupted by a brief positive deflection secondary to ventricular contraction called the c-wave (or notch). In this instance the x-wave is labeled x and x′ to signify the portion of the wave prior to and after a c-wave.

The next positive deflection following the x-decent is the v-wave, occurring near the end of ventricular systole (occurring shortly after the T-wave on the ECG). The negative deflection following the v-wave, termed the y-descent, occurs coincident with the LV pressure decline, or 40–100 ms after the LV pressure when measured by the PCWP due to delay of pressure transfer through the lungs. The magnitude of the v-wave is determined by the pressure–flow relationship of the atrial chamber. A low LA compliance (i.e. stiffness) may produce large v-waves on the PCWP tracing without significant mitral regurgitation. In

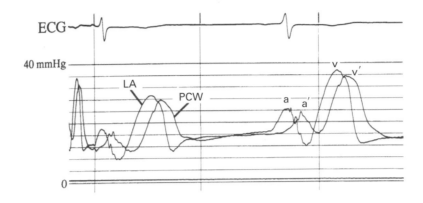

Figure 23.1

Hemodynamic tracings of the left atrium (LA) and pulmonary capillary wedge (PCW) pressure demonstrating precise a- and v-waves. The a'- and v'-waves are those of the PCW, which is delayed by approximately 120 ms. The time lines are 1 s. The pressure scale is 0–40 mmHg. (Reproduced from Kern MJ (ed). The Cardiac Catherization Handbook, 4th edn. St Louis, MO: Mosby, 2003.[3])

patients in atrial fibrillation, the c-notch may be confused with an a-wave (Figure 23.3).

PCWP versus direct LA assessment

In most circumstances, the PCWP can be used to approximate the LA pressure. Comparing PCWP and LA pressure tracings shows that the a- and v-waves on the PCWP tracings are delayed by 40–120 ms (Figure 23.1). Moreover, the peak LA v-wave occurs within the downstroke of the LV pressure, whereas the peak v-wave using the PCWP is delayed and falls outside the LV down-slope. For precise calculations of mitral pressure gradients using the PCWP compared with the LA pressure tracing, phase-shifting of the pressure v-wave to correspond to the LV pressure downstroke should be performed prior to planimetering the mitral valve gradient area.

The PCWP can be used as a reliable alternative to direct LA pressure when the pressures are low and the waveforms are normal in appearance. Several techniques are available to determine if the PCWP is accurate.[2,3] The easiest and most common is to confirm the presence of the a- and v-waves and that the v-wave corresponds to the T-wave on the ECG. Furthermore, the pulmonary artery diastolic pressure should be greater than the mean wedge pressure. An O_2 saturation drawn in the wedge position should return a value >95% (or similar to the arterial oxygen saturation) in normal individuals. In most circumstances the PCWP and the measured LA pressure should not differ by more than 2–5 mmHg.[1,3]. The PCWP may not be a reliable indicator of LA pressure in patients with elevated wedge pressures, severe pulmonary hypertension, pre-existing rheumatic mitral valve disease, significant lung disease, patients on ventilators, with prosthetic mitral valves, or with congenital anomalies.

In those cases when the PCWP is inadequate, direct LA pressure assessment is required and is obtained via a trans-septal puncture. There are multiple trans-septal techniques for crossing the atrial septum, and each physician will select a method best suited for his or her laboratory, skills, and background.

In brief, one method of trans-septal catheterization starts by visualizing the heart in an antero-posterior (AP) projection, and placing a pigtail catheter in the aorta at the sinus of Valsalva to serve as an anatomic reference point and source for aortic pressures.[3] A Mullins sheath with a Brockenbrough catheter (or the Brockenbrough catheter alone) is advanced over a guidewire to the level of the superior vena cava (SVC) via the right femoral vein. The guidewire is removed and the sheath is flushed. Next, the trans-septal needle is advanced through the catheter to the SVC. Continuous pressure monitoring is used during septal puncture through the trans-septal needle. The catheter/needle assembly is retracted

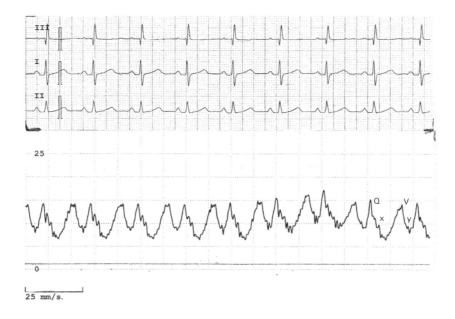

A

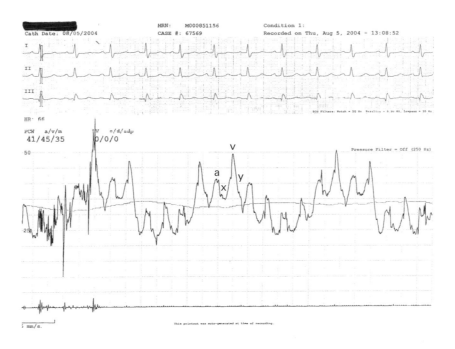

B

Figure 23.2

(A) Hemodynamic tracing of right atrial (RA) pressure. The time lines are 25 mm/s and the scale is 0–50 mm. Precise a- and v-waves can be seen in this RA pressure. The timing of the waveforms is provided from the ECG. (B) Pulmonary capillary wedge pressure (PCWP), demonstrating respiratory variation of the pressure waveform and a- and v-waves. Note that the v-wave is greater in the PCWP than in the RA pressure. The pressure scale is 0–50 mmHg.

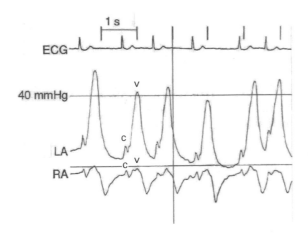

Figure 23.3

Simultaneous left atrial (LA) and right atrial (RA) pressures in a patient in atrial fibrillation. Note the large v-wave in the LA pressure, which is not present in the RA pressure. In addition, the LA pressure waveform demonstrates a c-notch which can be mistaken for an a-wave, which is absent since this patient is in atrial fibrillation. The v-wave in the RA pressure is minimal and the prominent y-descent can be appreciated in both the LA and RA pressures. The pressure scale is 0–40 mmHg.

caudally into the right atrium, sequentially crossing the aortic root and the ridge of the foramen ovale, and finally with clockwise rotation, seating in the fossa ovale. The assembly is advanced slightly, making secure purchase on the atrial septum.

Viewing the needle location in a right anterior oblique (RAO) projection will insure that the trans-septal needle is positioned in the middle of the atrial septum (Figure 23.4). The needle should not be pointing too far posteriorly. Of importance, a patent foramen ovale is present in 15–20% of patients, allowing passage into the left atrium without puncture.

While monitoring the hemodynamic tracings, the catheter/needle assembly is advanced, observing the change from RA to LA pressures. Confirmation by hemodynamic waveforms and blood oxygen saturation should be performed. Once the position has been confirmed, the sheath can be advanced into the LA over the catheter.

Complications of trans-septal catheterization have been reported to be low (<3%); they include needle-tip perforation and tamponade.[4,5] Atrial septal puncture can lead to a defect in 19–62% of

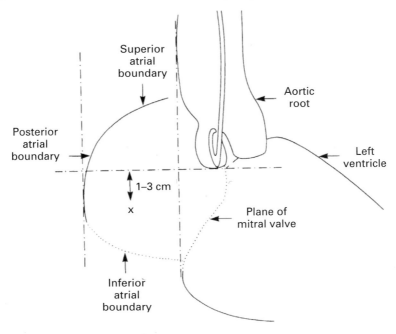

Figure 23.4

Diagrammatic representation of cardiac anatomy for trans-septal puncture. 'x' marks the mid-atrial point, at which atrial puncture would be optimal. (Reproduced from: Kern MJ (ed). The Cardiac Catheterization Handbook, 4th edn. St Louis, MO: Mosby, 2003.[3])

patients, depending on the methods used to assess atrial septal defect. A more significant and potentially lethal complication results from puncture of the aortic root, coronary sinus, or the posterior free wall of the atrium. Almost all deaths related to trans-septal catheterization are as a result of cardiac tamponade.

Pressure wave artifacts

Waveform artifacts may interfere with appropriate interpretation of the hemodynamic assessment. Accurate pressure tracings should have appropriate fidelity without underdamping or overdamping. Underdamped signals (Figure 23.5A) have exaggerated peaks representing rapidly transmitted pressure waves with sudden sharp accelerations and decelerations that create multiple oscillatory waves on the pressure tracing (also known as ringing).[3,6] An underdamped tracing can be corrected by increasing fluid path viscosity by filling the catheter with blood or contrast.

An overdamped pressure wave (Figure 23.5B) produces rounded waveforms and is often due an air bubble or contrast within the catheter or pressure tubing. Flushing the catheter, manifold, and transducer with saline, clearing air bubbles, will generally alleviate this artifact. Under- and overdamping are exaggerated with smaller-caliber catheters.

Other common hemodynamic artifacts include improper pressure recording scales, paper speed, and time lines. Loose electrical or fluid connections will also produce erroneous pressure waveforms.

Mitral valve pathology

Mitral regurgitation

Mitral regurgitation (MR) is commonly encountered in current clinical practice, representing up to 30% of patients being evaluated for bypass surgery.[7] The most common etiologies of MR include mitral valve prolapse, ischemic papillary muscle dysfunction, ruptured chordae tendinae, infective endocarditis, rheumatic heart disease, and annular dilatation secondary to a dilated cardiomyopathy. Abnormal coaptation of the mitral valve apparatus results in a regurgitant ori-

fice that remains open during systole, allowing the pressure gradient between the LV and LA to drive flow into the LA.

Normally, pulmonary venous efflux is the sole contributor to filling of the LA. With significant regurgitation of the mitral valve, atrial filling is markedly increased in late systole as the atrium receives volume from both the pulmonary veins and the LV, which is reflected hemodynamically as the v-wave (Figure 23.6). In fact, the regurgitant flow can be estimated based on the Torricelli principle, which states that the flow is proportional to the square root of the gradient across the orifice. The driving pressure gradient in MR begins with mitral valve closure and persists until mitral valve opening. However, varying causes of MR have been shown to result in varying flow patterns across the regurgitant orifice during systole.[8] Specifically, the orifice area is at its greatest during mid-systole and small during early and late systole in patients with mitral valve prolapse.[9] Patients with dilated cardiomyopathy have been shown to have a progressively decreasing orifice area throughout systole,[10] while those with rheumatic MR have a constant orifice area during systole. These differences in regurgitant flow patterns contribute to the varying murmurs auscultated in these patients and flow patterns observed on color flow Doppler examinations, but do not substantially change the invasive hemodynamic profile of these patients.

The size of the v-wave does not uniquely reflect the degree of MR.[11,12] Rather, compliance and the pressure–volume (P–V) properties of the LA determine the v-wave amplitude (Figure 23.7). Four principal factors acting on the LA P–V relationship can influence the morphology of the v-wave: (1) the value of blood entering the atrium during ventricular systole (i.e. mitral regurgitation), (2) the rate of forward flow into the atrium, (3) systemic afterload, and (4) LV contractile force. Severe MR can produce a normal v-wave tracing in the face of a compliant atrium. In addition to mitral regurgitation, large v-waves are also seen in mitral stenosis (low compliance) and high-volume states (e.g. patients with a ventricular septal defect). LA stiffening secondary to ischemia, hypertrophy, or tachycardia with decreased diastolic emptying (shorter PR interval) can result in large v-waves.

Mitral regurgitation can occur acutely, resulting in a sudden rise in LA volume and a fall in

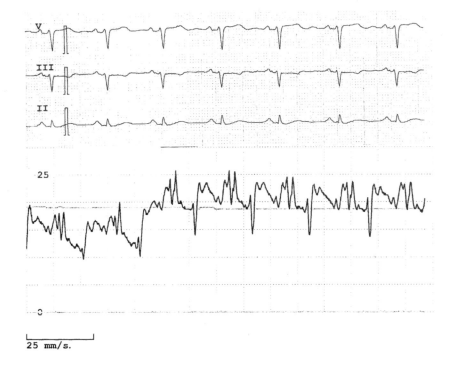

A

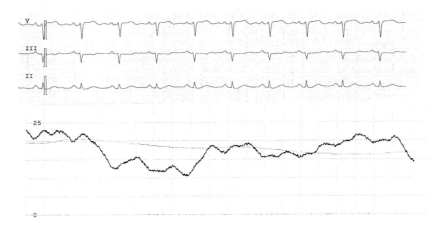

B

Figure 23.5

(A) Underdamped right atrial pressure waveform. (B) Overdamped pressure wave in the same patient. Compare these tracings with Figure 23.2(A).

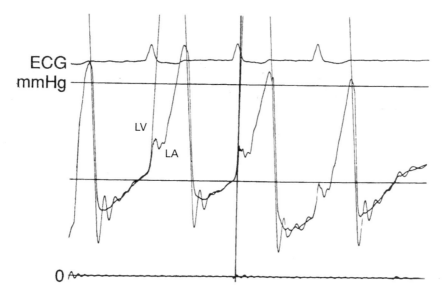

Figure 23.6

Left ventricular (LV) and left atrial (LA) pressures on a 0–40 scale demonstrating correspondence of LA and LV pressures across diastole. Note the large v-wave beginning just after isovolumetric contraction and the lack of gradient between the LA and LV pressure on the initiation of diastole. There is no narrowing to cause a pressure gradient and the severe mitral regurgitation demonstrates complete chamber equilibration between LA and LV in diastole. (Reproduced from: Kern MJ (ed). The Cardiac Catheterization Handbook, 4th edn, St Louis, MO: Mosby, 2003.[3])

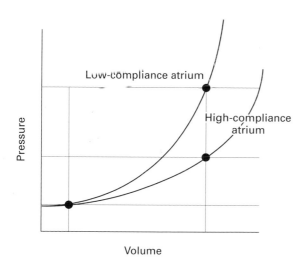

Figure 23.7

Pressure–volume curves of two patients who have low- and high-compliance atria, respectively. In the case of high-compliance atrium, a large increase in volume produces only a small increase in pressure, whereas on a low-compliance atrium, the same increase in volume produces a doubling of the pressure waveform.

forward stroke volume and cardiac output. Because of the rapidity of the increase in volume, the only way in which the LA can accommodate the increase in volume is the rapid development of pulmonary congestion. As a result, large v-waves may be more prominent in these patients, along with elevated PCWP and pulmonary arterial pressures. These features appear in contrast to patients with chronic MR, where the LA dilates, accommodating the increase in volume. This compensation also increases LA compliance, which often blunts the transmission of v-waves in the PCWP tracing. Often, the PCWP and pulmonary pressures remain nearly normal in patients with chronic MR.

Mitral stenosis

The incidence of mitral stenosis (MS) in the USA has changed over the last century, with a dramatic decline in rheumatic heart disease. Other causes of MS remain rare, but include mitral annular calcification, in elderly patients, resulting in reduced mitral valve leaflet mobility. Despite the etiology of MS, the hallmark of the disease is a reduced orifice area for blood flow from the LA to the LV, resulting in a pressure gradient between these two chambers (an LA-to-LV gradient). To maintain cardiac output in the face of a reduced orifice area, larger and larger pressure gradients are required. The relationship between flow and pressure as described in the Gorlin formula is used to calculate an estimated mitral valve area using standard hemodynamic measurements (equation 1). A simplified version of this formula (Hakke) is also used commonly in clinical practice (equation 2):

$$MVA = \frac{CO/DFP}{K \times \sqrt{MVG}} \qquad (1)$$

$$MVA = \frac{CO}{\sqrt{MVG}} \qquad (2)$$

where CO is the cardiac output (in ml/min), DFP is the diastolic filling period (in s), K (= 37.9) is a constant for mitral valve assessment, MVA is the mitral valve area (in cm^2), and MVG is the mean valve gradient (in mmHg). Because the heart rate and diastolic filling period are not included in equation (2), this simplified formula is less accurate with atrial fibrillation, tachycardia, bradycardia, and low-output states. In patients with concomitant MR, both formulae underestimate the valve area, because neither calculation can account for the regurgitant flow. However, quantitative angiographic assessment of the LV stroke volume can be performed and has been utilized in the calculation of cardiac output to more accurately measure the valve area in the setting of coexisting MR.

Clinical decision-making in MS is based primarily on the estimated valve area computed from echocardiography or from catheterization. The normal mitral valve area generally exceeds 4 cm^2. Mild MS is characterized by a valve area of 1.5–2 cm^2, moderate MS by an area between 1 and 1.5 cm^2, and severe MS by an area of less than 1 cm^2.[7]

Calculation of the mitral valve area as part of routine catheterization in patients with MS often utilizes the PCWP in place of direct LA pressure

assessment. It must be noted that investigators have found that the transmitral gradient can be slightly overestimated when using the PCWP (Figure 23.1).[13] Thus, care must be taken to assure that the PCWP is accurate (as previously described) before calculating the valve area in these patients, and trans-septal techniques to directly assess the LA pressure should be utilized if there are concerns.

In patients with MS in sinus rhythm, mean LA pressure is elevated and characterized by a prominent v-wave with a gradual pressure decline after mitral valve opening (y-descent). The a-wave is also exaggerated during atrial contraction. Measurement of the mitral valve gradient is performed by simultaneously recording the LV and PCW (or LA) pressures. As seen in Figure 23.8, the area between the pressure tracings during diastole can be calculated and the mean mitral valve gradient subsequently derived. Pulmonary pressures become elevated with more significant elevations in LA pressure and therefore have been used as a marker for the hemodynamic consequences of MS. However, in the early stages of the disease, LA and pulmonary arterial pressures are often normal or nearly normal. If the patient's symptoms are prominent in this situation, hemodynamic measurements during exercise provocation are indicated (Figure 23.9). A subset of patients will have significant elevations in pulmonary arterial pressure accompanied by an increase in the transmitral gradient in response to exercise, indicating a more severe form of the disease than the resting hemodynamics would suggest.[14]

Occasionally, there is a subset of patients with significant symptoms limiting activity but in whom, upon initial evaluation with non-invasive testing or invasive hemodynamics, there is little gradient across the mitral valve. In these patients, it has been found that this discrepancy can be further evaluated with exercise testing or dobutamine administration. In this way, the exercise tolerance transmitral gradient response to exercise and pulmonary artery pressures can be obtained in a serial fashion. With exercise evaluation, patients with pulmonary arterial pressure elevation greater than 60 mmHg, mean transmitral gradient greater than 15 mmHg or PCWP greater than 25 mmHg with exertion have been found to have significant mitral stenosis and should be considered for treatment.[15–17]

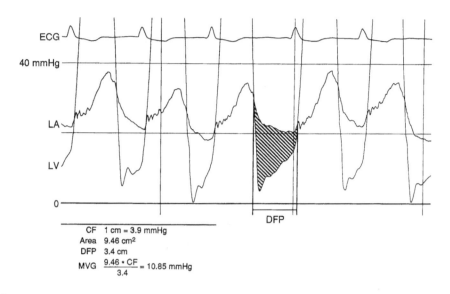

CF   1 cm = 3.9 mmHg
Area 9.46 cm²
DFP   3.4 cm
MVG $\dfrac{9.46 \cdot CF}{3.4}$ = 10.85 mmHg

Figure 23.8

Left atrial (LA) and left ventricular (LV) pressure tracings in a patient with mitral stenosis. The diastolic filling period (DFP) is shaded, a factor for calculation (CF) is provided, and the mitral valve gradient (MVG) from the traditional Gorlin formula is also provided. Mitral stenosis in this case involves the patient in atrial fibrillation. There is no a-wave and the c-notch can be really appreciated. (Reproduced from Kern MJ (ed). The Cardiac Catheterization Handbook, 4th edn, St Louis, MO: Mosby, 2003.[3])

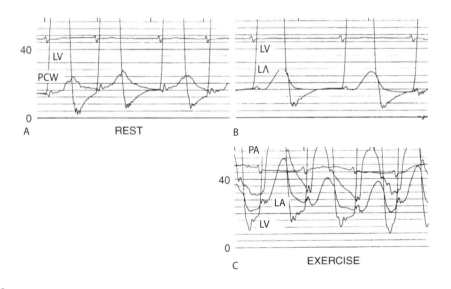

Figure 23.9

A: Left ventricular (LV) and pulmonary capillary wedge (PCW) pressures in a patient with a low mitral valve gradient. Note the end-equilibration of LV and PCW pressures. The scale is 0–40 mmHg. B: Left atrial (LA) and LV pressures in the same patient. Note the improved LA pressure v-wave with equilibration of the pressure gradient at mid-diastole. C: With exercise, the LA and LV pressures now demonstrate a significant diastolic gradient of at least 8 mmHg. This example demonstrates the added information obtained by exercise hemodynamics in patients with mild mitral stenosis. (Reproduced from: Kern MJ (ed). The Cardiac Catheterization Handbook, 4th edn. St Louis, MO: Mosby, 2003.[3])

Bioprosthetic valve assessment

Diagnosis of prosthetic valve dysfunction often proves challenging, as there are frequently discordant data obtained from different testing modalities.[18,19] Prosthetic valves have varying natural histories due to their individual characteristics, such as durability, thrombogenicity, and orifice area. Mechanical valves, and in particular the dual-leaflet metallic valves, have been widely accepted as the standard because of their durability. However, the use of bioprosthetic valves has recently been increasing. Clinical and hemodynamic evaluation for recurrent symptoms must be performed to exclude bioprosthetic failure.

Complete assessment of a mechanical or bioprosthetic mitral valve requires both echocardiography and catheterization. Transesophageal echocardiography assesses valve ring stability, leaflet motion, and valve surface and orifice areas. Transvalvular hemodynamic data from catheterization continues to represent the gold standard for the assessment of the effective orifice area in prosthetic valves, and often requires trans-septal approach to assess direct LA pressure. Depending on the type of prosthetic valve, different expected effective orifice areas are seen (Table 23.1).

Specific considerations regarding the invasive hemodynamic assessment of a prosthetic mitral valve center around accurate estimation of the LA pressure. Specifically, the PCWP may be erroneously high in these patients, leading to an overestimate of the mitral gradient. Therefore, operators should carefully evaluate the accuracy of the wedge tracing. Trans-septal catheterization should be performed in those patients with discordant hemodynamic data or significant clinical symptoms.

Table 23.1 Expected hemodynamic characteristics of prosthetic mitral valves

Valve type	Effective orifice area (cm^2)
Caged ball	1.4–3.1
Single tilting disk	1.9–3.2
Bileaflet tilting disk	2.8–3.4
Heterograft bioprosthesis	1.7–2.5

From: Otto CM (ed). Textbook of Clinical Echocardiography, 2nd edn. Philadelphia: WB Saunders, 2000.[19]

Hemodynamics of mitral balloon valvuloplasty

The hemodynamics of mitral balloon valvuloplasty can be appreciated by a clinical case example. A 49-year-old woman has progressive dyspnea on exertion. She recalls a prolonged 'febrile' childhood illness associated with joint aches and rash. A heart murmur was found on high school physical examination. Her echocardiogram suggested mitral valve disease. Cardiac catheterization provided the initial hemodynamic tracing (Figure 23.10). Based on the mitral hemodynamics obtained with the PCW, one might conclude that there is a mitral valve gradient. However, this tracing is of poor quality and thus may not reflect the exact valvular gradient. An LA trans-septal puncture was performed. The PCW pressure and direct LA pressure from the trans-septal technique are compared in Figure 23.11 and show that the mean pressures of the PCW and LA are equal but the phasic natures of the waveforms do not correspond. Because of the poor fidelity, the PCWP here should not be used for valve assessment in this patient. Before balloon valvuloplasty, the direct LA pressure by the trans-septal approach and the LV pressure was recorded (Figure 23.12). From these hemodynamics, it is easy to appreciate that the there is normal sinus rhythm, with a mean LA–LV gradient of approximately 14 mmHg. Note that the LA v-wave is larger than the a-wave. Mitral balloon valvuloplasty is hemodynamically indicated, provided that the clinical and echocardiographic findings are concordant and the echocardiographic score is favorable. Mitral balloon valvuloplasty was then performed (Figure 23.13).

After balloon valvuloplasty, the PCWP demonstrated a residual significant gradient and indicated that the procedure, based on hemodynamics, appeared to be incomplete (Figure 23.14). Since the PCWP was not a reliable tracing to gauge mitral gradients initially, the direct LA pressure is again needed (Figure 23.15). Using the LA pressure, there is no significant residual gradient, nor is there any hemodynamically important mitral regurgitation. The procedure is finished.

The initial poor-quality PCWP did not clearly delineate the a- or v-waves. A mitral gradient cannot be precisely determined based on the quality

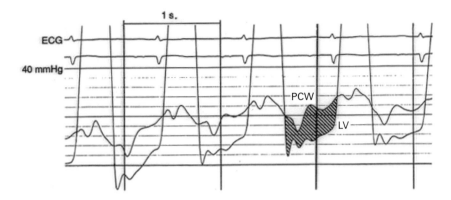

Figure 23.10

Pulmonary capillary wedge (PCW) and left ventricular (LV) pressures in a patient with suspected mitral stenosis. The poor fidelity of the PCW waveform limits the ability to appreciate the true gradient. (Reproduced from: Kern MJ (ed). The Cardiac Catheterization Handbook, 4th edn. St Louis, MO: Mosby, 2003.[3])

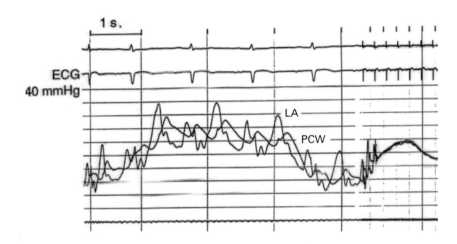

Figure 23.11

Simultaneous left atrial (LA) and pulmonary capillary wedge (PCW) pressure recordings on a 0–40 scale. The mean pressures are equal, but the phasic components of each pressure demonstrate superior fidelity of the LA pressure. (Reproduced from: Kern MJ (ed). The Cardiac Catheterization Handbook, 4th edn. St Louis, MO: Mosby, 2003.[3])

of this tracing. However, because the LA and PCW mean pressures match, the estimate of the valve gradient would not likely exceed 16 mmHg from this tracing. One might infer that the patient probably does not have significant MR, since there is no v-wave. A normal mitral valve gradient with this PCWP wave artifact is a possibility, but is inconsistent with the physical examination.

On consideration of the LA and PCW, the two mean pressures are the same, although the fidelity of the LA waveform is obviously much better than that of the PCWP. If the fidelities of the tracings were the same, either could be used to assess MS. The mean LA–LV pressure gradient is approximately 14 mmHg, which can be estimated by counting the number of 4 mmHg divisions across the diastolic period. An estimation of the mitral valve area can be made using the quick formula or (Hakke) formula (MVA = cardiac output divided by the square root of the mean gradient).

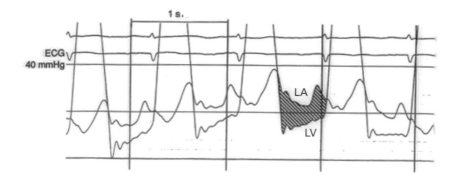

Figure 23.12

Left atrial (LA) and left ventricular (LV) pressures in the same individual demonstrating a good-fidelity LA pressure waveform and a significant mitral valve gradient of approximately 14 mmHg. Note that the a-wave and v-wave are easily identified in this particular patient, who is in sinus rhythm. (Reproduced from: Kern MJ (ed). The Cardiac Catheterization Handbook, 4th edn. St Louis, MO: Mosby, 2003.[3])

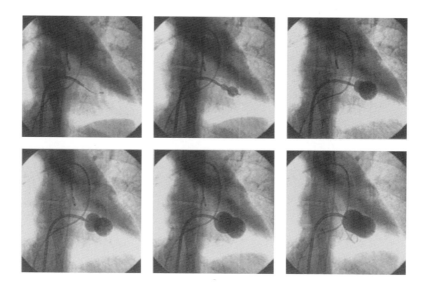

Figure 23.13

Sequential inflations of the Inoue valvuloplasty balloon for mitral valve stenosis. (Reproduced from Kern MJ (ed). The Cardiac Catheterization Handbook, 4th edn. St Louis, MO: Mosby, 2003.[3])

This quick formula does not apply for heart rates >100 or <60 beats/min. As discussed earlier, a large v-wave alone does not necessarily indicate severe MR in patients with low atrial compliance.

After the valvuloplasty procedure, based on direct LA and LV tracings, there is no significant v-wave or suggestion that MR occurred. There is little potential for an erroneous gradient unless major zeroing errors have occurred. Erroneous assumptions regarding the presence or absence of gradients can be made if one relies on PCWP tracings with poor fidelity.

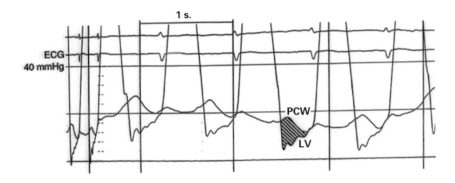

Figure 23.14

Following balloon valvuloplasty, the pulmonary capillary wedge (PCW) and left ventricular (LV) pressures were recorded. Note the significant residual mitral valve gradient. Based on the fidelity of the initial PCW pressure recordings, this gradient may be in question. (Reproduced from: Kern MJ (ed). The Cardiac Catheterization Handbook, 4th edn. St Louis, MO: Mosby, 2003.[3])

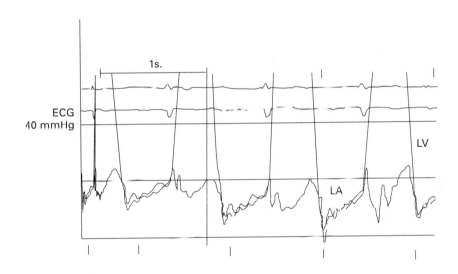

Figure 23.15

Left atrial (LA) and left ventricular (LV) pressures following mitral valvuloplasty, demonstrating complete elimination of mitral valve gradient and no significant v-waves, indicating a successful procedure without mitral regurgitation. (Reproduced from: Kern MJ (ed). The Cardiac Catheterization Handbook, 4th edn. St Louis, MO: Mosby, 2003.[3])

Conclusion

Hemodynamic assessment of the mitral valve supports echocardiographic and clinical findings with regard to MS and MR. Discrepancies in clinical and echographic findings can be resolved by accurate hemodynamic assessment across the mitral valve using either good-fidelity PCWP tracings or LA pressure directly after trans-septal access. The accurate calculation of cardiac output and hemodynamic data provide the best result for calculation of mitral valve area using either the standard Gorlin or Hakke formulae. Examples of hemodynamic tracings provided in this chapter should assist the physician in determining optimal hemodynamic assessment of the mitral valve.

References

1. Lange RA, Moore DM, Cigarroa RG, Hillis LD. Use of pulmonary capillary wedge pressure to assess severity of mitral stenosis: is true left atrial pressure needed in this condition? J Am Coll Cardiol 1989; 13: 825–9.

2. Rapaport E, Dexter L. Pulmonary 'capillary' pressure. Meth Med Res 1958; 7: 85–93.

3. Kern MJ (ed). The Cardiac Catheterization Handbook, 4th edn. St Louis, MO: Mosby, 2003.

4. Clugston R, Lau FYK, Ruiz C. Transseptal catheterizations update 1992. Cathet Cardiovasc Diagn 1992; 26: 266–74.

5. Roelke M, Smith AJ, Palacios IF. The technique and safety of transseptal left heart catheterization and the Massachusetts General Hospital experience with 1279 procedures. Cathet Cardiovasc Diagn 1994; 32: 332–9.

6. Lambert CR, Pepine CJ, Nichols WW. Pressure measurements. In: Pepine CJ (ed). Diagnostic and Therapeutic Cardiac Catheterization. Baltimore: Williams and Wilkins, 1989: 283–93.

7. Rahimtoola SH, Durauraj A, Mehra A, Nuno I. Current evaluation and management of patients with mitral stenosis. Circulation 2002; 106: 1183–8.

8. Schwammenthal E, Chen C, Benning F, et al. Dynamics of mitral regurgitation flow and orifice area. Physiologic application of the proximal flow coverage method: clinical data and experienced testing. Circulation 1994; 90: 307–22.

9. Enriquez-Sarano M, Sinak L, Tajik A, et al. Changes in effective regurgitant orifice throughout systole in patients with mitral valve prolapse: a clinical study using the proximal isovelocity surface area method. Circulation 1995; 92: 2951–8.

10. Yim SF, Enriques-Sarano M, Tribouilloy C, et al. Determinants of the degree of mitral regurgitation in patients with systolic left ventricular dysfunction. Circulation 2000; 102: 1400.

11. Pichard AD, Kay R, Smith H, et al. Large V waves in the pulmonary wedge pressure tracing in the absence of mitral regurgitation. Am J Cardiol 1982; 50: 1044–50.

12. Fuchs RM, Menser RR, Yin FCP, et al. Limitations of pulmonary wedge V waves in diagnosing mitral regurgitation. Am J Cardiol 1982; 49: 849–54.

13. Nishimura RA, Rihal CS, Tajik AJ, Holmes DR. Accurate measurement of the transmitral gradient in patient with mitral stenosis. A simultaneous catheterization and Doppler echocardiographic study. J Am Coll Cardiol 1994; 24: 152–8.

14. Gorlin R, Sawyer CG, Haynes FW, et al. Effects of exercise on circulatory dynamics in mitral stenosis. Am Heart J 1951; 41: 192–203.

15. Cheriex EC, Pieters FA, Janssen JH, et al. Value of exercise Doppler echocardiography in patients with mitral stenosis. Int J Cardiol 1994; 45: 219–26.

16. Tamai J, Nagata S, Akaike M, et al. Improvement in mitral flow dynamics during exercise after percutaneous intravenous mitral commissurotomy: noninvasive evaluation using continuous-wave Doppler technique. Circulation 1990; 81: 46–51.

17. Leavitt JI, Coats MH, Falk RH. Effects of exercise on transmitral gradient and pulmonary artery pressure in patients with mitral stenosis or in prosthetic mitral valve: a Doppler echocardiographic study. J Am Coll Cardiol 1991; 17: 1520–6.

18. Vongpatanasin W, Hillis LD, Lange RD. Prosthetic heart valves. N Engl J Med 1996; 335: 407–16.

19. Otto CM (ed): Textbook of Clinical Echocardiography, 2nd edn. Philadelphia: WB Saunders, 2000.

24

Impact of emerging percutaneous techniques of mitral valve repair on cardiology and cardiac surgical practice

Peter C Block

Mitral valve surgery is the second most common valvular surgery performed in the USA,[1] and over the last decade its volume has doubled (Figure 24.1). In the USA, rheumatic disease is an increasingly uncommon indication for mitral valve surgery, and most mitral valve operations are performed for other etiologies of mitral regurgitation. Mitral valve replacement with or without associated coronary artery bypass surgery totaled more than 65 000 cases in 2003.[1] Mitral valve repair has had a similar dramatic increase in volume over the same time period. In 2003, mitral valve repair was performed in approximately 20 000 patients, and repair associated

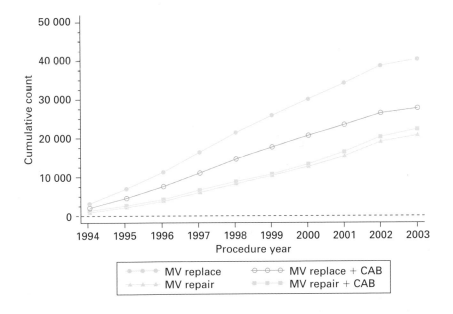

Figure 24.1

Number of mitral valve (MV) operations performed in the USA in 1994–2003.[1] CAB, coronary artery bypass surgery.

with coronary artery bypass surgery accounted for an additional 20 000 cases. Length of stay in hospital over the last decade has slowly declined (Figure 24.2), but still averages from approximately 1 week for mitral valve repair surgery alone to almost 2 weeks for mitral valve replacement combined with coronary artery bypass surgery.[1]

The surgical mortality for first-time elective mitral valve repair is low (2.5% in males, 3.9% in females), but there is an overall complication rate of 35%, including infectious, neurologic, pulmonary, and renal complications.[2] When combined with coronary artery bypass surgery, the morbidity and mortality rates for mitral valve surgery increase to 6.1% for males and 12.2% for females. Patients undergoing a second thoracic operation also have higher mortality. Thus, although surgical mitral valve repair and replacement are common, there are still risks associated with the surgery.

The most common causes of mitral regurgitation (MR) can be classified into four categories: ischemic, degenerative, cardiomyopathic, and rheumatic.[3] However, to discuss patient selection for treatment of MR, it is recommended to focus on leaflet dysfunction as opposed to etiology.[4] This classification is based on the opening and closing motions of the mitral leaflets. Patients with type I dysfunction have normal leaflet motion. MR in these patients is due to annular dilatation or leaflet perforation. There is increased leaflet motion in patients with type II dysfunction, with the free edge of the leaflet overriding the plane of the annulus during systole (leaflet prolapse). The most common lesions responsible for type II dysfunction are chordal elongation or rupture and papillary muscle elongation or rupture. Patients with type IIIa dysfunction have restricted leaflet motion during both diastole and systole. The most common lesions are leaflet thickening/retraction, chordal thickening/shortening or fusion, and commissural fusion. The mechanism of MR in type IIIb dysfunction is restricted leaflet motion during systole. Left ventricular enlargement with apical papillary muscle displacement due to ischemic or idiopathic cardiomyopathy causes this type of valve dysfunction. Thus, consideration of both leaflet pathology and abnormalities of the mitral supporting apparatus must be taken into account when any type of repair procedure is contemplated.

The importance of the mitral valve's papillary muscle architecture to left ventricular function has shifted the preferred surgical approach to MR from replacement to repair.[1,2] In general, mitral valve repair is superior to replacement for MR, with lower operative mortality, improved late sur-

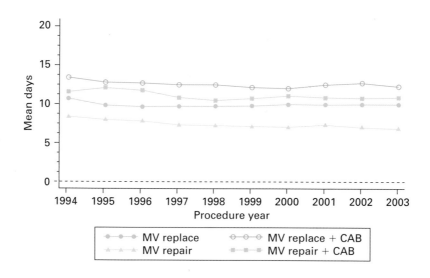

Figure 24.2

Length of stay for patients undergoing mitral valve surgery in the USA in 1994–2003.[1] CAB, coronary artery bypass surgery.

vival, a reduced risk of endocarditis, fewer thromboembolic complications, and better preservation of left ventricular function.[1,2,5–8] However, not all patients are candidates for valve repair. Successful mitral valve repair is dependent on individual valve anatomy and pathology, and many patients require valve replacement instead. Thus, for rheumatic MR, the distorted leaflet anatomy secondary to fibrosis, the associated subvalvular fibrosis, and calcification rarely allow valve repair. Annular dilatation, alteration of the subvalvular apparatus, and distorted leaflet tissue also present special challenges to successful valve repair. For these reasons, most surgeons attempt a complete repair, combining direct valvular restoration with an annuloplasty device. In the evaluation of patients for possible percutaneous transcatheter repair or replacement, these valuable lessons learned over many years of surgical experience must not be forgotten. The challenges are magnified severalfold in percutaneous approaches.

The long-term experience of open annuloplasty repair provides valuable lessons in applying percutaneous technology indiscriminately to all patients with MR caused by annular dilatation. Recent evidence would suggest that: (a) the trigone-to-trigone area is not a rigid fixed structure, as previously thought, and dilatation also occurs in this area;[9,10] (b) significant leaflet tethering caused by papillary displacement may not be correctable by annuloplasty alone;[11,12] and (c) patients with ischemic MR may have an earlier return of regurgitation when a flexible posterior annuloplasty device is used rather than a more rigid, complete remodeling ring.[13,14] Similarly, despite favorable reports from Alfieri et al,[14] the use of the edge-to-edge technique as a standalone procedure remains a source of debate in the surgical literature. The best results using the Alfieri technique are produced when the procedure is performed with an associated annuloplasty. Midterm results have demonstrated suboptimal results of the edge-to-edge technique for MR repair when performed without an annuloplasty, and in patients with ischemic MR.[15,16] Coupling percutaneous annular remodeling with percutaneous edge-to-edge technology may address some of these concerns,[17] although undoubtedly there are patients who can be treated with the production of a double-orifice valve alone.

Surgical approaches to cardiac valve repair and replacement require the use of cardiopulmonary bypass, usually in association with cardioplegic cardiac arrest. However, the trend in all of cardiac surgery is to minimize the extent of intervention, particularly with respect to thoracotomy and its associated morbidities. Percutaneous delivery of cardioplegia solution via coronary and coronary sinus catheters now allows valvular cardiac surgery through minithoracotomies. Robotic surgery and less invasive techniques for minimizing the invasiveness of cardiac valvular surgery are in development. It is clear that the future of cardiac surgery is in optimizing a minimalist approach.[1,2,5–8] The logical progression of this goal is the development and appropriate use of percutaneous endovascular techniques for the treatment of cardiac valvular disease. Thus, both interventional cardiologists and cardiac surgeons are approaching the same goal, although from opposite directions.

Systems for percutaneous mitral valve repair incorporate two primary approaches: (1) mitral annuloplasty[18] and (2) anterior and posterior leaflet attachment using an edge-to-edge clip or suture.[19,20] Posterior annuloplasty can be accomplished by device placement in either the coronary sinus or the left atrium (or a combination) or by device placement behind the posterolateral wall of the left ventricle. All are designed to reduce the circumference of the posterior mitral annulus or to move the posterior annulus toward the anterior leaflet, thereby improving mitral valve coaptation. The concept faces multiple anatomic challenges very much like surgical repair. These include dilatation of the trigone-to-trigone area, leaflet tethering by papillary muscle displacement, mitral annular calcification, inability to fix the annuloplasty to the fibrous trigone, and the potential for compromise of the circumflex coronary artery as it passes beneath the coronary sinus. Newer concepts include intra-atrial devices that mimic surgical annuloplasty devices more closely. These might circumvent some of the potential pitfalls of coronary sinus devices. Despite the fact that the coronary sinus lies adjacent to the annulus, anatomic variability of their relation is great. In some patients, the sinus lies below the posterior annular plane, and although a 'cinching' device might constrict the posterior annulus and/or move it forward relative to the anterior leaflet of the mitral valve, if atrial muscle alone transmits the effect of the device, then dilatation of the relatively thin atrial muscle may occur over time and the desired effect may be lessened or lost. However, if the relationship of the sinus to the posterior annulus is such that the device exerts an effect on the annulus directly, or if adequate forward positioning of the posterior annulus is produced, the effect may be salutary and permanent. The effects of a chronic foreign body device within the coronary sinus are not known, although long-term experience with transvenous left ventricular pacemakers placed in a similar position is comforting.

To circumvent the potential inability to use the coronary sinus as a conduit in all patients, some devices might be placed directly onto the anterior and posterior fibrous annulus via a trans-septal approach, or a percutaneous transmyocardial cinching device placed within the pericardium might be an alternative solution. All of these and more are under consideration, and will have to await proof-of-principle demonstrations and ultimately phase I and phase II trials in humans.

The edge-to-edge repair concept has been used extensively in surgically treated patients, but the best results have been obtained when combined with an annuloplasty.[14] The results of edge-to-edge repair have been suboptimal in patients with restricted leaflet motion (type III dysfunction), including a recent surgical series where it was used in combination with a partial band posterior annuloplasty in patients with ischemic regurgitation.[12] However, in phase I trials (EVEREST), percutaneous repair has effectively reduced the severity of MR, albeit in highly selected patients who have either mitral valve prolapse involving the A2/P2 region of the valve or in patients with ischemic MR who have slight restriction of leaflet motion but still enough depth of coaptation to allow clip attachment. A more precise duplication of the Alfieri procedure will be produced by the placement of a transcatheter stitch to join the anterior and posterior mitral leaflets, thereby mimicking the open surgical technique. It is anticipated that these and possibly other techniques will be studied in both phase I and phase II trials to determine safety and efficacy in the long term.

How will all of these developments – and, in some cases, clashing ideas – affect the care of cardiac patients with valvular heart disease? Undoubtedly, there will be controversy, but this should be coupled with the realization that the new percutaneous techniques will allow us to better understand valvular heart disease and the effects of intervention (both surgical and percutaneous). Most importantly, it will give cardiologists and cardiac surgeons the opportunity to collaborate in the design of trials that will help develop the best strategies for patient care. Some patients with MR will be best served by a percutaneous approach. Others will still need surgical correction, and a third group may need a form of 'hybrid' therapy in which minimally invasive surgical and percutaneous transcatheter techniques are used concomitantly. An example of such a patient might be one with a complex atherosclerotic lesion at the take-off of the left anterior descending (LAD) coronary artery (possibly best treated with off-pump robotic or minimally invasive LIMA/LAD surgery (LIMA = left internal mammary artery)) associated with severe MR, which could be treated with a percutaneous repair. Catheterization laboratories will begin to look more like operating rooms with appropriate support facilities, and operating rooms will begin to look like catheterization laboratories with fluoroscopy and cineangiographic capability. Cardiac surgical and interventional cardiology teams will likely combine to map out the best strategies for individual patients and use their combined skills in the same setting. This will minimize hospital stays and patient care costs.

The treatment strategies for patients with MR are already changing, with a shift toward earlier intervention. Current guidelines[21] point out that, for the patient with MR, the onset of symptoms, atrial arrhythmias (especially atrial fibrillation), presence of pulmonary hypertension, or onset of left ventricular decompensation heralded by a left ventricular ejection fraction (LVEF) of <60% and a left ventricular end-systolic dimension (ESD) of >45 mm, repair or replacement should be considered. In addition, in patients in whom repair is highly likely, operation at present should be considered for the following groups: (1) acute symptomatic MR for which repair is likely; (2) patients with New York Heart Association (NYHA) II–IV symptoms and normal left ventricular function (LVEF >0.60 and ESD <45 mm); (3) symptomatic or asymptomatic patients with LVEF 0.50–0.60 and ESD 45–50 mm; (4) symptomatic or asymptomatic patients with moderate left ventricular dysfunction (LVEF 0.30–0.50 and/or ESD 50–55 mm).

Lastly, the guidelines note that in an asymptomatic patient with severe MR and normal left ventricular function, mitral repair may be contemplated to preserve left ventricular size and function and prevent the sequelae of chronic MR. When percutaneous technologies can be used routinely, earlier treatment of MR will become standard and early intervention might well result in better long-term outcome with regard to left ventricular function and the other deleterious results of chronic left ventricular volume overload. It is difficult to imagine that percutaneous technologies will allow repair of MR of all causes. As percutaneous techniques improve, certainly more patients will be candidates for treatment, but it is unlikely that in the near future, flail leaflet segments due to ruptured chordae, complex chordal shortening, and similar conditions will not still require surgery. Percutaneous technology is new, and should proceed cautiously. Patients should be carefully chosen so as to minimize risk and maximize the chance for success. This, at first, will limit candidates for percutaneous repair.

Finally, how should the new percutaneous technologies be tested? A major problem with all new devices is how to evaluate a first-generation product against the established 'gold standard' (in this case, a cardiac surgical procedure). How should a new device that avoids cardiac surgery but is less efficacious – especially initially – be best evaluated? Randomized controlled trials must be used to evaluate the superiority or clinical equivalence of the percutaneous device(s). It is important to point out that it is statistically impossible to demonstrate equivalence between two treatments. Therefore, a 'clinically acceptable' difference ('delta') between the two treatments must be specified at the outset. Safety and efficacy must be evaluated separately, although each endpoint may best be evaluated with either trial design. For some patients, a comparison of percutaneous technology with medical therapy might be needed (for example, a comparison between standard medical therapy and percutaneous repair of MR in patients with cardiomyopathy and severe mitral regurgitation). To make evaluation more difficult, in any trial designed to evaluate an intervention, 'crossovers' in patient care will occur and will have to be taken into account in evaluating the outcome of the trial.

The design of a phase II trial evaluating percutaneous mitral repair (annular- or leaflet-based) will depend on safety and durability data from a phase I study. Safety data will have to be accumulated for up to at least 1 year. Additionally, one will need to know the capacity of a successful repair in salvage or 'rescue' operations in the event of device failure or a procedural complication, documenting whether the device negatively altered the open surgical procedure. All of these issues will have to be carefully thought out by those participating in trial design and in reviewing the outcome. This will present a unique opportunity for cardiologists and cardiac surgeons to interact and collaborate so as to maximize the knowledge gained from, and utilization of, the results.

References

1. Society of Thoracic Surgeons Adult Cardiovascular National Database, Spring 2004 executive summary contents: www.sts.org.
2. Enriquez-Sarano M, Schaff HV, Orszulak TA, et al. Valve repair improves the outcome of surgery for mitral regurgitation. Circulation 1995; 91: 1022–8.
3. Otto CM. Evaluation and management of chronic mitral regurgitation. N Engl J Med 2001; 335: 740–6.
4. Carpentier A. Cardiac valve surgery – the "French connection". J Thorac Cardiovasc Surg 1983; 86: 323–37.
5. Fucci C, Sandrelli L, Pardini A, et al. Improved results with mitral valve repair using new surgical techniques. Eur J Cardiothorac Surg 1995; 9: 621 6.
6. Maisano F, Torraca L, Oppizzi M, et al. The edge-to-edge technique: a simplified method to correct mitral insufficiency. Eur J Cardiothorac Surg 1998; 13: 240–5.
7. Maisano F, Schreuder JJ, Oppizzi M, et al. The double-orifice technique as a standardized approach to treat mitral regurgitation due to severe myxomatous disease: surgical technique. Eur J Cardiothorac Surg 2000; 17: 201–5.
8. Cohn LH. Mitral valve repair for ischemic mitral regurgitation. Adv Cardiol 2002; 39: 153–6.
9. Heub AC, Jatene FB, Moreira LF, et al. Ventricular remodeling and mitral valve modifications in dilated cardiomyopathy: new insights from anatomic study. J Thorac Cardiovasc Surg 2002; 124: 1216–24.
10. McCarthy PM. Does the intertrigonal distance dilate? Never say never. J Thorac Cardiovasc 2002; 124: 1078–9.
11. Calafiore AM, Gallina S, Di Mauro, et al. Mitral valve procedure in dilated cardiomyopathy: repair or replacement? Ann Thorac Surg 2001; 71: 1146–53.

12. Bhudia SK, McCarthy PM, Smedira NG, et al. Edge-to-edge (Alfieri) mitral repair: results in diverse clinical settings. Ann Thorac Surg 2004; 77: 1598–606.

13. Gorman JH 3rd, Gorman RC, Jackson BM, et al. Annuloplasty ring selection for chronic ischemic mitral regurgitation: lessons from the ovine model. Ann Thorac Surg 2003; 76: 1556–63.

14. Alfieri O, Maisano F, De Bonis M, et al. The double-orifice technique in mitral valve repair: a simple solution for complex problems. J Thorac Cardiovasc Surg 2001; 122: 674–81.

15. Gillinov M, Cosgrove DM, Blackstone EH, et al. Durability of mitral valve repair for degenerative disease. J Thorac Cardiovasc Surg 1998; 116: 734–48.

16. Maisano F, Schreuder JJ, Oppizzi M, et al. The double-orifice technique as a standardized approach to treat mitral regurgitation due to severe myxomatous disease: surgical technique. Eur J Cardiothorac Surg 2000; 17: 201–5.

17. Dieter RS. Percutaneous valve repair: update on mitral regurgitation and endovascular approaches to the mitral valve. Applications in imaging. Cardiac Intervent 2003; October 2003: 11–14.

18. Maniu CV, Jeetendra BP, Reuter DG, et al. Acute and chronic reduction of functional mitral regurgitation in experimental heart failure by percutaneous mitral annuloplasty. J Am Coll Cardiol 2004; 44: 2652–61.

19. Fann JI, St Goar FG, Komtebedde J, et al. Beating heart catheter-based edge-to-edge mitral valve procedure in a porcine model: efficacy and healing response. Circulation 2004; 110: 988–93.

20. St Goar FG, Fann JI, Komtebedde J, et al. Endovascular edge-to-edge mitral valve repair. Short-term results in a porcine model. Circulation 2003; 108: 1990–3.

21. Bonow RO, Carabello B, de Leon ACJ, et al. ACC/AHA Guidelines for the Management of Patients with Valvular Heart Disease. J Am Coll Cardiol 1998; 32: 1486–588.

25

Established methods of surgical mitral valve repair and replacement

A Marc Gillinov, Delos M Cosgrove

Introduction

Mitral valve surgery is indicated in patients with severe mitral regurgitation or stenosis and in those with moderately severe mitral valve dysfunction who require cardiac surgery for other reasons. In general, mitral valve repair is preferred to mitral valve replacement.[1–6] Advantages of mitral valve repair over replacement include improved survival, better preservation of left ventricular function, and increased freedom from thromboembolism, anticoagulant-related hemorrhage, and endocarditis.[7–15] In spite of these advantages, mitral valve repair is relatively underutilized in the USA, with less than 40% of patients with mitral valve dysfunction undergoing repair.[16] The feasibility and advicability of mitral valve repair depend upon the etiology of mitral valve dysfunction and the pathology encountered, and understanding the importance of these factors aids in the selection of appropriate candidates for repair.[17]

Commonly encountered etiologies of mitral regurgitation include degenerative disease (also known as myxomatous disease or floppy mitral valve), rheumatic disease, endocarditis, and left ventricular dilatation and dysfunction associated with ischemic and non-ischemic cardiomyopathies. In the last of these conditions, termed functional mitral regurgitation, changes in left ventricular and annular function and geometry cause incomplete mitral leaflet coaptation, resulting in mitral regurgitation.[8] Mitral valve repair is possible in 95% of patients with degenerative mitral valve disease and in the majority of patients with endocarditis or functional mitral regurgitation caused by ischemic or non-

ischemic cardiomyopathy.[17] In contrast, mitral valve repair is less applicable to those who present for surgical treatment of rheumatic mitral valve disease. In rheumatic patients with pure mitral regurgitation or mixed mitral stenosis and regurgitation, repair durability is limited. Most rheumatic patients with pure mitral stenosis and pliable leaflets undergo percutaneous balloon valvotomy, a procedure that is associated with good results.[2]

Surgical treatment of mitral valve disease requires mastery of both mitral valve repair and replacement, with the particular approach being tailored to the patient's pathology. The most common categories of mitral valve dysfunction are degenerative disease and functional regurgitation, the two entities most amenable to repair and the two conditions for which new percutaneous approaches are likely to succeed. The purpose of this chapter is to present contemporary options for mitral valve repair and replacement, with particular emphasis on surgical technique and long-term durability in patients with degenerative and functional mitral regurgitation.

Surgical approach

Surgical mitral valve repair or replacement may be accomplished using a variety of chest wall incisions. The median sternotomy incision is most commonly employed (Figure 25.1). This incision facilitates access to the mitral valve and to all other cardiac structures, and is therefore favored in patients who require concomitant coronary artery bypass grafting. In patients with isolated valvular heart disease (mitral valve disease with

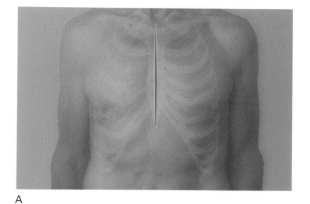

A

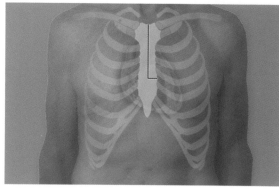

B

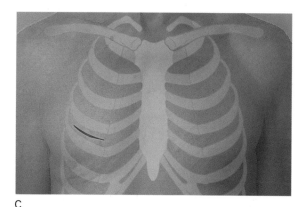

C

Figure 25.1

Chest wall incisions used for mitral valve surgery. (A) Median sternotomy. (B) Minimally invasive approach: partial upper sternotomy. (C) Minimally invasive approach: small right thoracotomy.

or without other valvular lesions), minimally invasive approaches are employed. Excellent mitral valve exposure can be achieved through a 6–8 cm incision (Figure 25.1), and experience at the Cleveland Clinic with more than 3000 mitral valve operations has validated this approach.[18] Others have reported excellent results with robotically assisted and port-access mitral valve procedures.[19–21]

No matter what chest wall incision is chosen, the surgeon must employ cardiopulmonary bypass and cardioplegic arrest to perform the mitral valve operation. This is extremely well tolerated, and even complex mitral valve repairs rarely require more than 60 minutes of cardiopulmonary bypass. With minimally invasive approaches, the hospital mortality rate is less than 1%, blood transfusions are infrequent, and the median length of hospital stay is 6 days.[18,22]

Repair techniques

Annuloplasty

Annuloplasty is the cornerstone of mitral valve repair. It is included in all mitral valve repairs, and, in the case of functional mitral regurgitation, generally constitutes the entire repair. The functions of an annuloplasty include (1) correction of annular dilatation, (2) increase in leaflet coaptation by decreasing the anterior–posterior dimension of the annulus, (3) reduction of tension on suture lines, and (4) prevention of future annular dilatation.[23,24]

Mitral annuloplasty may be achieved using prosthetic annuloplasty devices (Figure 25.2), suture alone, or suture with another buttressing material (e.g. pericardium or Dacron). It is generally accepted that the best results are achieved

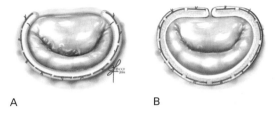

Figure 25.2

Prosthetic annuloplasty devices. (A) Cosgrove–Edwards annuloplasty band. (B) Carpentier–Edwards annuloplasty ring.

with a prosthetic annuloplasty. Commercially available prosthetic annuloplasties may be configured as rings or bands and may be flexible or rigid. All function well, increasing leaflet coaptation by reducing mitral annular diameter. The choice of annuloplasty technique is currently a matter of controversy among surgeons.[25–28] However, clear clinical differences between different prosthetic annuloplasties have not been identified.[1,25]

In degenerative mitral valve disease, most annular dilatation occurs along the posterior annulus,[17,24] and equivalent results have been achieved with annuloplasty bands and rings.[1] In functional mitral regurgitation, there is dilatation along the entire annulus, although the dilatation is most pronounced posteriorly.[27] The concept of a flexible annuloplasty is appealing, as it pre-

serves mitral annular motion; however, a relationship between annular flexibility and standard measures of clinical outcome has not been established.[23,29,30]

Prosthetic annuloplasty rings and bands are implanted by passing sutures through the mitral annulus and then through the annuloplasty device. As each suture is tied, the annulus is plicated, reducing the annular circumference and increasing leaflet coaptation. With annuloplasty bands, sutures are placed about the posterior annulus, extending from fibrous trigone to fibrous trigone. With ring annuloplasties, sutures are placed around the entire annulus. In patients with degenerative disease, the annuloplasty is sized according to the surface area of the anterior mitral leaflet. In contrast, in patients with functional mitral regurgitation, the annuloplasty is typically undersized to optimize leaflet coaptation.

In patients with degenerative mitral valve disease, the annuloplasty is added to other repair techniques that correct leaflet prolapse; annuloplasty alone does not correct leaflet prolapse. Failure to incorporate an annuloplasty in these patients jeopardizes repair durability (Figure 25.3).[1]

As noted above, in patients with functional mitral regurgitation caused by ischemic and non-ischemic cardiomyopathies, mitral annuloplasty generally constitutes the entire repair procedure. Such patients have left ventricular dilatation and

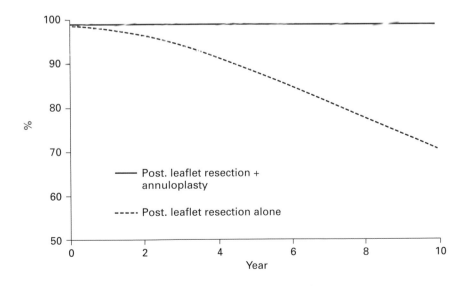

Figure 25.3

Freedom from reoperation after mitral valve repair. Annuloplasty improves repair durability.

dysfunction; the valve leaflets and chordae are normal, but leaflet motion is restricted, preventing coaptation and allowing mitral regurgitation. By reducing the anterior–posterior diameter of the valve, an undersized annuloplasty increases leaflet coaptation and reduces mitral regurgitation. In the past, hospital mortality in these patients with heart failure was excessive. However, in recent years, the hospital mortality rate for mitral valve surgery in such patients has dropped to 3–5%.[8,25,26] While initially successful in the majority of patients with functional mitral regurgitation, annuloplasty is associated with important recurrent mitral regurgitation in 20–30%.[25,31] Patients with complex regurgitant jets and severe tenting of both leaflets are particularly prone to repair failure; in these patients, mitral valve replacement may be a better option.[25]

Correction of posterior leaflet prolapse

Posterior leaflet prolapse is the most common pathologic finding in patients with degenerative mitral valve disease, affecting 70%.[1] In 49% of these patients, it is the primary cause of mitral

regurgitation. The prolapse is caused by elongated or ruptured chordae, and usually affects the middle scallop, or P2 segment, of the mitral valve. On echocardiography, an anteriorly directed jet of mitral regurgitation is identified.

Repair of posterior leaflet prolapse is achieved by quadrangular resection. Described by Carpentier,[17] this technique includes resection of the segment of posterior leaflet subserved by the pathologic chordae. After leaflet resection, the repair is completed by plication of the annulus, suture of the free edges of the leaflets, and placement of a prosthetic annuloplasty. The hospital mortality rate for this sort of procedure is less than 1%. This repair technique is highly reproducible and is associated with excellent long-term durability, including a 10-year freedom from reoperation of 98% (Figure 25.3).[1,5-7] Published 20-year results confirm excellent repair durability[5,6] and demonstrate that successful valve repair restores these patients to a survival curve similar to that of the general population.[5]

In the setting of excess leaflet tissue, quadrangular resection for posterior leaflet prolapse has been associated with left ventricular outflow tract obstruction caused by systolic anterior motion (SAM) of the anterior leaflet of the mitral valve.[32-34] In patients who develop SAM, the pos-

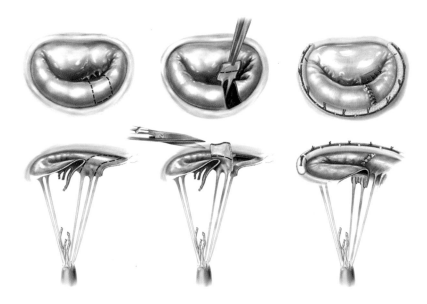

Figure 25.4

Chordal transfer to correct anterior leaflet prolapse. Posterior leaflet chordae are transferred to the unsupported free edge of the anterior leaflet. The posterior leaflet is repaired as after a quandrangular resection.

terior leaflet is tall, and the point of coaptation is displaced anteriorly toward the left ventricular outflow tract.[32] This complication can be avoided by performing a sliding repair in conjunction with quadrangular resection. With this technique, a segment of posterior leaflet with abnormal chordae is resected as for a standard quadrangular resection. In order to move the point of leaflet coaptation posteriorly, the height of the remaining posterior leaflet is reduced. This is accomplished by detaching the posterior leaflet from the annulus and then resuturing the leaflet to the annulus, taking deep bites to reduce its height. The sliding repair is only slightly more complex than a standard quadrangular resection, and it virtually eliminates the risk of SAM.[32,33] Occasionally, other techniques are used to correct posterior leaflet prolapse. These include the Alfieri edge-to-edge repair and the creation of artificial chordae. However, these approaches are most commonly employed for correction of anterior leaflet prolapse (see below).

Correction of anterior leaflet prolapse

Traditionally, correction of anterior leaflet prolapse has been more challenging than correction of posterior leaflet prolapse, and anterior leaflet prolapse has been associated with greater probability of initial mitral valve replacement and a lower durability of mitral valve repair.[1,7] However, with increased experience and application of new techniques, repair of anterior leaflet prolapse is now feasible in the majority of cases.[35-39] A variety of techniques may be used to correct anterior leaflet prolapse. The most commonly employed include chordal transfer, creation of artificial chordae, and the Alfieri edge-to-edge repair.

Chordal transfer provides durable repair of anterior leaflet prolapse.[36,37] Chordal transfer entails relocation of normal chordae to the segment of anterior leaflet that prolapses due to chordal elongation or rupture. Occasionally, normal secondary anterior leaflet chordae may be detached from the undersurface of the leaflet and sutured to the free edge of the prolapsing anterior leaflet. More commonly, a segment of posterior leaflet with its attached chordae is detached from the posterior annulus and sewn to the prolapsing

segment of anterior leaflet (Figure 25.4). The posterior leaflet is then repaired as after a quadrangular resection. Because normal, autologous chordae are used to support the anterior leaflet with this approach, there is no need to perform complex measurements or calculations to determine proper chordal length. However, correction of anterior leaflet prolapse with chordal transfer requires that the surgeon operate on both leaflets. Although chordal transfer is associated with excellent repair durability, surgeons employ a variety of other techniques to correct anterior leaflet prolapse.

There is currently great enthusiasm for the creation of artificial chordae to treat anterior leaflet prolapse. These chordae are usually constructed from Gore-Tex sutures. With this approach, one end of the Gore-Tex suture is attached to a papillary muscle head, and the other end is sutured to the unsupported free edge of the anterior leaflet (Figure 25.5).[35] This technique requires that the

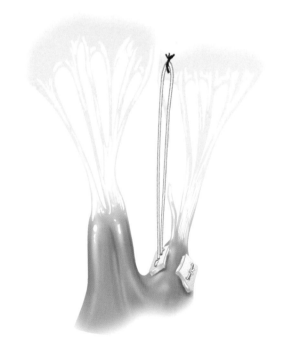

Figure 25.5

Gore-Tex chord for correction of anterior leaflet prolapse. A premeasured loop of Gore-Tex is affixed to the papillary muscle with a pledgetted suture. The loop is then attached to the free edge of the unsupported anterior leaflet, providing support.[40]

surgeon determine the appropriate length of the new chordae; recent developments have facilitated this.[40] The long-term durability of this technique is excellent; the new chordae do not rupture or elongate.[35] Artificial chordae may also be used to correct posterior leaflet prolapse, although this is an uncommon strategy.

The Alfieri technique for the correction of leaflet prolapse involves suturing the free edge of the anterior mitral leaflet to the free edge of the posterior mitral leaflet (Figure 25.6).[38] This technique is simple and rapid, and it may be used to correct anterior leaflet prolapse, posterior leaflet prolapse, or bileaflet prolapse. When placed in the middle of the valve, the stitch produces a valve with two orifices. The stitch may also be used to close a commissure when there is prolapse of either or both leaflets at the commissure.[36] The durability of this repair technique is highest for degenerative disease and is enhanced by the addition of an annuloplasty.[41,42] In current clinical practice, the edge-to-edge repair is most commonly employed in patients with anterior leaflet prolapse, and it is supplemented by an annuloplasty to optimize results. Although this technique narrows the mitral orifice, it is unlikely to cause stenosis in patients with degenerative disease.

Special situations

Annular calcification

Occasionally, degenerative mitral valve disease is accompanied by severe mitral annular calcification (MAC). In most instances, the calcium must be removed, and this greatly complicates mitral valve repair, increasing operative time and risk. Once the calcium has been removed, care must be taken to ensure that the atrioventricular groove is intact; if there is atrioventricular dissociation, it is repaired primarily or, more commonly, with a pericardial patch. In spite of this complexity, if the calcium does not extend into the leaflets, mitral valve repair is feasible in many patients with MAC.[43]

In selected cases, repair may be achieved without addressing the annular calcium. Both anterior leaflet and posterior leaflet prolapse may be corrected by creation of artificial chordae or by an

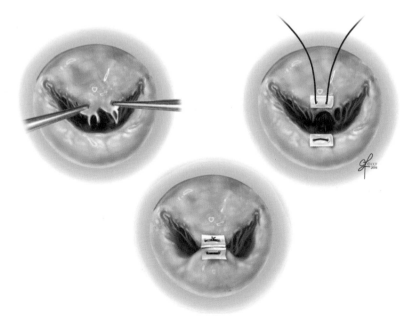

Figure 25.6

Alfieri edge-to-edge repair for anterior leaflet prolapse. A pledgetted stitch is used to affix the unsupported portion of the anterior leaflet to the normal free edge of the posterior leaflet. An annuloplasty completes the repair.

Alfieri edge-to-edge repair, obviating the need to remove the annular calcium. However, retained annular calcium may jeopardize durability.[41]

Endocarditis

Endocarditis affecting the native mitral valve is associated with chordal rupture, leaflet perforation, vegetations, and abscess formation.[2] Radical debridement is the cornerstone of the operative treatment of endocarditis. All infected material must be removed. If there are ruptured chordae to the posterior leaflet, quadrangular resection is performed. Anterior chordal rupture is repaired with standard techniques. Anterior leaflet perforations are repaired with autologous pericardial patches. Abscess cavities are debrided and excluded with a pericardial patch. We favor posterior autologous pericardial annuloplasty in patients with endocarditis in order to avoid implantation of prosthetic material.[2]

Eighty percent of infected mitral valves are amenable to repair, and recurrent endocarditis is rare. When compared with replacement, repair of infected mitral valves results in greater freedom from recurrent infection and higher early and late survival.[2]

Mitral valve replacement

While mitral valve repair is generally preferable to mitral valve replacement, not all mitral valves are amenable to repair. Replacement may be indicated for extremely diseased degenerative valves with severe annular calcification, rheumatic valves with leaflet calcification or mixed regurgitation and stenosis, infected valves with extensive tissue destruction, and valves with functional regurgitation characterized by bileaflet restriction and/or complex regurgitant jets. In most cases, when valve replacement is necessary, some or all of the leaflet tissue and attached subvalvular apparatus can be preserved. Preservation of the subvalvular apparatus is associated with better long-term left ventricular function and should therefore be a consideration when the mitral valve is replaced.[44]

Commonly employed mitral prostheses include mechanical and bioprosthetic valves (Figure 25.7). Mechanical valves require lifelong anticoagulation but are not subject to structural valve degeneration. In patients with normal sinus rhythm, bioprostheses do not require anticoagulation; however, the durability of bioprostheses in young patients is limited. Bioprostheses are preferred in patients aged 65 years or beyond,

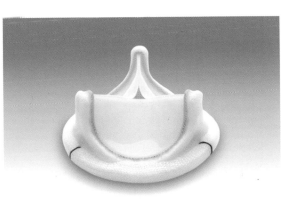

A

B

Figure 25.7

Prosthetic mitral valves. (A) Carpentier–Edwards pericardial valve (courtesy of Edwards Lifesciences, LLC, Irvine, CA). (B) St Jude mechanical valve (courtesy of St Jude Medical, Minneapolis, MN).

patients with concomitant coronary artery disease, and those with reduced left ventricular function and functional mitral regurgitation; such patients are unlikely to outlive the bioprosthetic valve. In addition, bioprostheses should be employed in patients who have contraindications to anticoagulation.

Implantation techniques are similar for both bioprosthetic and mechanical valves. With bioprosthetic valves, the struts should be positioned so that they do not obstruct the left ventricular outflow tract. With mechanical valves, care must be taken to ensure that retained subvalvular apparatus does not interfere with the valve mechanism.

Conclusions

MItral valve repair is the preferred treatment for mitral valve disease. In the most common causes of mitral valve dysfunction – degenerative disease and functional mitral regurgitation associated with left ventricular dysfunction – valve repair is possible using standardized techniques. Annuloplasty is a critical component of virtually all mitral valve repairs, and, in patients with functional mitral regurgitation, it is usually the only repair technique employed. The surgical risk is low, and long-term results, particularly with degenerative disease, are excellent. In patients with isolated valve disease, minimally invasive approaches reduce surgical trauma and speed recovery. It is likely that advances in percutaneous approaches to heart valve repair will enable the extension of this therapy to large numbers of patients.

References

1. Gillinov AM, Cosgrove DM, Blackstone EH, et al. Durability of mitral valve repair for degenerative disease. J Thorac Cardiovasc Surg 1998; 116: 734–43.
2. Gillinov AM, Cosgrove DM III. Current status of mitral valve repair. Am Heart Hosp J 2003; 1: 47–54.
3. Gillinov AM, Cosgrove DM. Mitral valve repair for degenerative disease. J Heart Valve Dis 2001; 11(Suppl 1): S15–S20.
4. Gillinov AM, Cosgrove DM. Mitral valve repair. Op Tech Thorac Cardiovasc Surg 1998; 3: 95–108.
5. Braunberger E, Deloche A, Berrebi A, et al. Very long-term results (more than 20 years) of valve repair with Carpentier's techniques in non-rheumatic mitral valve insufficiency. Circulation 2001; 104(Suppl I): I-8–I-11.
6. Mohty D, Orszulak TA, Schaff HV, et al. Very long-term survival and durability of mitral valve repair for mitral valve prolapse. Circulation 2001; 104(Suppl I): I-1–I-7.
7. Mohty D, Enriquez-Sarano M. The long-term outcome of mitral valve repair for mitral valve prolapse. Curr Cardiol Rep 2002; 4: 104–10.
8. Gillinov AM, Wierup PN, Blackstone EH, et al. Is repair preferable to replacement for ischemic mitral regurgitation? J Thorac Cardiovasc Surg 2001; 122: 1125–41.
9. Gillinov AM, Blackstone EH, Cosgrove DM III, et al. Mitral valve repair with aortic valve replacement is superior to double valve replacement. J Thorac Cardiovasc Surg 2003; 125: 1372–87.
10. Gillinov AM, Faber C, Houghtaling PL, et al. Repair versus replacement for degenerative mitral valve disease with coexisting ischemic heart disease. J Thorac Cardiovasc Surg 2003; 125: 1350–62.
11. Lawrie GM, Mitral valve repair vs replacement. Cardiol Clin 1998; 16: 437–48.
12. Lee EM, Shapiro LM, Wells FC. Superiority of mitral valve repair in surgery for degenerative mitral regurgitation. Eur Heart J 1997; 18: 655–63.
13. Perier P, Deloche A, Chauvaud S, et al. Comparative evaluation of mitral valve repair and replacement with Starr, Björk, and porcine valve prostheses. Circulation 1984; 70(Suppl I): I-187–I-192.
14. Ren JF, Aksut S, Lighty GW Jr, et al. Mitral valve repair is superior to valve replacement for the early preservation of cardiac function: relation of ventricular geometry to function. Am Heart J 1996; 131: 974–81.
15. Grossi EA, Galloway AC, Miller JS, et al. Valve repair versus replacement for mitral insufficiency: when is a mechanical valve still indicated? J Thorac Cardiovasc Surg 1998; 115: 389–96.
16. Savage EB, Ferguson TB Jr, DiSesa VJ. Use of mitral valve repair: analysis of contemporary United States experience reported to the Society of Thoracic Surgeons National Cardiac Database. Ann Thorac Surg 2003; 75: 820–5.
17. Carpentier A. Cardiac valve surgery – the "French correction". J Thorac Cardiovasc Surg 1983; 86: 323–37.
18. Gillinov AM, Banbury MK, Cosgrove DM. Is minimally invasive heart valve surgery a paradigm for the future? Curr Cardiol Rep 1999; 1: 318–22.
19. Nifong LW, Chu VF, Bailey BM. Robotic mitral valve repair: experience with the da Vinci system. Ann Thorac Surg 2003; 75: 438–43.

20. Mohr FW, Falk V, Diegeler A, et al. Computer-enhanced 'robotic' cardiac surgery: experience in 148 patients. J Thorac Cardiovasc Surg 2001; 121: 842–53.

21. Gallaway AC, Shemin RJ, Glower DD, et al. First report of the Port Access International Registry. Ann Thorac Surg 1999; 67: 51–8.

22. Cosgrove DM, Gillinov AM. Partial sternotomy for mitral valve operations. Op Tech Card Thorac Surg 1998; 3: 62–72.

23. Gillinov AM, Cosgrove DM III, Shiota T, et al. Cosgrove–Edwards annuloplasty system: midterm results. Ann Thorac Surg 2000; 69: 717–21.

24. Carpentier A, Cauptain J, Blondeau P, Dubost Ch. A new reconstructive operation for correction of mitral and tricuspid insufficiency. J Thorac Cardiovasc Surg 1971; 61: 1–13.

25. McGee EC, Gillinov AM, Cohen G, et al. Recurrent mitral regurgitation after annuloplasty for functional ischemic mitral regurgitation. J Thorac Cardiovasc Surg 2004; 128: 916–24.

26. Adams DH, Filsoufi F, Aklog L. Surgical treatment of the ischemic mitral valve. J Heart Valve Dis 2002; 11(Suppl 1): S21–S25.

27. Gorman JH III, Gorman RC, Jackson BM, et al. Annuloplasty ring selection for chronic ischemic mitral regurgitation: lessons from the ovine model. Ann Thorac Surg 2003; 76: 1556–63.

28. Miller DC. Ischemic mitral regurgitation redux – to repair or to replace? J Thorac Cardiovasc Surg 2001; 122: 1059–62.

29. Raffoul R, Uva MS, Rescigno G, et al. Clinical evaluation of the physio annuloplasty ring. Chest 1998; 113: 1296–301.

30. David TE, Komeda M, Pollick C, Burns RJ. Mitral valve annuloplasty: the effect of the type on left ventricular function. Ann Thorac Surg 1989; 47: 524–8.

31. Tahta SA, Oury JH, Maxwell JM, et al. Outcome after mitral valve repair for functional ischemic mitral regurgitation. J Heart Valve Dis 2002; 11: 11–18.

32. Jebara VA, Mihaileanu S, Acar C, et al. Left ventricular outflow tract obstruction after mitral valve repair. Results of the sliding leaflet technique. Circulation 1993; 88: 30–4.

33. Perier P, Clausnizer B, Mistarz K. Carpentier 'sliding leaflet' technique for repair of the mitral valve: early results. Ann Thorac Surg 1994; 57: 383–6.

34. Gillinov AM, Cosgrove DM III. Modified sliding leaflet technique for repair of the mitral valve. Ann Thorac Surg 1999; 68: 2356–7.

35. David TE. Artificial chordae. Semin Thorac Cardiovasc Surg 2004; 16: 161–8.

36. Gillinov AM, Cosgrove DM. Chordal transfer for repair of anterior leaflet prolapse. Semin Thorac Cardiovasc Surg 2004; 16: 169–73.

37. Perier P. Surgical repair of the prolapsing anterior leaflet with chordal shortening. Semin Thorac Cardiovasc Surg 2004; 16: 174–81.

38. Alfieri O, De Bonis M, Lapenna E, et al. 'Edge-to-edge' repair for anterior mitral leaflet prolapse. Semin Thorac Cardiovasc Surg 2004; 16: 182–7.

39. Saunders PC, Grossi EA, Schwartz CF. Anterior leaflet resection of the mitral valve. Semin Thorac Cardiovasc Surg 2004; 16: 188–93.

40. von Oppell UO, Mohr FW. Chordal replacement for both minimally invasive and conventional mitral valve surgery using premeasured Gore-Tex loops. Ann Thorac Surg 2000; 70: 2166–8.

41. Maisano F, Caldarola A, Blasio A, et al. Midterm results of edge-to-edge mitral valve repair without annuloplasty. J Thorac Cardiovasc Surg 1987; 126: 1987–97.

42. Bhudia SK, McCarthy PM, Smedira NG, et al. Edge-to-edge (Alfieri) mitral repair: results in diverse clinical settings. Ann Thorac Surg 2004; 77: 1598–606.

43. Carpentier AF, Pellerin M, Fuzellier JF, Relland JYM. Extensive calcification of the mitral valve annulus: pathology and surgical management. J Thorac Cardiovasc Surg 1996; 111: 718–30.

44. David TE, Burns RJ, Bacchus CM, Druck MN. Mitral valve replacement for mitral regurgitation with and without preservation of chordae tendinae. J Thorac Cardiovasc Surg 1984; 88: 718–25.

26

Percutaneous leaflet repair for mitral regurgitation using the Evalve edge-to-edge clip technique

Ted Feldman, Ottavio Alfieri, Fred St Goar

Introduction

Edge-to-edge mitral valve repair for mitral regurgitation was first described by one of the present authors (Ottavio Alfieri).[1-3] In 1991 he was performing a surgical closure of an atrial septal defect (ASD) in a 29-year-old woman. He observed that the patient, along with her ASD, had a well-functioning double-orifice mitral valve – a rare but well-described congenital abnormality. He carefully inspected the unusual valve finding and left it alone. Later that day, he was operating on a patient suffering from severe mitral regurgitation due to segmental prolapse of the anterior leaflet secondary to chordal rupture. When traditional mitral repair techniques were ineffective in resolving the patient's valvular insufficiency, in lieu of replacing the valve, based on his observations from the earlier case, he approximated the free edges of the leaflets at the site of regurgitation with a suture and re-established functional coaptation. The patient had an excellent outcome with an uncomplicated postoperative recovery.

Surgical edge-to-edge repair

The long-term results using this surgical technique in patients with mitral regurgitation due to anterior leaflet prolapse are compelling. In a recent review of 160 consecutive patients, the rate of freedom from reoperation was 96.6±1.74% at 12 years.[4] These long-term results are similar to those obtained in patients with posterior leaflet prolapse who undergo quadrangular resection. The majority of the patients in this series received a prosthetic ring in addition to the edge-to-edge repair. Results of mitral valve repair for anterior leaflet prolapse compared with posterior leaflet prolapse are consistently worse in terms of freedom from reoperation. Thus, in selected patients, use of the edge-to-edge repair has effectively removed anterior leaflet prolapse as an incremental risk factor for suboptimal outcome following mitral valve reconstructive surgery.

Barlow's disease (severe global myxomatous degeneration of the mitral valve with bileaflet prolapse) is another condition for which the edge-to-edge repair has been used extensively with good outcomes. A series covering a 10-year period of 423 consecutive Barlow's disease patients treated with a double-orifice repair was recently reviewed (unpublished data). During that time span, no patient with Barlow's disease received a valve replacement, regardless of the presence of extensive annular calcification. The rate of freedom from reoperation was satisfactory: 90.0±4.48% at 7 years. No patient developed mitral stenosis as a result of the operation, and good functional capacity was documented on postoperative exercise testing.

The edge-to-edge technique has been recently applied to patients with commissural prolapse. This lesion is difficult to treat using conventional methods of mitral repair. Results are less predictable and satisfactory than those obtained when prolapse affects the central part of the valve. Over a 5-year period, 32 patients with severe mitral insufficiency due to commissural prolapse have been treated with edge-to-edge repair. Under these circumstances, the procedure does not result in a double-orifice mitral valve, but in a valve with a single orifice that is slightly smaller than the original one. After a mean follow-up period of 2.4 years, 31 patients have been found with no or minimal mitral regurgitation on echocardiographic study, while moderate mitral incompetence was documented in one patient (unpublished data).

The edge-to-edge technique in conjunction with annuloplasty has also been used in patients with severe mitral regurgitation in the context of dilated cardiomyopathy, either ischemic or idiopathic. The rate of freedom from failure of mitral repair was $95 \pm 3.4\%$ at 3 years, significantly higher than that obtained with annuloplasty alone. By logistic regression analysis, absence of the edge-to-edge repair was identified as the only predictor of mitral valve repair failure.[5] Since recurrence of mitral regurgitation in dilated cardiomyopathy is mostly due to progressive remodeling, the edge-to-edge suture is possibly effective by counteracting the remodeling process.

The edge-to-edge repair is a relatively simple surgical procedure, but there are a few pitfalls to take into account. The approximating suture must be located exactly at the site of regurgitation. The site of regurgitation corresponds to the prolapsing portion of the leaflets in degenerative mitral disease and it is easily identifiable by the surgeon at operation. In idiopathic or ischemic cardiomyopathy, the mitral valve appears morphologically normal, and therefore the location of the edge-to-edge suture should be echo-guided to match the origin of the regurgitant jet. The extension of the suture should be enough to correct valve insufficiency, but not too long to avoid valve stenosis. When great redundancy of the leaflets is present, as in Barlow's disease, the stitches should be passed away (at least 1 cm) from the free edge of the leaflet, in order to reduce redundancy of the valve tissue and prevent postoperative systolic anterior motion.

It is important to emphasize that the surgical edge-to-edge technique has not been used in patients suffering from isolated posterior leaflet prolapse – a population who constitute the majority of the patients requiring mitral valve repair.

This is due to the fact that excellent and predictable results have been obtained with quadrangular resection, with up to 30-year follow-up. However, edge-to-edge repair is potentially quite applicable to this patient population and similar results should be expected.

In surgical experience, the edge-to-edge repair has almost invariably been associated with a ring annuloplasty. In the surgical candidate, the annulus is often dilated because the operation is usually carried out rather late in the course of the disease. Even when the operation is performed before the occurrence of annular dilatation, a prosthetic ring is implanted to 'stabilize the repair'. In this latter situation, however, annuloplasty could well be unnecessary. Satisfactory results have been reported after edge-to-edge repair when annuloplasty was intentionally avoided due to a normal annular size,[6] and thus a free-standing technique has applicability in a select and (as yet) not well-defined group of patients.

Results of conventional surgery for mitral regurgitation

Outcomes from surgical therapy have not been characterized in detail with prospective trials. The traditional endpoint for evaluation of the results of mitral repair surgery has been freedom from reoperation. The reported rate of freedom from reoperation after annuloplasty and leaflet resection for degenerative mitral regurgitation is about 95% at 5 years. These same populations of patients have mortality rates between 4% and 8% over the same period of time. Since mortality is not included in the endpoint freedom from reoperation, this endpoint creates a false impression that does not reflect the true clinical outcomes for these patient groups. Furthermore, very few studies have prospectively evaluated the rate of recurrent mitral regurgitation after annuloplasty and leaflet resection.

In a study by Flameng[7] et al from Belgium with prospective echocardiographic follow-up in 242 patients, significant recurrence of mitral regurgitation was observed after 5 and 7 years following repair. By 7 years, three-quarters of patients had some mitral regurgitation, and almost one-third had regurgitation severe enough to be considered by the authors to be clinically significant.

These benchmark results are representative of the bar to which percutaneous mitral repair for similar patients will ultimately be compared.

Another surgical option is valve replacement. When surgical valve repair is technically feasible, it results in superior hemodynamics and in lower morbidity and mortality than prosthetic valve replacement surgery. Chronic anticoagulation is also avoided. Repair techniques include relatively complex leaflet resection, repositioning and reshaping techniques for the mitral annulus, and chordal repair techniques. Repair is not feasible in all patients, and even when it is the intended therapy, mitral valve replacement is sometimes performed. Even the best centers where there is a strong bias for performing mitral valve repair, replacement is the resultant form of management in up to 10% of patients.

Development of percutaneous edge-to-edge mitral valve repair

In his initial description of edge-to-edge repair, Alfieri noted that the surgical method was suited to adaptation as a percutaneous approach. The simplicity and potential of the Alfieri repair technique was noted by the cardiology community. In 1999, Fred St Goar focused on developing a method to accomplish edge-to-edge repair via a percutaneous approach. The initial endeavors were directed towards mimicking the surgical procedure, i.e. a suture-based repair (Figure 26.1). Investigational work was performed on a sophisticated bench model of mitral valve regurgitation. The model was created by removing the left atrium of an isolated pig heart and transecting the primary chordae of the middle scallop of the posterior leaflet. The heart was placed in a warm bath and, using a catheter introduced through the apex, the left ventricular pressure was varied to

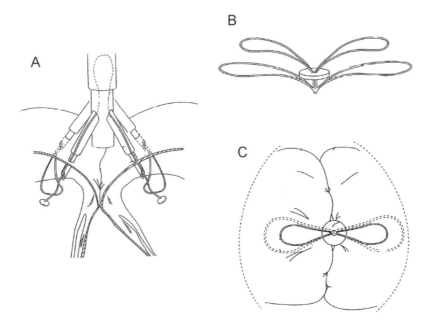

Figure 26.1

(A) Suture delivery system to duplicate the surgical edge-to-edge surgical leaflet repair. It was quickly recognized that stabilizing elements to hold the leaflets steady were necessary. (B) Leaflet-stabilizing elements were developed to hold the leaflets in place, with the concept that stabilization of the leaflets was a necessary component of suturing. (C) It was recognized that stabilizing elements without sutures were adequate to grasp and fixate the leaflets, duplicating the surgical repair without the need for sutures.

mimic the cardiac cycle and create physiologic mitral leaflet motion and regurgitation.

In the process of evaluating various suture-based approaches, it became evident that to successfully place sutures in a controlled fashion, the leaflets needed to be stabilized and immobilized. A series of various stabilizing concepts were investigated. It became clear that a wire figure-of-eight open loop could be oriented in the left atrium orthogonal to the line of leaflet coaptation and then advanced through the valve into the ventricle. When the loops were pulled back up to the level of the annulus, they not only captured and stabilized the leaflets but also resolved the mitral insufficiency. Through multiple iterations, this concept evolved into what is now the Evalve clip and catheter-based mitral valve repair system (Figures 26.2 and 26.3).[8–11]

It is important to note that the late results of clip placement in the animal model exactly mimic the results of the surgical approach for the creation of a double-orifice mitral valve. Fann et al[9,10] evaluated the healing response to placement of the Evalve clip in a porcine model. The clip was placed transatrially in the beating heart, and follow-up studies were then performed at intervals out to 1 year. Gross inspection showed that by 6 months there was complete incorporation of the clip into a tissue bridge. This mimics the gross

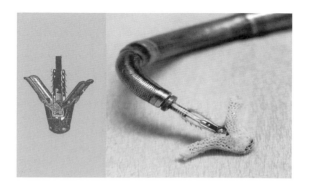

Figure 26.3

The Evalve clip is shown on the left. The two clip arms are partially open. Barbed gripping elements can be seen parallel to the central portion of the clip. The mitral valve leaflets are grasped between the gripping elements and the clip arms, and then the clip is closed over them. On the right is a photograph of the clip with its polyester covering. The clip is attached to the clip delivery catheter. The gripping elements can be seen clearly adjacent to the central portion of the clip at its attachment to the clip delivery system

pathologic and histopathologic findings observed in patients after standard suture material is used to create a double orifice via a surgical approach. The duplication of the surgical repair using this percutaneous method is the foundation for the application of this device in patients.

Technique for Evalve edge-to-edge repair

Percutaneous edge-to-edge repair is accomplished using the trans-septal approach to the left atrium. A guide catheter is placed across the atrial septum into the mid-left atrial cavity. A clip delivery system is introduced through the guide into the left atrium, above the mitral valve (Figure 26.4). The delivery system helps navigate the clip toward the mitral leaflets. The clip is opened above the leaflets, angulated so that it is perpendicular to the line of leaflet coaptation, and then passed across the leaflets into the left ventricular cavity. The clip is pulled back and closed to grasp the free edges of the mitral leaflets at the central portion of the orifice. Once closed, an edge-to-edge repair with a double mitral orifice is created (Figure 26.5). The results can be evaluated using color Doppler, pulmonary vein flow Doppler

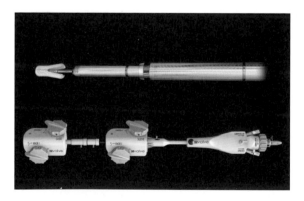

Figure 26.2

Schematic of the Evalve device. The Evalve clip is shown at the top; it is made of cobalt–chromium covered with Dacron fabric to aid in endothelialization. The clip is attached directly to a clip delivery system, which is placed through a guide catheter. At the bottom, from left to right, are shown the steering knobs for the guide catheter, the steering knobs for the clip delivery system, and the screw mechanism that opens and closes the clip.

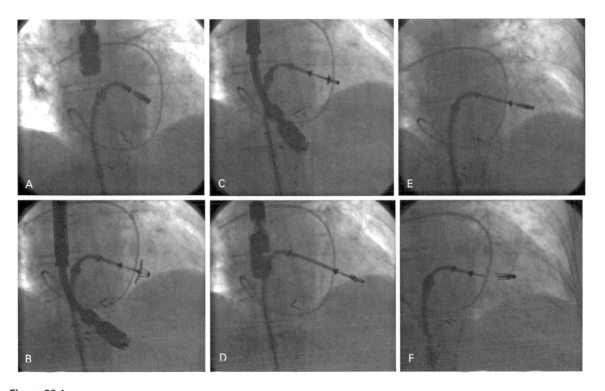

Figure 26.4

(A) Fluoroscopic images of the clip delivery system placed through the guide catheter. The clip is in the left atrium. A transesophageal echocardiographic probe is seen at the top of the picture. A pulmonary artery catheter is positioned in the distal right pulmonary artery. (B) The clip has been opened and advanced toward the mitral leaflets, but remains in the left atrium. (C) The clip has been rotated using transesophageal echocardiograhic guidance so that the arms of the clip are perpendicular to the long axis of the line of coaptation of the mitral leaflets, (D) The open clip has been advanced through the mitral leaflets into the left ventricular cavity. The clip is advanced across the valve in the open position in order to minimize the chance for entanglement of the chordae tendinae. (E) The clip has been pulled back to grasp the mitral leaflets, and closed, It remains attached to the clip delivery system. (F) After adequate control of mitral regurgitation has been verified using two-dimensional and Doppler echocardiographic assessment, the clip is released.

assessments, and angiography. After adequate reduction of mitral regurgitation has been achieved, the clip can be detached from the delivery system and left as a permanent implant.

The clip is a mechanical device with two arms that are opened and closed by a control mechanism on the clip delivery system. The two arms have an open span of 2 cm. The width of the clip is 4 mm. Inside the clip are two gripping elements on the superior side of the arms, with small barbs that close the arms after the mitral leaflets have been engaged by the clip. Leaflet tissue is captured between the closed arms and the grippers, and the clip is then locked to result in apposition or coaptation of the two leaflets. The clip is covered with polyester fabric to enhance endothelial overgrowth. The clip is attached to a clip delivery catheter system, which is passed through the guide catheter into the left atrium. Both the guide catheter and the clip delivery system are steerable using two-knob wire pulley systems. The clip delivery system is advanced through the guide catheter with the tip attached to the end of the delivery system and positioned so that the clip is oriented directly above the coaptation line of the mitral leaflets, centered in three planes.

The Evalve clip was initially evaluated in an acute and chronic porcine animal model, and resulted in an anatomic repair analogous to the surgical suture repair. Histology at 6 months showed complete encapsulation of the clip device in a fibrous tissue bridge.[8–11]

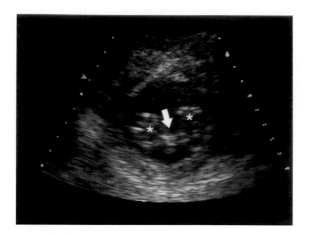

Figure 26.5

Transthoracic echocardiographic image recorded from the first patient treated in the EVEREST protocol in the USA. The image was obtained at the 1-month protocol-driven follow-up point. This is a short-axis image of the left ventricle at the level of the mitral orifice. The large arrow points at the clip in the center of the mitral leaflets. The asterisks denote the two orifices of the now double-orifice mitral valve.

In humans, the procedure is performed in the cardiac catheterization laboratory under general anesthesia using both fluoroscopic and transesophageal echocardiographic guidance. General anesthesia is indicated due to the relatively prolonged time with a transesophageal probe in place.

After anesthesia and preparation of the patient, a trans-septal puncture is performed using standard techniques. The intra-atrial septum is gently dilated and the guide catheter is then directed into the left atrium over a supportive guidewire. The guide catheter diameter is 24 Fr at the skin entry site and 22 Fr as it crosses the atrial septum. The guide is placed in the mid-left atrium, deaired, and then flushed. The clip delivery system is introduced into the guide catheter and the clip is advanced into the mid-left atrial chamber. With echocardiographic and fluoroscopic guidance, the clip is moved in multiple iterations until it is centered over the mitral orifice in three planes (Figure 26.4). The clip is opened so that the grasping elements are between 150° and 180°, and then the clip is turned perpendicular to the long axis of the leaflet edges. This requires either a transgastric short-axis transesophageal echocar-

diographic view, or, if this cannot be obtained, transthoracic echocardiography to demonstrate a proper orientation of the clip with reference to the long axis of the leaflet edges. The clip is advanced into the left ventricle just below the tips of the mitral leaflets and the perpendicular orientation of the arms is again verified. The clip is then pulled back until the mitral leaflets are captured in the clip arms. The gripping elements are lowered onto the atrial side of the leaflets, and the clip is closed to firmly grasp mitral leaflet tissue.

If both leaflets have been grasped successfully, a double orifice results from the edge-to-edge approximation of the leaflets. The degree of mitral regurgitation can then be reassessed using Doppler echocardiography. Both color Doppler and blood flow patterns in the pulmonary veins are critical to make an adequate assessment of the change in mitral regurgitation.

If the control of mitral regurgitation is not adequate, the clip can be opened, the mitral leaflets released, and the clip repositioned. When the clip must be withdrawn through the chordae back into the left atrium, the arms can be everted so that they may be retracted through the chordae without entanglement.

After the leaflets have been grasped, a double orifice formed, and adequate control of the mitral regurgitation achieved, the clip is released from the clip delivery system, and the delivery system and guide catheter are withdrawn (Figure 26.6). In some cases, it is apparent that one clip is not adequate to improve mitral regurgitation adequately, and a decision at that point must be made as to whether a second clip might be successful. The first clip could be released and the production repeated to place a second clip. The clip may be placed either adjacent to the first clip or at another point to create a triple-orifice mitral valve. Repeat hemodynamic, angiographic, and echocardiographic assessments are performed to verify the final results, and the catheters are removed using standard methods.

Because the procedure is performed under general anesthesia, the anesthesiologist plays a critical role. We have worked with a cardiovascular anesthesiologist who brings to the procedure familiarity with the assessment of mitral valve repair in the surgical setting. Cardiologists are well versed with echocardiographic quantification of mitral regurgitation in the conscious

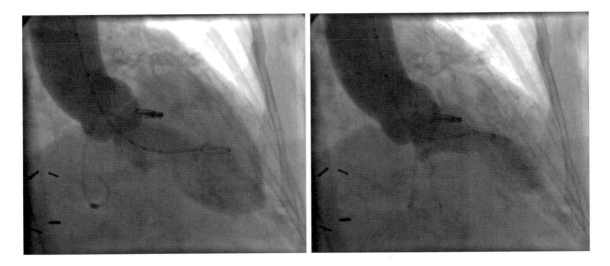

Figure 26.6

Fluoroscopic images of the valve during left ventriculography. On the left is a diastolic frame with the clip silhouette overlapping the aortic root. On the right is a systolic frame showing complete contraction of the left ventricle without any angiographic evidence of mitral regurgitation.

unsedated patient, but this is altered in the anesthetized patient. Changes in blood pressure, afterload, and vascular tone greatly complicate the evaluation of procedural results in this setting. Working with an anesthesiologist who is well versed in intraoperative echocardiographic interpretation greatly facilitates assessment of an adequate endpoint in terms of the degree of reduction of mitral regurgitation.

The role and insight of the cardiovascular surgeon are also important in the development of the percutaneous mitral valve repair procedure. The understanding developed in the field of cardiovascular surgery through many decades of experience with mitral valve repair is particularly critical in patient selection. The general classification of patients as having functional, ischemic, or degenerative mitral regurgitation is oversimplified for the adequate categorization of patients as ideal for percutaneous repair versus surgical repair at this early stage of the development of these procedures.

Results of the phase I trial to evaluate Evalve edge-to-edge repair

The first implant of an Evalve clip in a patient was successfully performed in June 2003 by Jose Antonio Condado, in Venezuela. To evaluate the feasibility of percutaneous repair using this device, a phase I safety trial was initiated, with the first patient being enrolled on 2 July 2003. The trial was a non-randomized registry involving up to 12 roll-in patients at six centers, and a maximum of 32 patients.

Inclusion criteria include age 18 years or older, candidacy for mitral valve surgery including cardiopulmonary bypass, and suitability for transseptal puncture. All patients met the guidelines for mechanical therapy of mitral regurgitation outlined in the American College of Cardiology/American Heart Association (ACC/AHA) Task Force Guidelines for Treatment of Valvular Heart Disease. Symptomatic patients with moderate to severe or severe mitral regurgitation were included (Tables 26.1 and 26.2). Asymptomatic patients with moderate to severe or severe mitral regurgitation and compromised left ventricular function were also included. Left

Table 26.1 Mitral regurgitant severity of moderate to severe or severe grade as defined by a minimum of 3 of the following criteria, one of which must be quantitative (i.e. 4, 5, or 6)

1. Color flow jet may be central and large (>6 cm^2 or >30% of left atrial area) or smaller if eccentric, encircling the left atrium
2. Pulmonary vein flow may show systolic blunting or systolic flow reversal
3. Vena contracta width >0.3 cm measured in the parasternal long-axis view
4. Regurgitant volume of >45 ml/beat
5. Regurgitant fraction >40%
6. Regurgitant orifice area >0.30 cm^2

Table 26.2 Inclusion criteria

1. Age 18 years or older
2. Moderate to severe or severe mitral valve regurgitation (MR):

   (a) Symptomatic moderate to severe or severe MR, or
   (b) Asymptomatic moderate to severe or severe MR with a compromised left ventricle (left ventricular ejection fraction <60% or left ventricular end-systolic dimension >45 mm)

3. The regurgitant jet originates from the central two-thirds of the line of coaptation of the mitral valve
4. The mitral valve coaptation depth is ≤11 mm
5. Candidate for mitral valve surgery including cardiopulmonary bypass
6. Female subjects of childbearing potential must have a negative pregnancy test
7. Trans-septal catheterization is determined to be feasible by the treating physician

ventricular ejection fraction less than 60% or left ventricular end-systolic dimension greater than 45 mm represented left ventricular dysfunction severe enough to warrant repair.

Patients with prior sternotomy for any reason were excluded from the phase I trial due to the concern that, in the event of emergency surgery, this would delay obtaining access for surgical mitral valve therapy.

Case selection requires a careful evaluation of the echocardiographic appearance of the valve. Patients with ischemic and functional mitral regurgitation were often not included. Mitral regurgitation due to severe ischemic disease is typically caused by leaflet tethering, which potentially limits the depth of leaflet available for

apposition with the clip. Functional mitral regurgitation, usually a consequence of severe left ventricular dysfunction, typically creates annular dilatation, which is best corrected with an annuloplasty. Patients suffering from degenerative mitral regurgitation thus represented the predominant group enrolled in the trial. To be included in the study, the regurgitation had to arise from the central two-thirds of the mitral leaflets. Large flail segments were considered an exclusion.

The primary endpoint for the EVEREST I trial (percutaneous edge-to-edge mitral valve repair using the Evalve clip) was safety at 30 days. Safety was defined as freedom from death, myocardial infarction, cardiac tamponade, cardiac surgery for failed clip or device, clip detachment, permanent stroke, or septicemia. Secondary safety endpoints included hospital vascular complications, 30-day and the 6-month bleeding, endocarditis, clip thrombosis, hemolysis, or mitral valve surgery, and the 6-month secondary safety endpoint was cardiac surgery for the failed clip or device.

The primary efficacy endpoint was reduction of mitral regurgitation to 2+ or less, which is the definition of successful therapy in the AHA/ACC Task Force Guidelines for Treatment of Valvular Heart Disease. Secondary efficacy endpoints included successful implantation of the clip and implantation without major adverse events in the hospital. The 30-day and 6-month secondary efficacy endpoints included mitral regurgitation severity determined by echocardiography and mitral valve function, including transvalvular pressure gradient, mitral valve area, and cardiac output. New York Heart Association (NYHA) functional class was also evaluated as a secondary efficacy endpoint.

An echocardiography core laboratory was used extensively in both patient selection and assessment of results. American Society of Echocardiography guidelines, with an emphasis on objective measurements, were strictly followed for classification of mitral regurgitation severity.[12]

At the TCT (Transcatheter Cardiovascular Therapeutics) Meeting on 30 September 2004, the results for the first 27 patients treated in the feasibility trial were reported.[13] The mean age was 67 years, 59% were male, and 44% were NYHA class III or IV, and 41% were in atrial fibrillation. The mitral regurgitation etiology was degenerative in 92% of patients, and ischemic in 2 patients (7%).

Ultimately, a clip was implanted in 24 of 27 patients. The 3 patients in whom a clip was not placed were among the first 7 patients treated and represent an important part of the early learning curve. All underwent elective surgery, 2 with repair and 1 with mitral valve replacement. Successful edge-to-edge leaflet coaptation with creation of a double orifice could be performed in all 27 patients. Of the 24 in whom a clip was deployed, 67% had resultant 2+ or less mitral regurgitation at discharge. Major adverse events occurred in only 4 patients.

A critically important part of the early learning curve was demonstrated by the average device time. First procedures in most institutions required over 3 hours, while sixth, seventh, and eighth procedures typically required less than 2 hours to perform.

The primary endpoint of major adverse events was noted in four patients. One patient had a neurologic deficit classified as a stroke, with full recovery later. A clip detached from one of the two mitral leaflets in 3 patients, without embolization in any cases. There were no cases of cardiac surgery for failed clip, myocardial infarction, cardiac tamponade, or septicemia.

Among patients who required surgery after clip placement, repair could be accomplished in 83%. One patient underwent late valve replacement. It is of critical importance that the option for surgical repair was preserved in all patients, even when surgery was performed for inadequate control of the mitral regurgitation greater than 30 days after clip implantation.

Echocardiographic core laboratory evaluation of mitral regurgitation showed a decrease from a severity of 3.7 at baseline to less than 2 after the roll-in patients had been considered. While this initial data is compelling, the strategy for application and indications for this procedure remain to be determined. The feasibility study included patients who were candidates for mitral repair surgery. This represents a broad spectrum. At one end are younger patients often with an age between 30 and 50 years, in whom the longer-term results of mitral valve repair surgery are relatively understood. At the other extreme are patients who are poor risk for surgery, often in their eighth decade or with significant comorbidity. These patients would do well with diminished

mitral regurgitation by any method, especially if the challenges of surgery in the elderly could be avoided. It is possible that in this latter group, a lesser degree of efficacy in terms of mitral valve regurgitation would be acceptable if the safety of the procedure were substantially greater. The ideal application of this procedure for these various patient subsets will depend entirely on the late results of the procedure as we come to learn more about it with further experience.

The success of the feasibility trial for the Evalve clip has led to the proposal of a pivotal phase II trial. This will be a randomized comparison by intention to treat of percutaneous mitral valve repair using the Evalve clip versus standard surgical repair. A number of important trial design considerations come into play. The long-term efficacy of surgical repair is not extensively documented. It is possible that the efficacy of a percutaneous procedure aimed only at edge-to-edge repair compares favorably with the combined approaches of annuloplasty and leaflet resection likely to be used in the surgical arm of the trial. In addition, crossover to mitral valve replacement in either arm, if successful, is still part of the intended therapy strategy. Thus, the strategy of mitral valve repair using edge-to-edge percutaneous repair as a first planned therapy has the potential for comparing well with surgery as a planned first therapy, and may offer significant clinical advantages.

The future of percutaneous mitral repair

A number of alternative percutaneous methods for mitral repair are under development. Edge-to-edge repair using a suture-based approach has been pilot-tested in animal models, and attempted in a few patients. Catheter-directed annuloplasty using either the coronary sinus or the left ventricular endocardial surface as delivery routes for annulus cinching devices are also in development, and phase 1 clinical trials have been initiated with these systems. Thus, while the Evalve clip is the first percutaneous technology undergoing active clinical evaluation, its exact role and niche remain to be defined and will depend on the balance of efficacy, safety, and long-term durability. At the very least, it will offer an alternative therapy to patients for whom surgical valve repair or replacement is not feasible. The degree to which the Evalve clip repair approximates surgical benchmark results will determine its place as primary therapy for the management of mitral regurgitation.

References

1. Alfieri O, Maisano F, De Bonis M, et al. The edge-to-edge technique in mitral valve repair: a simple solution for complex problems. J Thorac Cardiovasc Surg 2001; 122: 674–81.
2. Alfieri O, Elefteriades JA, Chapolini RJ, et al. Novel suture device for beating-heart mitral leaflet approximation. Ann Thorac Surg 2002; 74: 1488–93.
3. Maisano F, Schreuder JJ, Oppizzi M, et al. The double orifice technique as a standardized approach to treat mitral regurgitation due to severe myxomatous disease: surgical technique. Eur J Cardiothorac Surg 2000; 17: 201–15.
4. Alfieri O, De Bonis M, Lapenna E, et al. 'Edge-to-edge' repair for anterior mitral leaflet prolapse. Semin Thorac Cardiovasc Surg 2004; 16: 182–7.
5. De Bonis M, Lapenna E, La Canna G, et al. Mitral valve repair for functional mitral regurgitation in end-stage dilated cardiomyopathy; the role of edge-to-edge technique. Circulation 2005; 112 (Suppl): I 402–8.
6. Maisano F, Caldarola A, Blasio A, et al. Midterm results of edge-to-edge mitral valve repair without annuloplasty. J Thorac Cardiovasc Surg 2003; 126: 1987–97.
7. Flameng W, Herijgers P, Bogaerts K. Recurrence of mitral valve regurgitation after mitral valve repair in degenerative valve disease. Circulation, 2003; 107: 1609–13.
8. St Goar FG, Fann JI, Komtebedde J, et al. Catheter-directed mitral valve repair: acute results in a porcine model. Circulation 2003; 108(Suppl IV): 493.
9. Fann JI, St Goar FG, Komtebedde J, et al. Off-pump edge-to-edge mitral valve technique using a mechanical clip in a chronic model. Circulation 2003; 108(Suppl IV): 493.
10. Fann JI, St Goar FG, Komtebedde J, et al. Beating heart catheter-based edge-to-edge mitral valve procedure in a porcine model; efficacy and healing response. Circulation 2004; 110: 988–93.
11. St Goar FG, James FI, Komtebedde J, et al. Endovascular edge-to-edge mitral valve repair: short-term results in a porcine model. Circulation 2003; 108: 1990–3.
12. Zoghbi WA, Enriquez-Sarano M, Foster E, et al. American Society of Echocardiography. Recommendations for evaluation of the severity of native valvular regurgitation with two-dimensional and Doppler echocardiography. J Am Soc Echocardiogr 2003; 16: 777–802.
13. Feldman T, Herrmann HC, Wasserman HS, et al. Percutaneous edge-to-edge mitral valve repair using the Evalve clip: current status of the EVEREST phase I clinical trial. Am J Cardiol 2004; 94(Suppl 6A): 79E.

27

Available transcatheter mitral valve repair techniques: CS method

Junya Ako, Ali Hassan, Yasuhiro Honda, Peter J Fitzgerald

Introduction

The mitral valve apparatus consists of the mitral leaflets, chordae tendinae, papillary muscles, and mitral annulus. Mitral valve regurgitation (MR) is a common disease resulting from abnormalities of any of these structures. Structural (primary) causes of MR include myxomatous degeneration, rheumatic changes, calcified annulus, infective endocarditis, and chordal rupture of tethering. Functional (secondary) MR is primarily due to incomplete coaptation of normal mitral leaflets as a result of progressive mitral annular dilation, alterations in left ventricular (LV) geometry, and/or papillary muscle dysfunction.[1–4]

Secondary MR frequently accompanies acute ischemic or chronic heart failure[5] and triggers a vicious cycle of continuing volume overload, ventricular dilation, progression of annular dilation, increased LV wall tension, and thereby further worsening MR and heart failure.[6,7] In addition, this functional disorder can eventually lead to loss of systolic sphincteric contraction of the mitral annulus and chordae tendinae retraction with fibrosis. This functional MR secondary to LV dysfunction remains a significant clinical issue, representing an independent predictor of mortality in patients with ischemic or non-ischemic heart failure.[5,8–10] There are data suggesting that intervention on the mitral valve appears to benefit patients with symptomatic heart failure.[11]

In the absence of structural mitral valve abnormalities, the dimension of the mitral annulus determines mitral leaflet coaptation, regurgitant orifice area, and ultimately subsequent MR. Therefore, the dominant modality of current surgical approach is insertion of a mitral annulo-plasty ring that reduces the annular circumference and pushes the posterior leaflet forward for better coaptation, thereby decreasing MR.[1,4] This approach maintains the mitral valve and sub-valvular apparatus, which helps preserve overall LV function, thereby offering an advantage over valve replacement techniques in the treatment of MR in patients with heart failure.

However, the relatively high hospital morbidity and mortality rates associated with open-heart procedures in patients with heart failure have hindered their broader application.[11,12] This limitation has led to an increasing demand for less invasive approaches that are applicable even to patients with severely compromised LV function. Several percutaneous treatment modalities via the coronary sinus have come into focus.[13–16] The anatomic proximity of the coronary sinus to the posterior mitral annulus, coupled with relatively undemanding percutaneous accessibility to this large vein, offers a basis for the development of less invasive, catheter-based mitral annulo-plasty.[17,18] This chapter provides an overview of the rationale for using the coronary sinus for percutaneous mitral annuloplasty, current prototypes, and other percutaneous approaches to directly address mitral valvular pathology.

Anatomy of the coronary sinus

Location and major tributaries

The coronary sinus runs along the circumflex coronary artery in the atrioventricular groove parallel to the posterior mitral annulus (Figure 27.1).

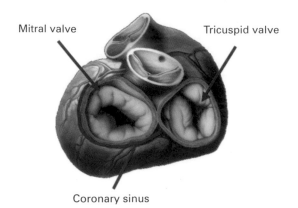

Mitral valve

Tricuspid valve

Coronary sinus

Figure 27.1

Location of the coronary sinus, which surrounds the mitral valve annulus.

It courses from the origin of the anterior interventricular vein, which runs adjacent to the left anterior descending coronary artery on the anterior surface of the heart. As the main channel of venous blood from the myocardium, the coronary sinus is drained into by a number of smaller veins: typically, from left to right along its course, the great cardiac vein, the oblique vein of Marshall, the posterior vein of the left ventricle, the posterior interventricular vein, the middle cardiac vein, and the small cardiac veins. The coronary sinus orifice, the aperture through which most of the venous drainage of the heart is returned to the circulation, lies anteroinferiorly of the tricuspid orifice in the right atrium.

Size, length, and shape

There are numerous variations in size, length, and shape of the coronary sinus. The diameter of the atrial ostium ranges between 7 and 16 mm.[19,20] The length is between 15 and 70 mm (median 37 mm).[21] A short coronary sinus has the length of a phalanx of a finger (7% of cases); a coronary sinus of medium length with its cylindrical form corresponds to two phalanges in 74% of cases; and an elongated coronary sinus has the length of three phalanges and exhibits a tubular, extended form in 18% of cases.

In a study by von Ludinghausen and Schott,[22] based on detailed dissections of 350 human cadaveric hearts, the coronary sinus in the left posterior coronary sulcus was coplanar to the mitral annulus in only 12% of the cases studied. In most specimens, the coronary sinus was in a displaced position toward the posterior wall of the left atrium. The displacement or elevation was slight (1–3 mm) in 16% of cases, moderate (4–7 mm) in 50%, and extreme (8–15 mm) in 22% (Figure 27.2).

Venous valves

The entrance of the coronary sinus into the right atrium is guarded by a fold – the Thebesian valve. The valve drops across the coronary sinus orifice whenever the pressure in the right atrium exceeds that in the vein (i.e. during atrial contraction). The types of valve shape have several patterns: incomplete (50%), crescentic (34%), cribriform (7%), semiannular (7%), and thread (2%). While 31% of hearts have a complete valve, the ostium is valveless in 19%.[22–24]

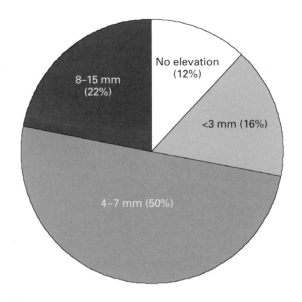

Figure 27.2

Degree of elevation of the coronary sinus from the posterior coronary sulcus.[22]

The anatomic marker dictating the site where the great cardiac vein widens to become the coronary sinus is Vieussens valve, which is present in 65–87% of hearts. Several morphologic types of valve can be distinguished: unicuspid (62%), bicuspid (25%), tricuspid (<1%), and multiple (<1%).[22]

Strategic imaging prior to catheter-based mitral annuloplasty

Due to significant anatomic variations in humans, prior assessment of venous anatomy as well as its adjacent structures is crucial for both patient triage and successful catheter-based mitral annuloplasty. First, the location, size, length, shape, and valves of the coronary sinus can directly influence the feasibility and efficacy of coronary sinus annuloplasty devices. In particular, the position of the coronary sinus relative to the mitral annulus holds the key to successful results. Second, the proximity of the coronary sinus to the circumflex coronary artery may pose a potential risk of distortion or damage to the artery by placement of an annuloplasty device. Thus, significantly calcified coronary lesions or previously implanted stents in the circumflex coronary artery should be pre-evaluated. Third, the presence and degree of mitral annular calcification are also important since the efficacy of annuloplasty via the coronary sinus depends partly on the rigidity of the mitral annulus.

Coronary angiography is the gold standard for the assessment of coronary artery lesions. With sufficient contrast for the venous follow-through phase, this conventional method can provide a venous road map as well as a visual correlation between the arterial and venous anatomies (Figure 27.3). In humans, the great cardiac vein generally crosses over the circumflex coronary artery in its distal portion at the transition into the coronary sinus. Pinching of the circumflex coronary artery by the coronary sinus annuloplasty device must be avoided. Direct venography by a retrograde injection into the coronary sinus with proximal balloon occlusion can offer the best method for the venous anatomy evaluation, allowing more precise morphologic and morphometric assessment of the coronary sinus. Currently, advanced non-invasive imaging tech-

niques using computed tomography (CT) or magnetic resonance imaging (MRI) technologies have been rapidly developed. Three-dimensional images of the heart are also useful to evaluate the geographic relationship between the coronary sinus and the mitral valve.

Devices addressing annular pathology via the coronary sinus

Percutaneous mitral annuloplasty devices (Figure 27.4)

Percutaneous catheter-based annuloplasty devices, the majority of which are 'ring-like' implants for insertion into the coronary sinus, are under development. By surrounding the anterolateral and posterior portions of the mitral valve annulus, these prototypes are designed to push the dislocated posterior annulus anteriorly for improved leaflet coaptation. One other approach does not use an implant device, but rather uses thermal energy to shrink the mitral annulus, thereby generating a similar effect. In animal studies, each device has shown promising acute results; some investigators have also reported chronic animal data or preliminary human experience.

Stent-like implant device

A stent-based approach is being tested as a partial annular ring implant device (Edwards Lifesciences, Irvine, CA). The 8 Fr prototype consists of three elements: two anchor stents to be deployed into the great cardiac vein and the coronary sinus, respectively, and the middle stent foreshortening to reshape the coronary sinus.

C-shaped implant device

A C-shaped annular ring implant device is being developed and has been tested (C-Cure, ev3, Plymouth, MN). The implant device is preloaded into a 10 Fr delivery catheter and is actuated via a handle on the catheter. Preliminary human experience of temporary C-Cure placement also showed a significant reduction of MR with no

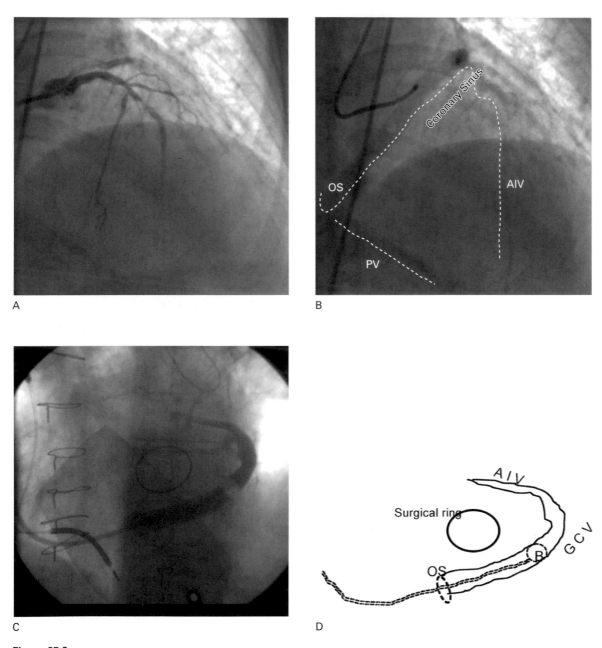

Figure 27.3

(A) Coronary angiography with the venous follow-through phase: left anterior descending coronary artery angiogram in the right anterior oblique projection. (B) Venous follow-through phase of coronary angiography. Contrast washout phase elucidative of the coronary vein. AIV, anterior interventricular vein; OS, ostium of coronary sinus; PV, posterior vein of the left ventricle. (C) Coronary sinus venography by retrograde contrast injection with proximal balloon occlusion: the coronary sinus and its major tributaries. (D) Relationship between the coronary sinus/great cardiac vein and a surgically implanted mitral annular ring. AIV, anterior interventricular vein; GCV, great cardiac vein; OS, ostium of coronary sinus; B, balloon.

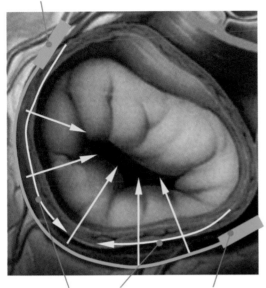

Distal anchor

Foreshortening   Proximal anchor

A

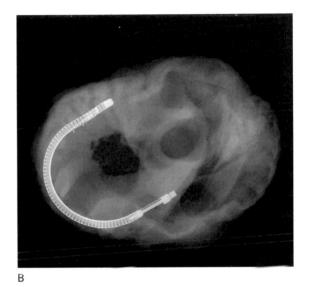

B

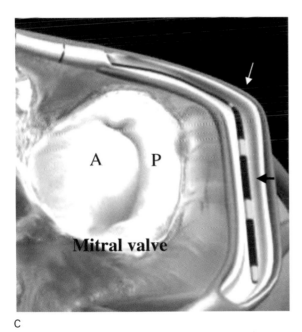

A   P

Mitral valve

C

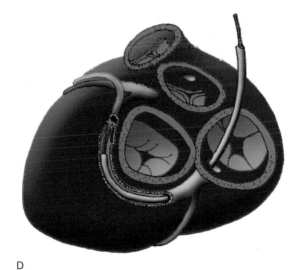

D

Figure 27.4

Mitral annuloplasty devices. (A) Stent-based percutaneous mitral annuloplasty device (Edwards Lifesciences, Irvine, CA). (B) C-shaped percutaneous mitral annuloplasty device (C-Cure, ev3, Plymouth, MN). (C) Straight percutaneous mitral annuloplasty device (A, anterior mitral leaflet; P, posterior mitral leaflet (Viacor, Wilmington, MA). (D) Wire-based percutaneous mitral annuloplasty device (Cardiac Dimensions Inc., Kirkland, WA). (Part (C) reproduced from: Liddicoat JR, MacNeill BD, Gillinov AM, et al. Catheter Cardiovasc Interv 2003; 60: 410–16.[17])

procedural complications. No data on permanent placement are available.

Straight implant device

A straight device is being developed as a temporary or permanent annuloplasty implant in the coronary sinus (Viacor, Wilmington, MA). The implant device consists of a composite nitinol and stainless steel construct, coated with medical-grade Teflon and polyethylene plastic. It comprises a substantially straight and rigid element, available in lengths ranging from 35 to 85 mm, which maintains its shape in the coronary sinus. This causes conformational changes in the mitral annulus, pushing forward the posterior annulus with an outward counterforce on the coronary sinus near commissures.[17] This device is designed to push the posterior leaflet forward, while minimizing potential damages to the circumflex coronary artery. In addition, this device exerts an outward counterforce on the parts of the coronary sinus near the commissures in order to improve coaptation.

As a preliminary human experience, 10 patients underwent temporary device placement immediately prior to the mitral valve repair surgery, confirming the feasibility of this technique in humans. No data on permanent placement are available.

Wire-based implant device

A wire-based implantable device has been tested in an animal model of heart failure-induced MR (Cardiac Dimensions Inc., Kirkland, WA). The device is constructed from nitinol wire, with distal and proximal anchors connected by an intervening cable sheath.[18]

Thermal energy approach

As an alternative to the implantable coronary sinus annuloplasty devices, a thermal energy technique is being developed (QuantumCor Inc., Irvine, CA). The principle of the mechanism is to shrink annular collagen by the heat generated with a coronary sinus probe, improving mitral competence without implanted materials. The prototype catheter has eight electrodes (approximately 1.5×2 mm), and the tip of the probe is malleable to conform to the annulus shape. Delivery of radiofrequency (RF) energy to the electrodes is computer-controlled by the maximum temperatures sensed by adjacent thermocouples.

Potential limitations

There are several potential issues particular to percutaneous coronary sinus repair of MR. Obviously, it is not possible to address valvular pathology with this technique. Thus, stand-alone use of this method is basically indicated only for secondary MR without significant valvular abnormality. Even in secondary MR, annuloplasty devices do not address the distorted left ventricle or displaced papillary muscle, and so there is only partial management of overall pathologic changes.[25] Therefore, the efficacy of this technique should be carefully assessed comparing with other modalities (Table 27.1).

As described previously, the position of the coronary sinus relative to the mitral annulus can significantly affect the effectiveness of this technique. As shown in Figure 27.2, the coronary sinus was in a displaced position toward the posterior wall of the left atrium in many cases.[22] Acceptable ranges of coronary sinus displacement for this technique remain to be investigated.

Other possible issues include the venous valves, which may make direct catheter cannulation difficult in some patients; potential damage, pinching, or stent deformation of the adjacent circumflex coronary artery; and significant mitral annular calcification that may limit the annuloplasty effect, as also discussed previously. Additionally, the congested coronary sinus space due to the implant device inside may affect the hemodynamics of cardiac circulation in the short or long term. The long-term risks of coronary sinus thrombosis/occlusion and erosion/perforation need to be determined as well.

Devices directly addressing annular pathology

Because the coronary sinus is not perfectly coplanar to the mitral annulus in most human cases,

Table 27.1 Comparison of mitral valve repair techniques

Method	Target disease	Advantage	Disadvantage	Complications	Companies
Coronary sinus	Secondary MR	Relatively feasible	Coronary sinus may not always be coplanar to mitral annulus	Damaging left circumflex, venous thrombosis, infection, coronary sinus rupture	Edwards Lifesciences, Viacor, Cardiac Dimensions, QuantumCor
Coronary sinus and trans-ventricular	Secondary MR	Ability to address the mitral annulus regardless of its relative position to the coronary sinus	Technically demanding	Not available	Mitralign
Edge-to-edge	Secondary and primary MR	Ability to treat primary MR	Technically demanding, high stress to valve components	Clip dislodgement, thrombosis, mitral stenosis, infection	E-valve, Edwards Lifesciences
Pericardial	Secondary MR	Ability to address ventricular remodeling	Thoracotomy necessary	Thrombosis, infection	MyoCor

devices that directly address annular pathology are also under development (Mitralign, MitralSolutions). These devices are only at a rudimentary stage, and no animal or clinical data are available.

Transluminal transventricular annuloplasty

A suture-based transventricular approach is being developed. Using magnetic guidance from another catheter in the coronary sinus, a suture is applied to the posterior mitral annulus by a transarterial–transventricular catheter (Mitralign, Salem, NH). No animal or human data are available.

Potential limitations

This approach may be technically more demanding than annuloplasty of the coronary sinus. Potential damage to the aortic valve, papillary muscle, and chordae tendinae may be of concern with this technology. Technical difficulties in effectively shortening dilated annulus, even by

surgical suture, pose concerns regarding the efficacy of this percutaneous technique.

Devices addressing valvular pathology

Percutaneous edge-to-edge mitral valve repair devices

Although mitral annuloplasty is effective for functional MR secondary to heart failure, the coexistence of primary valvular pathology, including structural leaflet changes and severely calcified annulus, can limit the number of candidates for this technique. To circumvent this limitation, several surgical methods addressing valvular pathology have been developed, one of which is the edge-to-edge or Alfieri technique, which creates a double-orifice mitral valve with central leaflet suturing ('bow-tie appearance').[26–28] The simplicity of this technique, as well as its clinical success,[29–31] have encouraged the development of less-invasive, catheter-based, edge-to-edge repair technologies. The initial results in a short-term animal model appear promising. Combined use of this method with a percutaneous annuloplasty device may offer further clinical benefit, particularly in high-risk patients with complex MR.[28]

Mitral valve edge-to-edge clipping device

A prototype system for percutaneous edge-to-edge repair consists of an implantable V-shaped clip attached to a delivery catheter, and a guide catheter with a bidirectional steering mechanism at the distal tip (Evalve, Redwood City, CA). The clip, constructed of implant-grade metals and covered with polyester, is a two-armed, soft tissue approximation device. It is designed to vertically coapt up to 8 mm of leaflet height and to promote leaflet-to-leaflet healing around and into the device to maintain a point of permanent leaflet approximation. The device is placed transseptally into the left atrium using femoral vein access. The implantable clip attached to the delivery catheter is opened, advanced through the mitral orifice, and then retracted to grasp the middle scallops of the anterior and posterior mitral leaflets during systole. If necessary, the clip can be opened and repositioned. After a functional double orifice has been confirmed by echocardiography, the clip is locked and detached from the delivery system. These manipulations of the clip are all controlled by the delivery catheter handle mechanisms.[32]

A phase I trial, EVEREST I (Endovascular Valve Edge-to-Edge Repair Study), has enrolled 27 patients to date. Of these 27 patients, clips have been deployed successfully in 24 (93%), and significant MR reduction has been observed in 18 (67%). A pivotal clinical trial is planned to follow.

Mitral valve edge-to-edge suture device

A percutaneous edge-to-edge suture device is also being developed and is undergoing preclinical testing (Edwards Lifesciences, Irvine, CA). The prototype utilizes a vacuum mechanism to capture the anterior and posterior mitral leaflets. A double orifice is created with needle stitches of the mitral leaflets, and the suture is fastened with a nitinol clip.

Potential limitations

Potential issues particular to percutaneous edge-to-edge repair include large device size, relatively technically demanding procedures, potential risk of endocarditis, leaflet degeneration, and uncertain long-term durability due to increased stress to valve components. Since the valve is exposed to increased stresses following edge-to-edge repair, a concomitant annuloplasty procedure may be required for the optimal long-term results.[33] In addition, the feasibility and efficacy of this technique are limited in subsets of patients with extreme valvular pathology, including rheumatic disease or a ruptured papillary muscle.

Future perspectives

Chronic heart failure is a major public health problem, affecting nearly five million people, with approximately half a million new cases diagnosed annually in the USA alone.[34] Despite mounting evidence of clinical benefits from surgical correction of secondary MR, patients with severe LV dysfunction are often considered poor operative candidates due to their high perioperative morbidity and mortality. With the advent of less-invasive catheter-based procedures, a paradigm shift in the management of functional MR may take place. In combination with percutaneous devices to address valvular pathology, catheter-based annuloplasty may also offer a therapeutic option for a certain subset of primary MR patients with coexisting comorbidities. Furthermore, ischemic MR, when considered reversible, may be managed successfully with temporary device placement. Although the experience described in this chapter is derived from first-generation devices, the promising results of preliminary animal studies encourage our future endeavor toward establishing safety and efficacy of these technologies in humans.

References

1. Miller DC. Ischemic mitral regurgitation redux – to repair or to replace? J Thorac Cardiovasc Surg 2001; 122: 1059–62.

2. Gillinov AM, Wierup PN, Blackstone EH, et al. Is repair preferable to replacement for ischemic mitral regurgitation? J Thorac Cardiovasc Surg 2001; 122: 1125–41.

3. Bolling SF, Pagani FD, Deeb GM, Bach DS. Intermediate-term outcome of mitral reconstruction in cardiomyopathy. J Thorac Cardiovasc Surg 1998; 115: 381–6; discussion 387–8.

4. Boltwood CM, Tei C, Wong M, Shah PM. Quantitative echocardiography of the mitral complex in dilated cardiomyopathy: the mechanism of functional mitral regurgitation. Circulation 1983; 68: 498–508.

5. Trichon BH, Felker GM, Shaw LK, et al. Relation of frequency and severity of mitral regurgitation to survival among patients with left ventricular systolic dysfunction and heart failure. Am J Cardiol 2003; 91: 538 43.

6. Lamas GA, Mitchell GF, Flaker GC, et al. Clinical significance of mitral regurgitation after acute myocardial infarction. Survival and Ventricular Enlargement Investigators. Circulation 1997; 96: 827–33.

7. Trichon BH, O'Connor CM. Secondary mitral and tricuspid regurgitation accompanying left ventricular systolic dysfunction: Is it important, and how is it treated? Am Heart J 2002; 144: 373–6

8. Robbins JD, Maniar PB, Cotts W, et al. Prevalence and severity of mitral regurgitation in chronic systolic heart failure. Am J Cardiol 2003; 91: 360–2.

9. Conti JB, Mills RM Jr. Mitral regurgitation and death while awaiting cardiac transplantation. Am J Cardiol 1993; 71: 617–18.

10. Blondheim DS, Jacobs LE, Kotler MN, et al. Dilated cardiomyopathy with mitral regurgitation: decreased survival despite a low frequency of left ventricular thrombus. Am Heart J 1991; 122: 763–71.

11. Harris KM, Sundt TM 3rd, Aeppli D, et al. Can late survival of patients with moderate ischemic mitral regurgitation be impacted by intervention on the valve? Ann Thorac Surg 2002; 74: 1468–75.

12. Bolling SF. Mitral reconstruction in cardiomyopathy. J Heart Valve Dis 2002; 11(Suppl 1): S26–S31.

13. Cazeau S, Leclercq C, Lavergne T, et al. Effects of multisite biventricular pacing in patients with heart failure and intraventricular conduction delay. N Engl J Med 2001; 344: 873–80.

14. Oesterle SN, Reifart N, Hauptmann E, et al. Percutaneous in situ coronary venous arterialization: report of the first human catheter-based coronary artery bypass. Circulation 2001; 103: 2539–43.

15. Thompson CA, Nasseri BA, Makower J, et al. Percutaneous transvenous cellular cardiomyoplasty. A novel nonsurgical approach for myocardial cell transplantation. J Am Coll Cardiol 2003; 41: 1964–71.

16. Herity NA, Lo ST, Oei F, et al. Selective regional myocardial infiltration by the percutaneous coronary venous route: a novel technique for local drug delivery. Catheter Cardiovasc Interv 2000; 51: 358–63.

17. Liddicoat JR, MacNeill BD, Gillinov AM, et al. Percutaneous mitral valve repair: a feasibility study in an ovine model of acute ischemic mitral regurgitation. Catheter Cardiovasc Interv 2003; 60: 410–16.

18. Kaye DM, Byrne M, Alferness C, Power J. Feasibility and short-term efficacy of percutaneous mitral annular reduction for the therapy of heart failure-induced mitral regurgitation Circulation 2003; 108: 1795–7.

19. Mohl W. Pressure controlled intermittent coronary sinus occlusion – an alternative to retrograde perfusion of arterial blood. In: Mohl W, Wonlner E, Glogar D (eds). The Coronary Sinus. Darmstadt: Steinkopff, 1984: 418–23.

20. Platzer W. Atlas der topographischen Anatomie. Thieme Verlag: Stuttgart, 1982: 108–9.

21. Mohl W (ed). Coronary Sinus Interventions in Cardiac Surgery. Georgetown, TX: Landes Bioscience, 2000.

22. von Ludinghausen M, Schott C. Microanatomy of the human coronary sinus and its major tributaries. In: Meerbaum S (ed) Myocardial Perfusion, Reperfusion, Coronary Venous Retroperfusion. Darmstadt: Steinkopff, 1990: 93–122.

23. Hellerestein HK, Orbison JL. Anatomic variations of the orifice of the human coronary sinus. Circulation 1961; 3: 1–35.

24. Marshall J. On the development of the great anterior veins in man and mammalia; including an account of certain remnants of foetal structure found in the adult, a comparative view of these great veins in the different mammalia, and an analysis of their occasional peculiarities in the human subject. Phil Trans R Soc Lond 1950; 140: 133–70.

25. Levine RA, Hung J. Ischemic mitral regurgitation, the dynamic lesion: clues to the cure. J Am Coll Cardiol 2003; 42: 1929–32.

26. Fucci C, Sandrelli L, Pardini A, et al. Improved results with mitral valve repair using new surgical techniques. Eur J Cardiothorac Surg 1995; 9: 621–6; discussion 626–7.

27. Galloway AC, Grossi EA, Bizekis CS, et al. Evolving techniques for mitral valve reconstruction. Ann Surg 2002; 236: 288–93; discussion 293–4.

28. Alfieri O, Maisano F, De Bonis M, et al. The double-orifice technique in mitral valve repair: a simple solution for complex problems. J Thorac Cardiovasc Surg 2001; 122: 674–81.

29. Maisano F, Torracca L, Oppizzi M, et al. The edge-to-edge technique: a simplified method to correct mitral insufficiency. Eur J Cardiothorac Surg 1998; 13: 240–5; discussion 245–6.

30. Maisano F, Schreuder JJ, Oppizzi M, et al. The double-orifice technique as a standardized approach to treat mitral regurgitation due to severe myxomatous disease: surgical technique. Eur J Cardiothorac Surg 2000; 17: 201–5.

31. Totaro P, Tulumello E, Fellini P, et al. Mitral valve repair for isolated prolapse of the anterior leaflet: an 11–year follow-up. Eur J Cardiothorac Surg 1999; 15: 119–26.

32. St Goar FG, Fann JI, Komtebedde J, et al. Endovascular edge-to-edge mitral valve repair: short-term results in a porcine model. Circulation 2003; 108: 1990–3.

33. Votta E, Maisano F, Soncini M, et al. 3-D computational analysis of the stress distribution on the leaflets after edge-to-edge repair of mitral regurgitation. J Heart Valve Dis 2002; 11: 810–22.

34. O'Connell JB, Bristow MR. Economic impact of heart failure in the United States: time for a different approach. J Heart Lung Transplant 1994; 13: S107–S112.

28

A hybrid approach to the mini-invasive replacement of the mitral valve

Younes Boudjemline, Emmanuelle Pineau, Philipp Bonhoeffer

Introduction

Extensive experimental work in transcatheter valve insertion is currently being undertaken to extend its indications to the whole spectrum of aortic and pulmonary valve diseases as well as to other cardiac valves.[1-6] Various approaches have been reported, in animals, to try to repair the mitral valve, including the edge-to-edge (Alfieri) repair using an intervascular clip, as well as annuloplasty through the coronary sinus.[7,8] However, to date, no transcatheter technique has been described to replace mitral valves. In surgical practice, semilunar heterograft or homograft valves have been used to replace the mitral valve.[9,10] Mitral substitutes require the reinsertion of papillary muscles, making their use impossible for transcatheter placement. Unfortunately, semilunar homograft or heterograft valves need to be sutured to a downsized annulus, which is not currently feasible with transcatheter techniques. In this chapter, we describe our ongoing work on this subject, and the future prospects of the described procedure.

Non-surgical replacement of the mitral valve

The lessons that we have learned from the tricuspid valve replacement experience are not directly applicable due to the close relationships between the atrioventricular annulus, the coronary artery circulation, and the aortic valve. The devices designed for the tricuspid valve are not likely to work in the mitral position. The mitral chordae and papillary muscles are more developed than in the tricuspid position. These particular features would hamper the complete opening of the ventricular disk, leading to a severe paravalvular leak. Even with appropriate opening of this part, subaortic obstruction and aortic insufficiency are potential complications linked to the particular anatomy of the left side and the size of the ventricular disk. To deal with these difficulties, we are developing modified devices with asymmetrical disks as designed for closure of perimembranous ventricular septal defect, together with alternative ways to fix the device to the annulus. To date, none of these developments have been tested in in vivo studies. Another difficulty is access to the diseased mitral valve. Given the weight of the device, it is likely that an arteriovenous loop between the femoral artery and vein after a transseptal puncture would be necessary. We have tested another way to overcome these difficulties. As for replacement of aortic valves, we have investigated the possibility of using the frame of a surgically implanted biological mitral valve as a support for a valved stent that we have attempted to implant though a transatrial approach.

Development of devices for transcatheter insertion of a semilunar valve in the mitral position

For this application, we used a currently available biological valve (Mosaic, Medtronic Inc., Atlanta, GA). This valve is a porcine valve that has a low profile, with flexible stent posts and a sewing ring. Stent design features include, in particular, markers allowing for radiographic visualization. Since radio-opacity was not sufficient with the fluoroscopic equipment in our animal catheterization laboratory, we sewed an additional radio-opaque ring onto a basic Mosaic aortic valve (Figure 28.1). This device was positioned surgically.

For transcatheter insertion, we modified the currently existing device available for human percutaneous pulmonary valve replacement (Numed Inc., Hopkinton, NY, and Medtronic Inc.). This device uses a CP stent with eight zigs and six rows, with lengths of 34 mm when crimped and 27.1 and 24.7 mm when dilated, respectively, to 18 and 22 mm in diameter. This is too long compared with the Mosaic valve, which has a length varying from 15 to 22 mm depending on the diameter (varying from 28 to 18 mm) and with the type (i.e mitral/aortic) of valve considered. The CP stent was shortened by reducing the number of rows from six to three because, for these experiments, the only available valves were 18 mm Mosaic aortic valves, which have a height of 15 mm (model 30502101). To avoid the creation of a tunnel after implantation, the venous wall of an 18 mm valve was dissected along the commissures as described previously for the device that we used for aortic valve replacement. Since the distance between leaflets is nearly equal (despite one leaflet usually being smaller than the other two), the number of zigs of the CP stents was made a multiple of three (i.e nine) to allow for sewing of the top commissures to the stent design. For practical reasons, the delivery system consisted of a custom-made front-loading long sheath identical to the one used for human percutaneous implantation of the pulmonary valve. Since the stent was made of an alloy of platinum and iridium, balloons were necessary to deploy the device. We employed 22 mm BIB balloon catheters (Numed Inc., Hopkinton, NY). It is obvious that for this application a modified delivery system with shorter cup, balloons, and overall length could have been employed.

Animal experience: study design

Six sheep weighing 35–70 kg were included in the study. We intended to replace the mitral valve surgically with a 21 mm Mosaic aortic valve sheltering an 18 mm porcine valve as a first step,

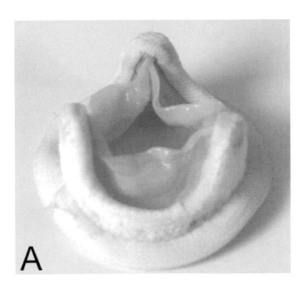 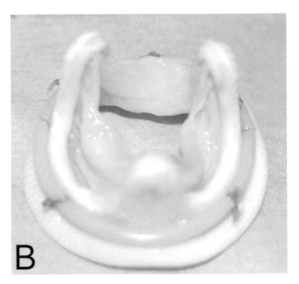

Figure 28.1

(A) A normal Mosaic valve. (B) The modified Mosaic valve: a radio-opaque ring was sewed onto its base to increase its visualization under fluoroscopy.

immediately followed by an off-pump transatrial implantation of a valved stent. The procedure was carried out under general anesthesia. The extracorporeal circulation was instituted between the femoral artery and the right atrium (RA) with a cannula introduced from the right jugular vein. A left thoracotomy was performed. The native mitral valve was excised through an opening of the left atrium (LA) and replaced by a Mosaic valve with a beating heart without any myocardial protection. After complete sewing of the heterograft, the LA opening was closed and the extracorporeal circulation stopped. Hemodynamic data (i.e right and left atrial and ventricular, pulmonary artery, and aortic pressures) and angiograms (i.e. left ventriculogram and aortogram) were acquired before and after the surgery. After a short incision (4 mm) on the left atrial wall distant to the previous opening and controlled by a purse-string on a 4.0 polypropylene suture, a wire was first introduced into the apex of the left ventricle (LV) through the previously placed heterograft. The valved stent loaded in the delivery system was then advanced over the wire under fluoroscopic guidance. The valved stent was then uncovered and positioned using the radio-opaque markers present on both devices (receivers and donor valves). When in position, balloons were subsequently inflated and deflated to deploy the valved stent. After insertion, the delivery system was carefully retrieved and the purse-string closed. Postimplantation assessment, including hemodynamics and angiograms, was performed prior to the completion of the protocol. Since the implanted Mosaic valve had a smaller diameter than the native annulus, we were aware of creating a significant gradient through the valve with high left atrial pressures that could potentially compromise the postoperative course. Because we did not have larger valves available at the time, we decided to conduct this study anyway to demonstrate that the approach was accurate. For these reasons, we expected to sacrifice all animals after the off-pump replacement of the mitral valve. Therefore, the procedure was considered successful if the following criteria were met: (1) successful delivery, (2) appropriate position and alignment, (3) absence of valvular regurgitation, and (4) absence of paravalvular leakage. High mean LA pressure and transprosthetic gradient were not considered, since we expected these numbers to be high due to the discrepancy between the native annulus and the diameter of the surgically valve implanted. Additional obstruction created by the valve implanted off-pump was considered to evaluate the success of the procedure.

Animal experience: study results

The Mosaic valve was replaced after a mean extracorporeal time of 65 minutes (Figure 28.2). Following its surgical insertion, the mean LA pressure was as high as 38 mmHg (ranging from 22 to 42 mmHg) with a mean LV end-diastolic pressure of 18.8 mmHg (ranging from 13 to 22 mmHg). Angiographic control showed perfectly functioning Mosaic valves without any subaortic valve obstruction and with a mild paravalvular leak in one animal. In the animal with the higher LA pressure, we were unable to control the bleeding from the atrial opening, and transatrial valved stent implantation was not attempted. In that animal, we tried and failed to insert the valve transseptally due to the acute angle between the puncture site and the Mosaic valve. The off-pump implantation of the valved stents was feasible in five out of six sheep. Implantations were performed easily in less than 10 minutes in all animals using fluoroscopic guidance only. No injection of radio-opaque dye was necessary during the positioning and delivery of the valve. Hemodynamic data did not change after the insertion of the valved stent. There was no significant gradient between the apex of the left ventricle, the subaortic region, and the aorta. Successfully implanted valves were all competent (Figure 28.3). Aortograms confirmed the absence of interference with the aortic valve (Figure 28.4). No migration occurred during the short follow-up. The animal with the smallest gradient and LA pressure was kept alive and is still alive after 2 months of implantation with a normally functioning heterograft and no systolic gradient between the LV and the aorta. At autopsy (four of five animals), all valved stents were sitting in the area of the Mosaic valves at a reasonable distance from the aortic valve. As expected, the valved stents were inactivating the leaflets of the Mosaic valves.

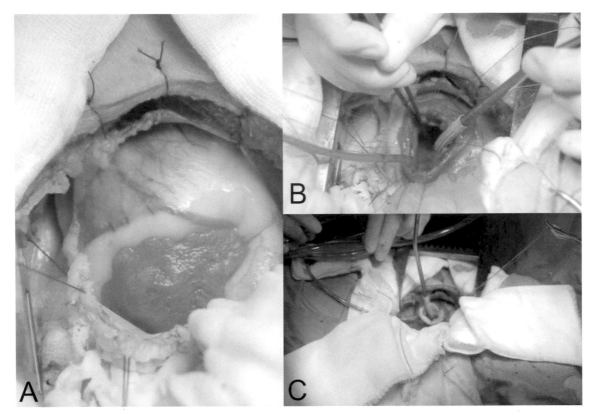

Figure 28.2

(A–C) Surgical views during the transatrial placement of the Mosaic valve.

Animal experience: study limitations and unanswered questions

The major limitation to the study is the use of a small Mosaic valve for the surgical replacement. As mentioned previously, this limitation prevents us from keeping the animals alive. Therefore, in five out of six animals, the study was performed acutely. However, there is no reason to think that the rate of success might be inferior. The only failure that we had was due to an uncontrolled bleeding secondary to high LA pressure. The use of appropriate valve size is likely to avoid this kind of complication, making the theoretical rate of success higher in the ideal situation. From an experimental point of view, a period of time between the surgical replacement and the off-pump implantation would ideally be better to allow for the recovery of the animal and to discriminate deaths linked to the surgical and off-pump procedures. For the reason detailed above, we were unable to wait for the recovery of the animals, but future studies might integrate this type of study design.

Another concern is the use of a venous valve in a systemic position. In vitro testing has shown that the competency of bovine jugular valves is maintained at back-pressures of 100 mmHg and higher. Long-term studies are, however, presently missing. We use this valve because of its availability, but, as mentioned previously, for transatrial insertion, the size of the delivery catheter is not a problem and so any valve substitute can be used for that indication. The only necessity is to have a valved stent that is no longer than the valve implanted surgically in order to avoid

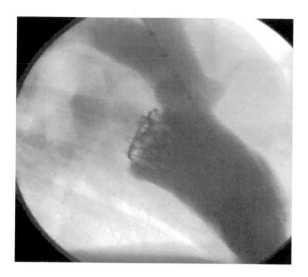

Figure 28.3

Left ventricular angiogram after transatrial insertion of the collapsible valved stent, showing good function of the surgically implanted valve and no subaortic stenosis.

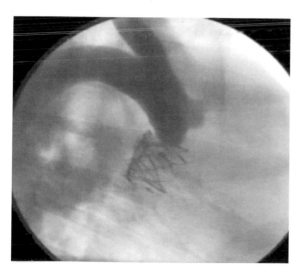

Figure 28.4

Aortography after transatrial insertion of the collapsible valved stent, showing no functional impairment of the aortic valve.

subaortic stenosis. As for mini-invasive aortic valve replacement, if the feasibility and efficacy of this type of technique can be demonstrated in the long term, this will lead to the consideration of biological valves as the first-line substitutes in patients for whom mechanical valves are often favored. The possibility of easily inserting, at low risk, a new valve using an off-pump technique might change the present view. The necessary technology is presently available to begin such a comparison. Before doing this, more animal studies with appropriate valve sizes and long-term follow-up need to be carried out. The heaviness of the present valved stent theoretically indicates its insertion via a transcatheter technique anterogradely or retrogradely after puncture of a peripheral vessel. But the demonstration remains to be done. As shown with tricuspid valve replacement, a specific device can be designed to allow for a 'complete' transcatheter replacement regardless of mitral valve anomalies. Further developments are, however, needed to manage the anatomic difficulties inherent with the mitral valve. There is no doubt in our mind that this step will come in the future.

Acknowledgments

We thank the British Heart Foundation for its financial support. We also acknowledge Numed Inc. and Medtronic Inc. for technical support and for providing us with Contegra conduits and Mosaic valves.

References

1. Bonhoeffer P, Boudjemline Y, Saliba Z, et al. Transcatheter implantation of a bovine valve in pulmonary position: a lamb study. Circulation 2000; 102: 813–16.

2. Boudjemline Y, Bonhoeffer P. Percutaneous implantation of a valve in the descending aorta in lambs. Eur Heart J 2002; 23: 1045–9.

3. Boudjemline Y, Bonhoeffer P. Steps toward percutaneous aortic valve replacement. Circulation 2002; 105: 775–8.

4. Bonhoeffer P, Boudjemline Y, Saliba Z, et al. Percutaneous replacement of pulmonary valve in a right-ventricle to pulmonary-artery prosthetic conduit with valve dysfunction. Lancet 2000; 356: 1403–5.

5.   Bonhoeffer P, Boudjemline Y, Qureshi SA, et al. Percutaneous insertion of the pulmonary valve. J Am Coll Cardiol 2002; 39: 1664–9.

6.   Cribier A, Eltchaninoff H, Bash A, et al. Percutaneous transcatheter implantation of an aortic valve prosthesis for calcific aortic stenosis: first human case description. Circulation 2002; 106: 3006–8.

7.   St Goar FG, Fann JI, Komtebedde J, et al. Endovascular edge-to-edge mitral valve repair: short-term results in a porcine model. Circulation 2003; 108: 1990–3.

8.   Liddicoat JR, MacNeill BD, Gillinov AM, et al. Percutaneous mitral valve repair: a feasibility study in an ovine model of acute ischemic mitral regurgitation. Catheter Cardiovasc Interv 2003; 60: 410–16.

9.   Salles CA, Buffolo E, Andrade JC, et al. Mitral valve replacement with glutaraldehyde preserved aortic allografts. Eur J Cardiothorac Surg 1998; 13: 135–43.

10. Kabbani SS, Ross DN, Jamil H, et al. Mitral valve replacement with a pulmonary autograft: initial experience. J Heart Valve Dis 1999; 8: 359–66.

Section 4

The tricuspid valve

29

Evaluation of the tricuspid valve using CMR

Mark A Fogel

Introduction

The use of cardiac magnetic resonance imaging (CMR) in the evaluation of valvar heart disease has played an increasingly important role in 21st century medicine. Although echocardiography is still utilized as a first-line imaging modality, CMR can offer a number of unique contributions to the assessment of both the atrioventricular and semi-lunar valves. This chapter will focus on these contributions as they apply to the tricuspid valve (TV) and congenital heart disease.

Advantages/disadvantages of CMR as it relates to the tricuspid valve

CMR is a broad-based non-invasive tool to assess the cardiovascular system and the TV specifically. Anatomy of valves can be easily assessed using either steady-state free-precession (SSFP) or spoiled gradient echo techniques both en-face or in long-axis views. In addition, valve function can be assessed utilizing cine CMR[1] and phase-encoded velocity mapping,[1,2] which is more robust and gives more useful and quantitative information than the information obtained using echocardiography or cardiac catheterization (see below). Gadolinium injection can create a three-dimensional (3D) image of the associated findings with TV pathology[3] and increased fibrous scar tissue in the valve;[4] however, the significance of the fibrous scar tissue in the valve remains unclear.

Besides being a non-invasive tool that does not expose the patient to ionizing radiation (which

places the patient at risk for future neoplastic disease[5,6]), CMR has the capability of assessing ventricular volumes and mass independent of geometric assumptions, because of its tomographic capabilities.[7] Indeed, multiple publications used to validate echocardiographic techniques take CMR as the 'gold standard'.[8,9] Another distinct advantage of CMR is that in nearly all imaging strategies, the picture is an average of many heart beats (unlike echocardiography and angiography), and therefore functional analysis by CMR can give a better handle on the long-term performance of the heart.[10] That is to say, the image itself is an average, embedding the function of the ventricle over the course of 15 seconds to 2 minutes in the image. The healthcare provider does not have to view many heart beats and do this averaging 'in his/her head', as in echocardiography and angiography.

Because of its tomographic nature, there are no overlapping structures to obscure the region of interest as is the case in angiography. CMR is not limited to acoustic windows as in echocardiography and patient size is nearly never a problem for imaging. There are no artifacts from calcifications, patches or prosthetic valves as in echocardiography, and 3D reconstruction of images is routine. In addition, no contrast agents are needed to visualize luminae, cavities, and valves as is the case, again, in angiography. Flow and velocity can be measured accurately without assumptions[11] (as opposed to echocardiography, for example, where velocity is measured and, with some geometric and physiologic assumptions, flow can be measured – but not routinely).

There are a few limitations to CMR that must be noted. Patients with pacemakers, pacemaker wires, and coils cannot be imaged because of the effects from and on the magnetic field. Sternal wires may give some artifacts near the region of interest. In addition, patients need to hold still in the scanner, so infants, small children, and unco-operative patients need to be sedated. For those who are not sedated, claustrophobia may be an issue, although this is rare. With new imaging sequences, arrhythmias generally are no longer a problem, but occasionally may preclude success-ful imaging.

Protocol and techniques utilized to evaluate the tricuspid valve

Any imaging technique requires a protocol to assess a disease state effectively, and CMR is no exception. Although each examination is tailored to the disease, a generalized method to approach CMR of the tricuspid valve has been developed and is outlined in this section.

After localizing the heart in the chest, acquiring anatomic data is the first procedure to be per-formed. This not only gives a basic survey of the cardiovascular system but also provides local-izers for future anatomic, physiologic, and func-tional imaging. A full, volumetric, contiguous axial dataset from the diaphragm to the thoracic inlet is obtained, generally using 'static' SSFP (e.g. true-FISP), which is a 'bright-blood' tech-nique' (Figure 29.1) where the cavities of the heart and blood vessels are signal-intense and the myocardium and other tissues are much less so (older spin echo or turbo spin echo techniques may also be used – Figure 29.1). SSFP is acquired in diastole, so the diastolic dimensions of the TV and the right ventricle (RV) can be assessed. These axial images form the basis of examining the anatomy and identifying the spectrum of dis-eases associated with TV pathology such as tri-cuspid atresia (TA) (Figure 29.1), pulmonary atresia with intact ventricular septum (PA-IVS), or Ebstein's anomaly.

Multiplanar reconstruction is then performed, where the axial images are stacked next to each other and any three planes can then be recon-structed. In this way, the exact slice orientation and positions can be obtained for any future imaging during the scan. In addition, it allows for inspection of the anatomy from multiple views from just the set of axial images.

Cine CMR, in the guise of SSFP or gradient echo sequences, is the next technique applied, and is tailored to the lesion under study (Figures 29.2 and 29.3). It is one of the 'workhorses' of CMR and is used to visualize cardiac motion and turbulent blood flow (causes a signal void in the image). In general, when examining the TV, a four-chamber view and an RV long-axis view through the valve are the first images obtained. From these images, evaluation of TV regurgita-tion or stenosis can be assessed as well as RV function. Cine CMR, especially SSFP, enables visualization of the leaflets and their attachments, which is especially important in cases of Ebstein's anomaly (Figure 29.2). To further evaluate TV anatomy, an en-face view of the valve is obtained; in general, the author has found that gradient echo images with a high flip angle to increase the signal of inflowing blood and highlight the leaflet edges works best. As a number of TV lesions have associated atrial septal defects (ASDs), cine CMR can be used to identify these defects; with the technique of presaturation tagging (where all the spins of the protons are destroyed in a region where a tag is laid down prior to imaging, and hence the signals from these protons are 'black' on the image), dark regions of flow across the ASD can be visualized in the bright areas of the atrial cavity. Quantitative pulmonary-to-systemic flow ratios in this instance can be obtained utiliz-ing velocity mapping (see below).[11]

Cine CMR is also used to evaluate RV volumes, mass, ejection fraction, and cardiac index[1,12–14] which are important in the physiologic assess-ment of various lesions associated with TV abnor-malities (e.g. PA-IVS and Ebstein's anomaly) and in quantifying the amount of TV regurgitation that is present (see below). After obtaining four–chamber and long-axis views of the RV, a set of cine CMR images are performed in short axis from the TV to the RV apex (usually 8–12 slices with the thickness depending upon the length of the RV) at a temporal resolution of 25–50 ms, depending upon the heart rate. By contouring the endocardial borders of each slice at end-diastole and end-systole and measuring the areas, the end-diastolic and end-systolic ventricular vol-umes can be obtained as the products of the measured areas and the slice thickness, with the results being summed across all slice levels. Multiplication of the stroke volume obtained by the heart rate during image acquisition yields the

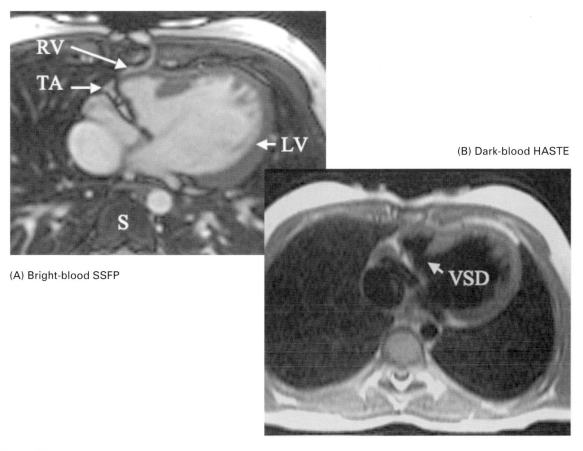

(B) Dark-blood HASTE

(A) Bright-blood SSFP

Figure 29.1

Static steady-state free-precession (SSFP; bright-blood) (A) and half-Fourier acquisition single-shot turbo spin echo (HASTE) (B) imaging of tricuspid atresia (TA). These axial images at approximately the same level demonstrate the atretic tricuspid valve and hypoplastic right ventricle (RV) along with a ventricular septal defect (VSD). LV, left ventricle; S, spine.

cardiac output. The ejection fraction is calculated in the usual fashion. By contouring the epicardial borders of the RV in the same way during end-diastole and subtracting the end-diastolic volume, the RV mass can be obtained. Regional ventricular wall motion can be visualized utilizing myocardial tagging, where, similar to the presaturation tag laid down to visualize an ASD, a series of parallel, thin, presaturation tags are laid down perpendicular to the longitudinal axis of the ventricle in the four-chamber and RV long-axis views (so-called 'one-dimensional' tagging). This divides the myocardium into 'cubes of magnetization', which can be seen to deform (Figure 29.2B). Regional shortening fractions can be obtained in this fashion. Two sets of parallel tags,

perpendicular to each other (so-called spatial modulation of magnetization, SPAMM), can be used in the left ventricle (LV) or the hypertrophied RV to measure strain and wall motion as well.

Velocity mapping is a CMR technique that uses the phase information in the image to measure velocity and flow[15–17] and is the next step in imaging the TV via CMR. In the through-plane version (Figure 29.4), velocity is measured into and out of the plane of the image and flow can then be calculated, while the in-plane version measures velocity in the plane of the image similar to echocardiography. On the image, directionality is encoded as either white or black and the amount of 'whiteness' or 'blackness' represents the degree of velocity and flow. Velocity mapping can

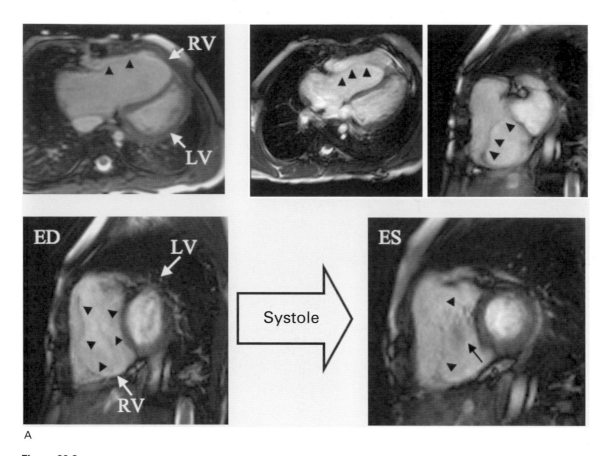

Figure 29.2

Static and cine steady-state free-precession (SSFP) (A) and gradient echo (B) imaging of Ebstein's anomaly (see next page). (A) The upper left image is a static SSFP axial image – note the dilated right ventricle (RV) and the bowing of the ventricular septum from RV to left ventricle (LV) in this diastolic image. Even in this static image, the elongated anterior leaflet can be seen (black arrowheads). The upper middle and right cine images are four-chamber and short-axis views at the level of the atrioventricular valve annulus, respectively, demonstrating the elongated anterior leaflet and the displacement of the septal leaflet (black arrowheads) towards the apex. The lower left and lower right images are end-diastolic (ED) and end-systolic (ES) short-axis cine frames in the mid ventricle demonstrating the anterior and posterior leaflets (black arrowheads) as well as tricuspid insufficiency (black arrow).

be used to obtain the TV inflow patterns as well as making RV pressure estimates with the TV regurgitation jet similar to Doppler echocardiography; however, the power of CMR lies in the fact that velocity mapping can quantitate TV forward and, in certain cases, reverse flow, which allows for calculation of the regurgitant fraction. TV regurgitant volumes can be measured by placing a velocity map across the pulmonary valve and measuring the forward flow, and subtracting this from the RV stroke volume as measured by cine CMR (see above). Alternatively, if the plane is positioned correctly, the regurgitant volume can be measured directly with a velocity map placed across the TV regurgitant jet (less commonly used because the angle is hard to determine). Since TV pathology may be associated with ASDs, velocity mapping can be used to determine the pulmonary-to-systemic flow ratio.[11]

Velocity mapping provides a very powerful tool, not only to measure flows but also as an internal check to validate the reliability of each CMR meas-

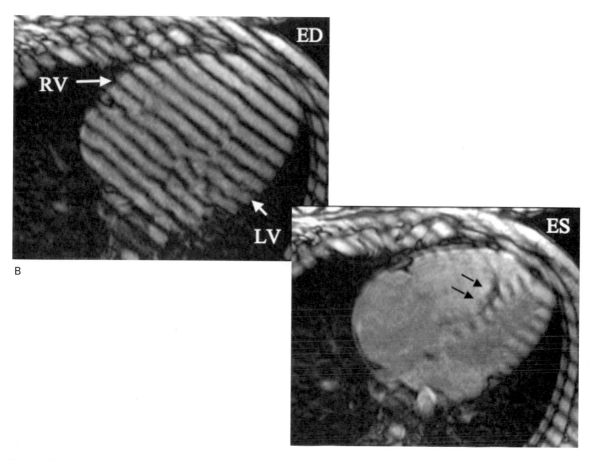

Figure 29.2 contd

(B) Gradient echo sequence in the four-chamber view in end-diastole (ED) (upper left) and end-systole (ES) (lower right), utilizing one-dimensional myocardial tagging. This divides the myocardium into 'cubes of magnetization', which can be seen to deform from ED to ES. Regional shortening fractions can be obtained in this fashion. A jet of tricuspid insufficiency in this patient with Ebstein's anomaly and marked displacement of the septal leaflet apically can be visualized near the apex (black arrows).

ure of cardiovascular performance. For example, in the absence of pulmonary or TV regurgitation, measurement of TV inflow utilizing velocity mapping should equal the stroke volume calculated by cine CMR and the flow in the main pulmonary artery as assessed using a velocity map across this vessel. This is routinely done in CMR.

Gadolinium is a magnetic contrast agent and, although it is not used directly in routine practice to image the TV, it is used to create 3D models of the associated abnormalities with TV pathology such as the branch pulmonary arteries in patients with either PA-IVS (Figure 29.5) or TA with normally related great arteries.[3] It is also useful in visualizing aortic-to-pulmonary collaterals. Gadolinium accumulates in scar tissue and, using a technique called delayed enhancement or viability CMR, this scar tissue can be visualized as a signal-intense region on the image.[18] A recent study[4] has demonstrated that in pathologic states

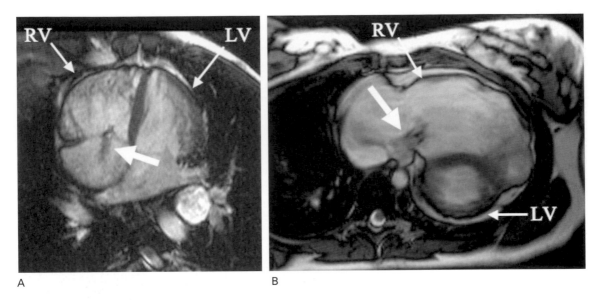

A   B

Figure 29.3

Cine steady-state free-precession (SSFP) imaging demonstrating tricuspid valve insufficiency (white arrows). (A) Static SSFP four-chamber view of a patient with tetralogy of Fallot with absent pulmonary valve leaflets. Note the right ventricular (RV) hypertrophy and dilation and the tricuspid insufficiency (thick white arrow). (B) A patient with a dilated RV cardiomyopathy with a severe, wide jet of tricuspid insufficiency (thick white arrow). LV, left ventricle.

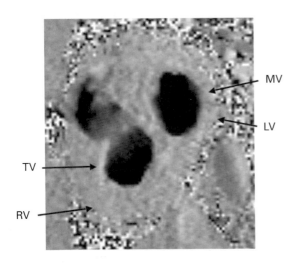

Figure 29.4

Through-plane velocity mapping in a patient with transposition of the great arteries. This image is taken at the level of the atrioventricular valve in diastole, with the leftmost black oval representing the tricuspid valve (TV) flow while the rightmost black oval represents mitral valve (MV) flow. In this image, black represents flow towards the apex and the degree of 'blackness' corresponds to the amount of flow and velocity. LV, left ventricle; RV, right ventricle.

such as hypoplastic left heart syndrome, delayed enhancement 'lights up' the TV as well, and although there is some speculation about the cause, it is unknown why this is the case (see below). This may also be used to evaluate for scar tissue in the myocardium in the associated lesions with TV pathology.[18] Specialized gadolinium techniques can also evaluate myocardial perfusion,[19] which may be important in lesions associated with TV pathology such as the RV-dependent coronary circulation in PA-IVS (see below).

CMR of specific tricuspid valve lesions

Tricuspid atresia

One of the more uncommon lesions, TA is found in 79 out of one million live births[20] and is typically divided into three major subgroups: normally related great arteries (I), which is the most common; D-transposition of the great arteries (II);

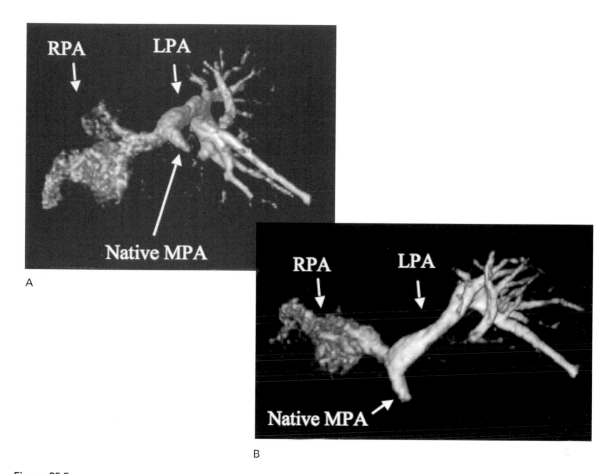

Figure 29.5

Three-dimensional (3D) shaded surface display of the main (MPA), right (RPA), and left (LPA) pulmonary arteries in a patient with pulmonary atresia and intact ventricular septum: coronal (A) and transverse (B) views in 3D. Note the small native MPA.

and L-transposition of the great arteries (III). Within each category, there are subdivisions labeled A, B, or C depending upon the presence or absence and size of the ventricular septal defect (VSD) and the presence or absence of pulmonary atresia or stenosis.[21] With obstruction to flow across the RV, the RV is hypoplastic and there is a requisite atrial septal communication. A persistent left superior vena cava is present in 12–15% of cases, which is important surgically because of the Fontan repair, and juxtaposition of the atrial appendage occurs in approximately 10%.

CMR imaging of TA begins with a set of contiguous axial static SSFP images through the thorax, which will identify not only the atretic valve

(Figure 29.1) but also the associated anomalies. Off-axis coronal static SSFP images through the long axis of the right atrium (RA) and RV confirm the diagnosis of TA. Cine CMR not only will demonstrate a lack of flow through the TV in the four–chamber and RV long-axis views but also is used to assess left ventricular (LV) function as well as flow across the atrial and ventricular septal (if present) communications. Velocity mapping is used to assess cardiac output. Throughout staged Fontan reconstruction, CMR is used to assess the various parts of the repair, including the systemic venous pathway (Fontan baffle), the pulmonary arteries, the ASD, the reconstructed aorta (if present), ventricular function, and regional lung perfusion (Figure 29.6).[7,22–26]

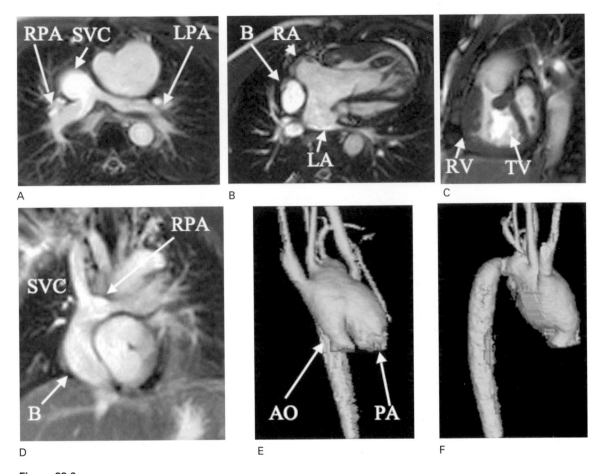

Figure 29.6

Cardiac magnetic resonance (CMR) of the Fontan operation. A selection of structures using various CMR techniques in evaluating the Fontan operation is presented. (A) Static steady-state free-precession (SSFP) image of the right (RPA) and left (LPA) pulmonary arteries along with the superior vena cava (SVC)–RPA connection. The aortic–pulmonary anastomosis is also seen in cross-section anterior to the LPA and to the left of the SVC (right on the image). (B, C) Cine still frames of the four-chamber (B) and short-axis (C) views of a patient with hypoplastic left heart syndrome. These cines were used to evaluate ventricular function, the presence of a fenestration, and atrioventricular or semilunar valve insufficiency. The systemic venous baffle (B) is seen in cross-section in (B) and the pulmonary venous pathway is seen in long axis. The tricuspid valve (TV) can be visualized en-face in (C). (D) Cine still frame of the long axis of the systemic venous baffle (B) and its connection to the SVC and RPA, with the atrium in cross-section. (E, F) Three-dimensional shaded-surface displays derived from gadolinium sequences of the aortic (AO)-to-pulmonary artery (PA) anastomosis (E) and the aortic arch (F). LA, left atrium; RA, right atrium.

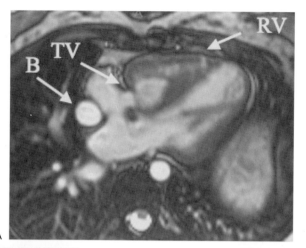

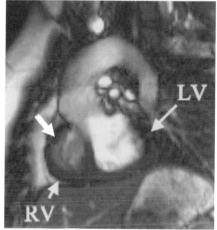

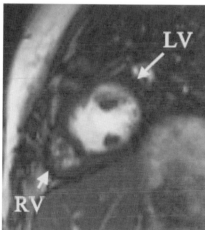

Figure 29.7

Steady-state free-precession (SSFP) imaging of pulmonary atresia with intact ventricular septum after the Fontan operation. (A) Cine SSFP frame of the four-chamber view demonstrating the hypoplastic tricuspid valve (TV), the hypoplastic and hypertrophied right ventricle (RV), the atrial septal defect, and the systemic venous baffle (B) in cross-section. (B) Cine SSFP frame in short axis below the atrioventricular valve annulus, where the TV leaflets can be seen (thick white arrow). This is also at the level of the left ventricular (LV) outflow tract. (C) Short-axis view in mid-ventricle demonstrating the relative sizes of the RV and LV.

Pulmonary atresia with intact ventricular septum (Figure 29.7)[27]

With almost double the incidence of TA, PA-IVS is still a very rare lesion, with an estimated incidence of 132 per million live births.[20] With obstruction to flow across the pulmonary valve, there is the requisite atrial septal communication, and varying degrees of TV dysplasia are seen; these include Ebstein's anomaly of the TV in approximately 5–10% of cases (see below), with annular size ranging from dilation to severe hypoplasia.[28] The RV is typically hypertrophied, with some decrease in cavity size in almost 90% of cases, although in a small number of cases, it can be dilated. The RV has been classically categorized as unipartite, bipartite, or tripartite, depending upon the presence of the inlet, outlet, or trabecular portions of the RV. Coronary abnormalities, including RV sinusoids, are common.

A set of contiguous axial static SSFP images through the thorax in PA-IVS will demonstrate hypoplasia of the TV if present, as well as atresia of the pulmonary valve and the size and geometry of the main and branch pulmonary arteries (Figure 29.7). A qualitative assessment of the size of the RV can be made at this time, along with how many sections it contains (unipartite, bipartite, or tripartite) as well as associated anomalies. Off-axis sagittal static SSFP images through the long axis of the RV outflow tract (RVOT) confirm the diagnosis of PA-IVS. Cine CMR in the RVOT will demonstrate lack of flow across the pulmonary valve. In the four-chamber and RV long-axis views, cine CMR can be used to visualize the anatomy of the TV, determine the presence of TV insufficiency, evaluate the atrial septal communication, and measure the diameter of the TV annulus, which has a bearing on the management and prognosis of the patient (Figure 29.7). A stack of short-axis images utilizing cine CMR can be used to measure RV size and function as well as LV function. In these views, the tricuspid valve anatomy can usually be visualized en face. Velocity mapping is used to assess cardiac output, and can also be used to obtain an RV pressure estimate from the TV regurgitant jet. Gadolinium techniques can be used to obtain 3D imaging of the branch pulmonary arteries and have the potential to evaluate RV myocardial perfusion with specialized CMR perfusion techniques (see above), which is important in those PA-IVS patients with an RV-dependent coronary circulation.

In both two-ventricle and single-ventricle repairs, CMR is also used in the postinterventional (catheterization or surgery) evaluation of this lesion. Static SSFP CMR can be used to evaluate the patency of the RVOT, whether an intervention on the native RVOT or an RV-to-pulmonary artery conduit has been performed. Dark-blood CMR can be used to anatomically visualize a systemic-to-pulmonary artery shunt if present. Cine CMR can be used for all of the pre-intervention evaluations as well as to determine the physiologic patency of the RVOT. Velocity mapping can be used for RV pressure estimation, pulmonary or tricuspid regurgitant fraction (in conjunction with RV volumes via cine CMR if needed), blood flow to the right and left lungs, pulmonary-to-systemic flow ratios, and, of course, cardiac output. Gadolinium techniques can be used for all of the pre-intervention evaluations, for 3D imaging of the Fontan baffle (if present) and the pulmonary arteries, and for determining RV viability and perfusion. Throughout a staged Fontan reconstruction, along with the gadolinium techniques mentioned, CMR is used to assess the various parts of the repair, including the systemic venous pathway (Fontan baffle), the pulmonary arteries, the ASD, ventricular function, and regional lung perfusion (Figure 29.6).

Ebstein's anomaly[29]

This disorder is also relatively rare, occurring in 114 out of one million live births.[20] There is a defect in delamination of the leaflets (nearly always the septal and posterior leaflets) causing 'atrialization' of the ventricle. The anterior leaflet is not displaced, but is usually enlarged and 'sail-like'. Pulmonary atresia can occur with this disease (see above), along with RV dysfunction and dilation as well as an atrial septal communication. The LV can be affected, with areas of fibrosis, hypertrophy, and dysplasia.

CMR of this disease[30] is striking, with a large dilated RV and a TV regurgitation jet seen on the initial contiguous axial static SSFP images (Figure 29.2). In some cases of severe TV regurgitation, little signal loss may be seen on static or cine CMR because of the free flow of blood from the RV to the atria or the atrialized portion of the RV (Figure 29.2). Pulmonary stenosis or atresia, as well as the atrial septal communication, can be visualized on static SSFP images as well. Cine CMR is used to visualize the leaflets (Figure 29.2) in both long axes (four-chamber view and RV long axis), and can occasionally be visualized en-face (which, because of the eccentric angle of the valve orifice, can be difficult). In addition, cine CMR can qualitatively (and sometimes quantitatively) assess RV function in this disease;[31] because of the eccentric angle of the functional valve annulus, it can sometimes be difficult to trace exactly what is functional RV and what is an atrialized portion on RV short-axis slices. TV regurgitation can also be assessed with cine CMR, along with pulmonary atresia or stenosis (if present, using an RVOT view) and atrial septal communication (again, if present). Velocity mapping can be used to assess forward cardiac output, which can be used in the quantitative assessment of TV regurgitation fraction. In addition, velocity mapping can be used to estimate the RV pressure via the Bernoulli equation and a pressure gradient across the pulmonary valve (if pulmonary stenosis is present) as well as to obtain velocity–time or flow–time curves across the valve if the angle is correct.[15,16] Gadolinium sequences can be used not only to create 3D models of the various associated lesions (e.g. the size of the pulmonary arteries in patients with

pulmonary valve stenosis) but also to assess myocardial scarring of the LV, which has been reported to occur by performing CMR viability imaging.

CMR can be used to follow the natural course of patients with Ebstein's anomaly as well as to assess intervention. This includes direct surgery on the valve, with the assessment of stenosis or insufficiency, as well as surgery on the associated malformations (e.g. pulmonary stenosis or atresia). Occasionally, a patient with Ebstein's anomaly will need to undergo a Fontan procedure, the assessment of which via CMR has already been outlined above.

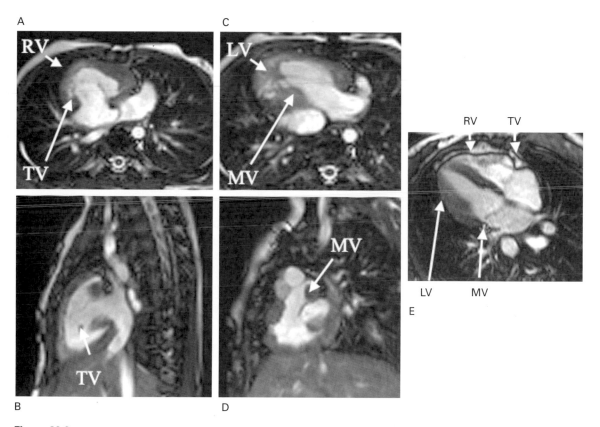

Figure 29.8

Steady-state free-precession (SSFP) imaging of the tricuspid valve (TV) in L-looped ventricles. (A–D) SSFP images of a patient with supero-inferior L-looped ventricles and criss-cross atrioventricular relations. The right ventricle (RV) is superior and communicates with the inferior left ventricle (LV) via a ventricular septal defect. (A, B) Orthogonal views of the TV: (A) more anteroposterior; (B) more sagittally oriented. (C, D) Orthogonal views of the MV: (C) more antero-posterior; (D) more sagittally oriented. Note how the MV and TV cross paths as they connect atria to ventricles – hence the name 'criss-cross atrioventricular relations'. (E) Still frame from a patient with situs inversus totalis with L-looped ventricles.

TV in L-loop ventricles[32]

The L-looping of the ventricles in the Van Praagh segmental approach indicates that the organization of the ventricles is left-handed, which is the reverse of the much more common right-handed normal organization of the ventricles (D-looping). So-called corrected transposition of the great arteries or transposition of the great arteries {S, L, L} is one type of L-looping. The TV valve in L-looped ventricles commonly has some type of abnormality, ranging from a very minor one such as elongation of the valve leaflets to a major structural anomaly such as Ebstein's anomaly. CMR is excellent for evaluating the TV in these lesions,[33] and its application is similar to that in PA-IVS, Ebstein's anomaly, and Fontan patients; however, slice positions and orientations will

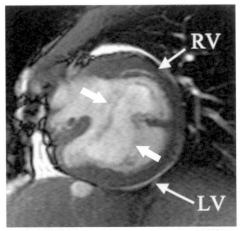

A

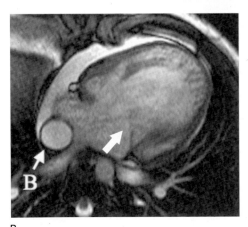

B

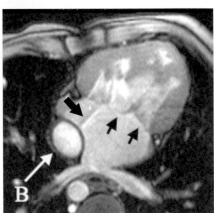

C

Figure 29.9

Steady-state free-precession (SSFP) and gradient echo imaging of endocardial cushion defect. (A) Cine SSFP frame in diastole of the common atrioventricular valve en-face (thick white arrows) in a short-axis view near the atrioventricular valve annulus in a patient with supero-inferior ventricles after Fontan repair. The morphologic right ventricle (RV) is superior and the morphologic left ventricle (LV) is inferior, with the interventricular septum horizontally oriented. Note that the superior leaflet does not have any attachments to the crest of the ventricular septum (Rastelli C). (B) Cine of the same patient in a four-chamber view where the systemic venous baffle (B) can be seen in cross-section as well as the valve leaflet (thick white arrow). (C) Gradient echo image in a four-chamber view of a patient with a malaligned atrioventricular canal over the LV after Fontan repair. The systemic venous baffle (B) can be seen in cross-section, as can the valve leaflets (black arrows). The thick black arrow points to the fenestration jet shunting from the systemic venous baffle to the pulmonary venous pathway.

be different because of the geometry of the ventricles (Figure 29.8).

Endocardial cushion defects

Although technically not TV defects, endocardial cushion defects and common atrioventricular canal defects encompass the region of the TV. These will not be elaborated upon in this chapter, but CMR, as with the other lesions, is an excellent modality to evaluate these patients (Figure 29.9).[34,35] It is useful in delineating the anatomy of the valve, whether it is malaligned or balanced over the ventricles, quantifying the common atrioventricular valve regurgitation and the ventricular function (using cine CMR and velocity mapping), and quantifying the pulmonary-to-systemic flow ratio (using velocity mapping across both the aorta and the pulmonary artery).[11]

Other imaging strategies and future directions

In the postoperative patient, it has been demonstrated (Figure 29.10) that in a wide variety of congenital heart lesions, the TV has a strongly increased signal on delayed-enhancement studies using CMR, as mentioned above.[4] The implications of this finding are unclear; however, the result is that the morphology of the TV can be visualized in diastole. This may be useful when other CMR techniques fail to visualize the valve.

CMR technology is advancing at a rapid pace. Techniques such as real-time CMR with real-time flow measurements are presently being developed. CMR will be able to place a velocity map across the TV and obtain a time–flow curve in real time instead of the velocity–time curve generated by Doppler echocardiography. In addition, interventional CMR is becoming increasingly important, with catheter based techniques being

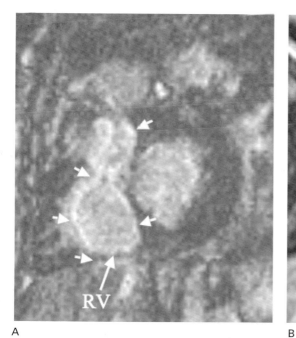

A

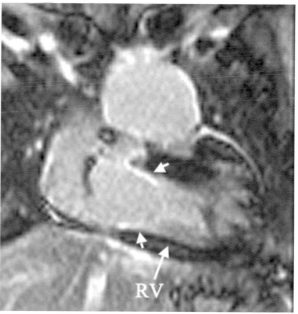

B

Figure 29.10

Viability studies utilizing gadolinium to image the tricuspid valve in postoperative patients. (A) Short-axis viability frame in diastole demonstrating the tricuspid valve en-face (arrowheads) in a postoperative patient, which 'lights up'. (B) Right ventricular (RV) long-axis view of a patient with hypoplastic left heart syndrome after Fontan operation: the arrowheads point to the tricuspid valve leaflets with increased signal intensity.

accomplished in the CMR suite rather than in the cardiac catheterization laboratory.[36] One can imagine a day when transcatheter intervention on the TV or on lesions associated with TV pathology (e.g. PA-IVS) will be a reality in the CMR suite, decreasing the risk of cancer in later life.

Conclusion

CMR of the TV offers imaging complementary to echocardiography and cardiac angiography, and often offers unique insights into the anatomy and atrioventricular valve function of the various TV lesions that present to the clinician. Quantification of TV insufficiency, and of myocardial perfusion and scarring, as well as 3D functional imaging of the ventricles and imaging of the associated abnormalities with the various TV lesions, are the added value CMR brings to the medical and surgical management of these patients.

References

1. Helbing WA, Rebergen SA, Maliepaard C, et al. Quantification of right ventricular function with magnetic resonance imaging in children with normal hearts and with congenital heart disease. Am Heart J 1995; 130: 828–37.
2. Helbing WA, Niezen RA, Le Cessie S, et al. Right ventricular diastolic function in children with pulmonary regurgitation after repair of tetralogy of Fallot: volumetric evaluation by magnetic resonance velocity mapping, J Am Coll Cardiol 1996; 28: 1827–35.
3. Neimatallah MA, Ho VB, Dong Q, et al. Gadolinium-enhanced 3D magnetic resonance angiography of the thoracic vessels. J Magn Reson Imaging 1999; 10: 758–70.
4. Harris MA, Ghoads G, Weinberg PM, Fogel MA. Magnetic resonance delayed enhancement for the detection of fibrous tissue in postoperative patients with various forms of congenital heart disease. J Am Coll Cardiol 2005; 45: abs.
5. Modan L, Keinan L, Blumstein T, Sedetzki S. Cancer following cardiac catheterization in childhood. Int J Epidemiol 2000; 29: 424–8.
6. Brenner DJ, Elliston CD, Hall EJ, Berdon WE. Estimated risks of radiation-induced fatal cancer from pediatric CT. AJR Am J Roentgenol 2001; 176: 289–96.
7. Fogel MA, Weinberg PM, Chin AJ, et al. Late ventricular geometry and performance changes of functional single ventricle throughout staged Fontan reconstruction assessed by magnetic resonance imaging. J Am Coll Cardiol 1996; 28: 212–21.
8. Papavassiliou DP, Parks WJ, Hopkins KL, Fyfe DA. 3-D echocardiographic measurement of RV volume in children with congenital heart disease validated by MRI. J Am Soc Echocardiogr 1998; 11: 770–7.
9. Nosir YF, Lequin MH, Kasprzak JD, et al. Measurements and day-to-day variabilities of LV volumes and EF by 3-dimensional echocardiography and comparison with MR. Am J Cardiol 1998 82: 209–14.
10. Fogel MA. CMR in congenital heart disease. In: Lardo AC, Fayad ZA, Chronos NAF, Fuster V (eds). Cardiovascular Magnetic Resonance. Established and Emerging Applications. London: Martin Dunitz, 2003: 201–30.
11. Hundley WG, Li HF, Lange RA, et al. Assessment of left-to-right intracardiac shunting by velocity-encoded, phase-difference magnetic resonance imaging. A comparison with oximetric and indicator dilution techniques. Circulation 1995; 91: 2955–60.
12. Boxt LM. Radiology of the right ventricle. Radiol Clin North Am 1999; 37: 379–400.
13. Boxt LM. MR imaging of pulmonary hypertension and right ventricular dysfunction. Magn Reson Clin North Am 1996; 4: 307–25.
14. Rebergen SA, Helbing WA, van der Wall EE, et al. MR velocity mapping of tricuspid flow in healthy children and in patients who have undergone Mustard or Senning procedure. Radiology 1995; 194: 505–12.
15. Nakagawa Y, Fujimoto S, Nakano H, et al. Magnetic resonance velocity mapping of transtricuspid velocity profiles in dilated cardiomyopathy. Heart Vessels 1998; 13: 241–5.
16. Nakagawa Y, Fujimoto S, Nakano H, et al. Magnetic resonance velocity mapping of normal transtricuspid velocity profiles. Int J Card Imaging 1997; 13: 433–6.
17. Mostbeck GH, Hartiala JJ, Foster E, et al. Right ventricular diastolic filling: evaluation with velocity-encoded cine MRI. J Comput Assist Tomogr 1993; 17: 245–52.
18. Kim RJ, Fieno DS, Parrish TB, et al. Relationship of MRI delayed constrast enhancement to irreversible injury, infarct age, and contractile function. Circulation 1999; 100: 1992–2002.
19. Nagel E, Klein C, Paetsch I, Hettwer S, et al. Magnetic resonance perfusion measurements for the non-invasive detection of coronary artery disease. Circulation 2003; 108: 432–7.
20. Hoffman JIE, Kaplan S. The incidence of congenital heart disease. J Am Coll Cardiol 200; 39: 1890–900.
21. Edwards JE, Burchell HB. Congenital tricuspid

atresia: a classification. Med Clin North Am 1949; 67: 530–42.

22. Graham TP Jr, Johns JA. Pre-operative assessment of ventricular function in patients considered for the Fontan procedure. Herz 1992; 17: 213–19.

23. Rebergen SA, Ottinkamp J, Doornbos J, et al. Postoperative pulmonary flow dynamics after Fontan surgery: assessment with nuclear magnetic resonance velocity mapping. J Am Coll Cardiol 1993; 21: 123–31.

24. Fellows KE, Fogel MA. MR imaging and heart function in patients pre- and post-Fontan surgery. Acta Paediatr Suppl 1995; 410: 57–9.

25. Fogel MA, Ramaciotti C, Hubbard AM, Weinberg PW. Magnetic resonance and echocardiographic imaging of pulmonary artery size throughout stages of Fontan reconstruction. Circulation 1994; 90: 2927–36.

26. Fogel MA, Weinberg PM, Fellows KE, Hoffman EA. A study in ventricular–ventricular interaction. Single right ventricles compared with systemic right ventricles in a dual-chamber circulation. Circulation 1995; 92: 219–30.

27. Freedom RM. Pulmonary Atresia with Intact Ventricular Septum. Mount Kisco, NY: Futura, 1989.

28. Freedom RM, Dische MR, Rowe RD. The tricuspid valve in pulmonary atresia and intact ventricular septum: a morphologic study of 60 cases. Arch Pathol Lab Med 1978; 102: 28–31.

29. Anderson KR, Zuberbuhler JR, Anderson RH, et al. Morphologic spectrum of Ebstein's anomaly of the heart: a review. Mayo Clin Proc 1979; 54: 174–80.

30. Choi YH, Park JH, Choe YH, Yoo SJ. MR imaging of Ebstein's anomaly of the tricuspid valve. AJR Am J Roentgenol 1994; 163: 539–43.

31. Eustace S, Kruskal JB, Hartnell GG. Ebstein's anomaly presenting in adulthood: the role of cine magnetic resonance imaging in diagnosis. Clin Radiol 1994; 49: 690–2.

32. Van Praagh, R. Segmental approach to diagnosis. In: Fyler DC (ed). Nadas' Pediatric Cardiology, 2nd edn. St Louis, MO: Mosby-Yearbook, 1992: 27–35.

33. Schmidt M, Theissen P, Deutsch HJ, et al. Congenitally corrected transposition of the great arteries (L-TGA) with situs inversus totalis in adulthood: findings with magnetic resonance imaging. Magn Reson Imaging 2000; 18: 417–22.

34. Parsons JM, Baker EJ, Anderson RH, et al. Morphological evaluation of atrioventricular septal defect by magnetic resonance imaging. Br Heart J 1990; 64: 138–45.

35. Jacobstein MD, Fletcher BD, Goldstein S, et al. Evaluation of atrioventricular septal defect by magnetic resonance imaging. Am J Cardiol 1985; 55: 1158–61.

36. Rickers C, Jerosch-Herold M, Hu X, et al. Magnetic resonance image-guided transcatheter closure of atrial septal defects. Circulation 2003; 107: 132–8.

30

Hemodynamic evaluation of tricuspid stenosis and regurgitation: Indications for repair and replacement

Alejandro J Torres, William E Hellenbrand

Introduction

In this chapter, we will consider the hemodynamic evaluation of the tricuspid valve and the indications for its repair or replacement.

The hemodynamic spectrum of the lesions afflicting the morphology of the tricuspid valve can be divided into four major entities:

- Tricuspid stenosis: congenital or acquired
- Tricuspid insufficiency: congenital or acquired
- Ebstein's anomaly
- Tricuspid valve as the systemic atrioventricular valve:
    - transposition of the great arteries, status post intra-atrial switch (Mustard– Senning procedures)
    - single ventricle (hypoplastic left heart syndrome)
    - congenitally corrected transposition of the great arteries.

Tricuspid stenosis

Cardiac catheterization provides information on tricuspid valve morphology and function from hemodynamic measurements as well as angiographic assessment. Tricuspid stenosis (TS) usually occurs as a component of multivalvular disease or other defects.

The diagnosis of TS is established when the mean pandiastolic gradient across the tricuspid valve is at least 2 mmHg. A diastolic pressure gradient of 5 mmHg between the right atrium (RA) and right ventricle (RV) is sufficient to elevate the mean RA pressure and cause symptoms of systemic venous hypertension. In most cases, pullback from RV to RA using a standard catheter confirms or excludes the presence of a gradient across the tricuspid valve. However, simultaneous recording of RA and RV pressures should be used if there is any doubt about the presence of TS. The diagnosis is also aided by the finding of a prominent a-wave and a blunted or absent y-descent on the atrial pressure tracing.

The transvalvular gradient increases during inspiration or exercise and decreases with expiration. In patients in whom sodium intake has been restricted or diuretics have been administered, TS can be partially 'masked' due to the low intravascular volume. Patients with echocardiographic features of TS without a resting valve gradient should undergo a hemodynamic study with provocative maneuvers.[1] A similar situation occurs in patients with a patent foramen ovale or an atrial septal defect with right-to-left shunting. In these patients, balloon occlusion of the atrial septum can 'unmask' a gradient across the tricuspid valve.

RV diastolic pressure is normal in patients with pure TS; coexisting tricuspid regurgitation (TR), pulmonary valve lesions, pulmonary hypertension, cardiomyopathy, and hypoplastic RV may all be responsible for elevations of RV diastolic pressure.

The tricuspid valve area can be calculated using the Gorlin formula,[2,3] but there is no general consensus as to what constitutes a critical orifice area for this valve.

Since the tricuspid valve annulus is easily measured, echocardiography can also assist with the quantitation of the severity of TS.[4,5] Some studies have attempted to correlate two-dimensional (2D) echocardiography findings with hemodynamically significant TS in patients with rheumatic fever, with contradictory results.[1,6,7] TS of different etiology than rheumatic fever has received less attention.

The Doppler techniques for TS are similar to those used with mitral stenosis. Calculation of peak and mean pressure gradients and pressure half-time provides valuable information regarding the severity of the obstruction and is used for TS of different etiologies and for serial follow-up evaluations. However, unlike the tricuspid valve area calculation, these measurements depend on the amount of transvalvular flow. The effective tricuspid valve area can be calculated from the continuity equation if no significant TR is present.

Patients with TS should be considered for an exercise stress echocardiogram to evaluate the gradient across the tricuspid valve with exercise and to assess functional capacity.

2D echocardiography is of particular significance when assessing patients with pulmonary atresia and intact ventricular septum. In these patients, tricuspid valve z-scores have been used to determine if a biventricular repair should be attempted. A tricuspid valve z-score of <3 has been reported to predict an unfavorable surgical outcome.[8–10]

Indications for intervention

Most isolated congenital tricuspid valve anomalies leading to TS present in infancy and childhood and require early intervention.

In older patients, management of the TS by itself almost always involves treating the patient symptomatically and repairing associated lesions. When severe TS accompanies mitral stenosis in patients with rheumatic fever, the tricuspid valve should be repaired. Correcting the mitral lesion alone rarely resolves the tricuspid lesion, and the patient's exercise capacity may remain markedly limited.[6] Tricuspid commissurotomy usually offers complete and safe correc-

tion of the stenotic valve. Percutaneous balloon valvuloplasty for both mitral and tricuspid valves as an alternative to surgical treatment has been described,[7] but has not been widely used.

Tricuspid insufficiency (tricuspid regurgitation)

Tricuspid insufficiency (tricuspid regurgitation) is defined as retrograde systolic flow from the RV to the RA. It is principally a volume-overload lesion of the RA and RV and is associated with enlargement of these chambers. If the lesion is severe, RV failure eventually develops, with chronically elevated venous pressure causing organ dysfunction, edema, and ascites. The volume overload causes the interventricular septum to flatten during diastole, indicating a reversed trans-septal pressure gradient (right > left).[11] During systole, the pressure in the left ventricle (LV) overcomes that of the RV, shifting the septum towards the right and restoring a more normal LV geometry. In patients with severe pulmonary hypertension, however, an abnormal septal position may be sustained through the entire cardiac cycle.

Hemodynamic assessment

The RA and RV end-diastolic pressures are elevated in TR, whether the condition is due to a primary lesion (i.e. a disease of the valve or its supporting structures) or is secondary to RV systolic overload (e.g. pulmonary valve stenosis or pulmonary artery hypertension). The hemodynamic distinction between primary and secondary TR is difficult. Generally, if the patient with severe TR has an RV systolic pressure equal to or less than 40 mmHg, the etiology is primary, whereas a systolic pressure greater than 60 mmHg suggests that TR is secondary.

The RA pressure recording reveals absence of the x-descent and a prominent v- or c–v-wave. However, the sensitivity of this measure can be reduced by other determinants of tricuspid valve function. For example, a highly compliant RA may diminish the appearance of the v-wave, despite severe valve regurgitation. Typically, there is a rise or no change on the RA pressure, instead of the usual fall, during inspiration. As the severity of tricuspid insufficiency progresses, the RA pressure wave increasingly resembles the RV pressure wave (ventricularization of the RA pressure). In the most severe cases, the RA and RV exhibit the pathophysiology of a common chamber and the pressure tracings are virtually identical.

Angiography

During cardiac catheterization, right ventriculography is performed to assess the severity of the regurgitation, but the fact that the catheter must be positioned across the tricuspid valve cannot exclude the possibility of 'catheter-induced' TR.[12] The use of special balloon catheters and low-rate injections minimizes the induction of spurious regurgitation. The degree of severity is estimated by noting the degree of opacification of the RA due to regurgitation back through the incompetent valve. With grade 1 (mild) regurgitation, the RA clears with each beat and is never entirely opacified. In grade 2 (moderate), the RA does not clear with one beat and is opacified, but the opacification does not equal that of the RV. In grade 3 regurgitation (moderately severe), the RA is completely opacified and the opacification is equal to that of the RV. In grade 4 regurgitation (severe), complete opacification of the RA occurs within one beat and becomes progressively more significant with each subsequent beat.

As with other valvulopathies, 2D-Doppler echocardiography has the potential to quantify the hemodynamic severity of TR non-invasively by methods similar to those used for mitral regurgitation.

The presence of a V notch on the slope of the deceleration phase in the continuous-wave Doppler of the TR jet is an indicator of severe regurgitation. The width of the vena contracta in patients with TR has been correlated well with the angiographically defined effective regurgitant orifice.[13] Visual estimates of the color Doppler signal by experienced readers also have shown good correlation with quantitative techniques.[14] The ratio of the maximal regurgitant jet area to the area of the corresponding atrium by a color Doppler technique, which has correlated well with the angiographic grading[15] of mitral insufficiency, can also be used for the grading of tricuspid insufficiency: a ratio less than 20% correlates

with an angiographic grade 1 regurgitation (mild), a ratio between 20% and 40% with grade 2 regurgitation (moderate), and a ratio greater than 40% with severe regurgitation.

Other Doppler techniques have been used to calculate regurgitant volume, regurgitant fraction, and effective regurgitant orifice.[16–19]

We need to stress that when TR is associated with residual shunts and pulmonary valve regurgitation, the above calculations have limited clinical application. In addition, the determination of the RV volume by 2D echocardiography is difficult, making the calculation of the effective regurgitant orifice less accurate.

The peak velocity of the TR jet has been used as a reliable indicator of the systolic RV-to-RA peak pressure gradient and is especially useful for assessing the degree of RV hypertension. The systolic RV pressure can be estimated by measuring the peak velocity of the jet and by using the simplified Bernoulli equation (pressure gradient $= 4 \times$ peak velocity^2).

Assessing the severity of TR by transesophageal echocardiography (TEE) is similar to the approach used in transthoracic imaging. The same Doppler techniques, such as the determination of the regurgitant orifice, can be obtained by TEE to quantify the degree of TR. The demonstration of systolic flow reversal in a hepatic vein by color Doppler and pulsed-wave Doppler is suggestive of severe TR. However, progressive RA dilation may eventually eliminate this finding.

In newborns with isolated severe tricuspid valve insufficiency, cyanosis and clinical findings of congestive heart failure appear early in life. Echocardiographic evaluation is likely to differentiate between functional and anatomic atresia of the pulmonary valve and estimate the systolic RV pressure by Doppler assessment of the TR jet.[20,21] Cardiac catheterization is unlikely to be necessary, but, if undertaken, it demonstrates an elevated RA pressure with a right-to-left shunt at the atrial level. The RV systolic pressure is usually not elevated.

Indications for intervention

The decision as to whether a patient should undergo tricuspid valve repair/replacement remains a challenge. Tricuspid valve disease is sometimes insidious in onset and may be well tolerated for long periods of time.

There are no standard guidelines on the timing of operation for patients with tricuspid insufficiency. In general, tricuspid valve repair or replacement should be considered for patients who develop dyspnea or fatigue thought to be due to tricuspid insufficiency, oxygen desaturation secondary to right-to-left shunting at the atrial level, progressive cardiomegaly on chest radiography or RV enlargement on echocardiography, RV dysfunction, poorly tolerated uncontrolled atrial arrhythmias, or deteriorating exercise capacity.

TR often accompanies other valvulopathies, particularly mitral stenosis in rheumatic valve disease. In these cases, even mild to moderate tricuspid valve insufficiency should be repaired during the initial operation for the associated valve lesions. Isolated tricuspid valve replacement in adult patients with previous mitral valve surgery has been associated with poor outcome.[22] Surgery is also indicated in patients with proven tricuspid valve endocarditis not responding to antibiotics or complicated by pulmonary embolism.

In patients with congenital heart disease, TR typically occurs after repair of right-sided obstructive lesions, most commonly tetralogy of Fallot.[23] An increased RV end-diastolic volume or an elevated residual RV systolic pressure after tetralogy repair has been associated with tricuspid insufficiency.[24] This leads to functional TR secondary to progressive tricuspid annulus dilatation. Some studies have suggested that in patients undergoing repair for residual RV outflow tract obstruction or insufficiency, tricuspid valve annuloplasty should be considered if moderate or severe tricuspid insufficiency is present.[25]

Congenital TR is an uncommon but well-recognized anomaly that usually results from tricuspid valve dysplasia and needs to be differentiated from Ebstein's anomaly. Surgical intervention may be needed if severe insufficiency persists and RV failure develops.[26,27] Transient severe tricuspid insufficiency, a condition often associated with perinatal stress, usually resolves spontaneously after several weeks and requires no intervention.

Acute onset of tricuspid insufficiency may be the result of endocarditis, blunt chest trauma, or ischemia. Without time to remodel, the RV may fail acutely. Likewise, the massive volume regurgitation into a non-compliant RA may result in significant venous hypertension. The decision-making in these acutely ill patients needs to be individualized.

Ebstein's anomaly

In Ebstein's anomaly, a wide spectrum of hemodynamic abnormalities occur at various ages. At one end of the spectrum are patients with mild anatomic abnormalities and relatively normal hemodynamics. At the other end are cyanotic newborns with severe TR and older children or young adults with late hemodynamic deterioration, possibly due to increased right-to-left shunting at the atrial level, right heart failure, progressive left heart dysfunction, or arrhythmias. Most patients with Ebstein's anomaly have significant TR, but in a minority TS can also be present. The hemodynamic characteristics of patients with Ebstein's anomaly also depend on the presence of other congenital heart defects. These may include a patent foramen ovale or an atrial septal defect, pulmonary valve stenosis or atresia, congenital pulmonary valve regurgitation, mitral stenosis, ventricular septal defects, tetralogy of Fallot, and corrected transposition of the great arteries.[28–30] Associated cardiac defects are more common in patients who present with hemodynamic deterioration early in life.

Historically, the diagnosis of Ebstein's anomaly can be made during cardiac catheterization, when an endhole catheter with an electrode at the tip is positioned just proximal to the tricuspid valve. The simultaneous recording of the intracavitary electrogram and pressure shows an RV type of complex, while the pressure tracing is that of the RA (atrialization of the RV).

The hemodynamic manifestations are usually secondary to the magnitude of the tricuspid insufficiency, although occasionally TS is also present. The RA pressure is usually elevated with a dominant v-wave and steep y-descent. However, if the RA is dilated, the RA pressure may be normal. A right-to-left atrial shunt resulting in systemic arterial desaturation is typically present. Balloon occlusion of the atrial septal defect may provide useful information when surgery is being contemplated. RA enlargement and leftward displacement of the tricuspid valve can make it very difficult to enter the functional RV. Catheter manipulation in the outflow tract to enter the pulmonary arteries is particularly difficult and may trigger serious arrhythmias. RV and pulmonary artery pressures are usually normal, as are left atrial (LA) and LV pressures. In patients with predominant tricuspid stenosis, RA pressure is elevated and a prominent a-wave and a diastolic atrioventricular pressure gradient are present. Patients with Ebstein's anomaly have a higher risk of developing significant arrhythmias during catheterization, particularly those with associated Wolff–Parkinson–White syndrome. The availability of more flexible, flow-directed balloon-tipped catheters has decreased the risk over the years.

RV contractile function is very difficult to assess by selective angiography because of the difficulty in defining RV borders and the presence of TR.

Newborns with Ebstein's anomaly and severe cyanosis represent a particular subgroup of patients. The TR is more pronounced, as pulmonary vascular resistance is high immediately after birth. Therefore, there may be little or no antegrade flow across the RV outflow tract during the first hours of life, even when the pulmonary valve is normal. The combination of TR and elevated pulmonary resistance can lead to volume-overload right heart failure and a significant right-to-left shunting at the atrial level. The distinction between anatomic and functional pulmonary atresia can usually be made by echocardiography. If cardiac catheterization is performed, a contrast injection in the aorta near the patent ductus arteriosus is likely to fill the pulmonary root and allow visualization of the pulmonary valve. A cardiothoracic ratio on chest X-ray of more than 85% has been associated with death in 100% of neonates.[31,32] Newborns with isolated Ebstein's anomaly usually show spontaneous improvement as the pulmonary vascular resistance decreases, and some of them develop enough antegrade flow across the RV outflow tract that no intervention is required during the neonatal period. Beyond infancy, the onset of symptoms has a more variable course. There are reports of patients living into their 70s and 80s with no symptoms, although the majority eventually present with some degree of dyspnea, fatigability, cyanosis, or palpitations[33,34] as RV dysfunction or paroxysmal arrhythmias develop. Some studies have found the presence and size of the intracardiac shunt to be the major factor

contributing to exercise intolerance in patients with unrepaired Ebstein's anomaly. RV dysfunction may be a contributing factor to lower cardiac output response relative to oxygen uptake in patients with non-significant intracardiac shunt.[35]

Echocardiography has become the procedure of choice for the diagnosis and assessment of patients with Ebstein's anomaly. The anatomic and functional severity do not always correlate. Patients with severe displacement of the tricuspid valve may have only mild dysfunction, and vice versa. In neonates, some echocardiographic findings have been correlated with poor prognosis. These include tethering to underlying myocardium of the anterosuperior tricuspid leaflet, RV dysplasia, and LV compression by the dilated LV. A group from the Great Ormond Street Hospital in London proposed the GOSE score,[36,37] which is defined as the ratio of the area of the RA and the atrialized RV to the combined area of the functional RV, LA, and LV, as a predictor of mortality. If this ratio is equal to or greater than 1.5 (grade 4), the observed mortality rate is 100%. A ratio of 1.1–1.4 (grade 3) was associated with a mortality rate of 10%, but a late mortality rate of 45% (usually in early childhood). Finally, a ratio of 1.0 or less (grade 1 or 2) was associated with 92% survival. The ratio between the area of the functional RV and the combined area of both the RA and the atrialized RV has also been described as an indicator of severity. Patients with a ratio of less than 0.35 have the poorest prognosis.[37,38]

Other echocardiographic findings that may indicate hemodynamic compromise in patients with Ebstein's anomaly are the magnitude of TR, an increase in RV dimension, paradoxical ventricular septal motion, and the presence of right-to-left shunting at the atrial level. The gradient across the regurgitant tricuspid valve estimated by continuous Doppler imaging is usually low.

Echocardiographic assessment of RV size and function is difficult, owing to the abnormal geometry of the cavity.[39] LV function is also difficult to assess, owing to the paradoxical motion of the interventricular septum, which influences the estimation of ejection fraction and shortening fraction. Some studies have found that LV systolic function may be decreased at rest and during exercise. Regional wall motion abnormalities have been demonstrated in different studies and may be secondary to an increased content of fibrous tissue in the LV myocardium.[40–43]

Indications for intervention

Patients with Ebstein's anomaly who require intervention can be divided into two groups. In the first group are those decompensated neonates with severe cyanosis and RV failure who will not survive unless urgent surgery is undertaken. However, surgical attempts at repairing these critically ill neonates have been uniformly unsuccessful in the past. Successful outcomes have been achieved with some procedures aimed at single-ventricle repair.[44,45] More recently, successful biventricular repairs have been performed in neonates with severe cyanosis and right heart failure.[46,47] The indication for early interventions was based on the identification of risk factors for early death. According to these studies, surgery within 2 weeks of life is recommended for asymptomatic neonates with a GOSE score grade 4, cardiothoracic ratio greater than 0.80, and severe TR. For symptomatic neonates, the criteria are severe cyanosis, mild cyanosis together with a GOSE score grade 3 or 4, a cardiothoracic ratio greater than 0.80, severe TR, and associated cardiac defects.

The second group includes those patients who survived the newborn period and present later in life with symptoms that typically represent the effects of progressive RV failure, and arrhythmias. Multiple operations for correction of the hemodynamic consequences of Ebstein's anomaly have been reported.[48–54] The common indications for operation include progressive cyanosis or symptomatic dyspnea and increasing RV size as assessed by echocardiography and radiographic cardiothoracic ratio. However, because of the less satisfactory operative outcome in patients in whom surgical intervention is performed with advanced hemodynamic and symptomatic deterioration, elective surgical therapy is now considered for patients still in New York Heart Association (NYHA) class I or II who present with progressive decline in RV function or develop significant intractable arrhythmias.

Tricuspid valve as the systemic atrioventricular valve

Tricuspid insufficiency after Mustard–Senning procedures

Mild to moderate TR is relatively common in patients after Mustard–Senning procedures. The reversal of the RV/LV pressure relationship results in a more rounded shape of the RV, which displaces the septal chordal attachments, decreasing leaflet coaptation. Moderate and severe tricuspid insufficiency have been observed in 27.5% and 7.4%, respectively, in a large cohort of patients.[55] Severe tricuspid insufficiency is more commonly found in patients with associated anomalies, particularly after ventricular septal defect repair. In other cases, severe tricuspid insufficiency develops as a consequence of RV dysfunction and dilatation.

After Mustard–Senning operation, patients usually undergo cardiac catheterization to assess pulmonary or systemic venous pathway obstruction. The hemodynamic consequences of TR in this setting are similar to those found in patients with mitral insufficiency, with the LV serving as the systemic ventricle. The RV end-diastolic pressure may be elevated, particularly in those patients in whom tricuspid insufficiency is associated with systolic or diastolic dysfunction. Tricuspid valve function needs to be evaluated along with RV function, since tricuspid insufficiency and RV dysfunction have been positively correlated.[55]

Complete echocardiographic evaluation of patients after an intra-atrial baffle procedure should include assessment of RV function and detection and grading of TR. However, echocardiographic quantitative evaluation of RV function in this situation has limitations. Because of its capacity to obtain anatomic and functional data, including RV systolic and diastolic volumes, ejection fraction, and quantification of TR, magnetic resonance imaging (MRI) has been regarded as the optimal imaging modality for these patients.[56–62] Equilibrium radionuclide ventriculography has been shown to be a good alternative for functional assessment of the systemic RV in patients for whom MRI is not available or appropriate.[57]

Indications for tricuspid repair/replacement in patients with a history of atrial switch remain controversial, and decision-making should be based not only on the degree of tricuspid insufficiency but also on RV function. Mild non-progressive tricuspid regurgitation is commonly seen. Most patients with moderate tricuspid regurgitation have some degree of RV dilatation. However, there is some overlap between the 'normal' systemic RV exhibiting physiologically mild dilatation and more significant degrees of dilatation with abnormal systolic function. Most patients with severe TR have concomitant RV dilatation and systolic dysfunction. In one study, the results of tricuspid intervention as an attempt to recover RV function in patients with tricuspid insufficiency have been disappointing.[63] Double-staged switch repair or heart transplantation should be considered as therapeutic options in patients with tricuspid insufficiency and moderate to severe RV dysfunction.

Tricuspid insufficiency after single-ventricle procedures

Surgical palliation for patients with hypoplastic left heart syndrome (HLHS) involves a three-staged approach leading to physiologic palliation by means of a modified Fontan operation. The presence of tricuspid insufficiency in these patients has been identified as a significant risk factor for reduced survival.[64–67] Tricuspid insufficiency may be present at birth or may develop during the stages of surgical reconstruction, and can result from either abnormal valve morphology or incomplete leaflet coaptation. The presence of moderate tricuspid insufficiency at birth or immediately after first-stage reconstruction presents a very poor long-term outcome. Until the second-stage operation, the RV carries an excess volume workload as a consequence of parallel pulmonary and systemic circuits. The combination of excess volume and increased afterload on the RV may result in cyclical worsening of the TR as ventricular volume loading leads to annular dilatation with further increase in valvular regurgitation. The increase in the pressure in the pulmonary venous atrium also impedes antegrade pulmonary flow, especially during systole.

Quantitative methods to accurately diagnose and follow up the degree of tricuspid insuffi-

ciency include quantitative echocardiographic techniques, radionuclide imaging, and MRI.[68,69]

Patients with moderate to severe tricuspid insufficiency should be considered for valve repair at the time of the bidirectional cavopulmonary anastomosis (BCA) or Fontan procedures.[70,71] However, the decrease in RV volume load provided by the BCA alone could result in significant improvement in the degree of tricuspid insufficiency and ventricular dysfunction in patients with mild and moderate TR.[72,73] These considerations are important in patients undergoing second-stage repair, since BCA can be performed without the requirement for cross-clamping or even cardiopulmonary bypass. Because of the improvement in tricuspid valve function observed after second-stage palliation, an expectant management is sometimes undertaken, with hopes of improvement with the reduction in volume overload. If moderate to severe insufficiency persists at the time of the Fontan procedure, tricuspid valve repair is performed at that time.

Tricuspid insufficiency associated with congenitally corrected transposition of the great arteries

Tricuspid valve abnormalities have been reported in 14–56% of patients with congenitally corrected transposition of the great arteries (CCTGA). Although Ebstein-like malformations are seen more frequently (15–45%), dysplasia of the valve and abnormal ventricular attachments are also common. In addition to the stress caused by the systemic systolic pressure, tricuspid insufficiency can be worsened by RV dilatation secondary to systolic dysfunction or volume overload when a ventricular septal defect is present.[74] Clinically significant tricuspid insufficiency is usually associated with RV dysfunction and has been reported in 20–50% of patients with CCTGA.[74–77] The question whether TR is a cause or a consequence of RV dilatation and dysfunction remains unanswered. Tricuspid insufficiency has been found to be an independent risk factor for death when compared with age at presentation, RV dysfunction, history of open-heart surgery, complete heart block, and presence of pulmonary over-circulation.[78] Interestingly, tricuspid insufficiency tends to worsen after ventricular septal defect repair and to improve after pulmonary artery banding. The most likely explanation for this finding is that the fall in LV pressure after ventricular septal defect closure modifies the geometry of the ventricular septum, resulting in lack of coaptation of the tricuspid valve leaflets.

In most cases, the assessment of the degree of TR as well as the quantification of RV function can be performed by Doppler echocardiography. MRI can be used to quantify volume, mass, and ejection fraction.[79] However, a complete heart catheterization and angiography are indicated to assess left and right heart pressures, systolic function, and valvular regurgitation before surgical procedures. Because of the anterior location of the atrioventricular (AV) node, patients with CCTGA are at higher risk to develop complete AV block during cardiac catheterization, particularly when a catheter is manipulated at the right-sided ventricular outflow track.

Management of patients with CCTGA and tricuspid insufficiency is difficult. In considering surgical intervention of the tricuspid valve, RV function should be assessed carefully. Attempts at tricuspid valve repair or replacement have mostly been unsuccessful.[78–84] In patients with severe tricuspid insufficiency associated with RV dysfunction, other options such as the double-switch operation or transplantation should be considered.

References

1. Ribeiro PA, Zaibag MA, Kasab SA, et al. Provocation and amplification of the transvalvular pressure gradient in rheumatic tricuspid stenosis. Am J Cardiol 1988; 61: 1307–11.
2. Gorlin R, Gorlin SG. Hydraulic formula for calculation of area of the stenosis mitral valve, other cardiac values, and central circulatory shunts. Am Heart J 1951; 41: 1–29.
3. Cohen MV, Gorlin R. Modified orifice equation for the calculation of mitral valve area. Am Heart J 1972; 84: 839.
4. Parris TM, Panidis IP, Ross J, Mintz GS. Doppler echocardiographic findings in rheumatic tricuspid stenosis. Am J Cardiol 1987; 60: 1414.
5. Ribeiro PA, Al Zaibag M, Al Kasab S, et al. Provocation and amplification of the transvalvular pressure gradient in rheumatic tricuspid stenosis. Am J Cardiol 1988; 61: 1307.
6. Georgeson S, Panidis IP, Kleaveland IP, et al. Effect of percutaneous balloon valvuloplasty on pulmonary hypertension in mitral stenosis. Am Heart J 1993; 125: 1374–9.
7. Sancaktar O, Deniz Kumbasar S, Semiz E, Yalçinkaya S. Late results of combined percutaneous balloon valvuloplasty of mitral and tricuspid valves. Cathet Cardiovasc Diag 2004; 45: 246–50.
8. Giglia TM, Jenkins KJ, Matitiau A, et al. Influence of right heart size on outcome in pulmonary atresia with intact ventricular septum. Circulation 1993; 88: 2248–56.
9. Bull C, Kostelka M, Sorenesen K, de Leval M. Outcome measures for the neonatal management of pulmonary atresia with intact ventricular septum. J Thorac Cardiovasc Surg 1994; 107: 359–66.
10. Choi YH, Seo JW, Choi JY, et al. Morphology of tricuspid valve in pulmonary atresia with intact ventricular septum. Pediatr Cardiol 1998; 19: 381–9.
11. Louie EK, Lin SS, Reynertson SI, et al. Pressure and volume loading of the right ventricle have opposite effects on left ventricular ejection fraction. Circulation 1995; 92: 819–24.
12. Pepino, CJ, Nichols, WW, Selby, JH. Diagnostic tests for tricuspid insufficiency: How good? Cathet Cardiovasc Diagn 1979; 5: 1.
13. Silver MD, Lam JHC, Ranganathan N, Wigle ED. Morphology of the human tricuspid valve. Circulation 1971; 43: 333–48.
14. Rivera JM, Vandervoort PM, Morris E, et al. Visual assessment of valvular regurgitation: comparison with quantitative Doppler measurements. J Am Soc Echocardiogr 1994; 7: 480–7.
15. Helmcke F, Nanda NS, Hsiung MC, et al. Color Doppler assessment of mitral regurgitation with orthogonal planes. Circulation 1987; 75: 175.
16. Spain MG, Smith MD, Grayburn PA, et al. Quantitative assessment of mitral regurgitation by Doppler color flow imaging: angiographic and hemodynamic correlations, J Am Coll Cardiol 1989; 13: 585.
17. Rokey R, Stoling LL, Zoghbi WA, et al. Determination of regurgitant fraction by pulsed Doppler two-dimensional echocardiography, J Am Coll Cardiol 1986; 7: 1273.
18. Enriquez-Sarano M, Bailey KR, Seward JB. Quantitative Doppler assessment of valvular regurgitation. Circulation 1993; 87: 841.
19. Enriquez-Sarano M, Seward JB, Bailey KR, Tajik AJ. Effective regurgitant orifice area: a noninvasive Doppler development of an old hemodynamic concept. J Am Coll Cardiol 1994; 23: 443–51.
20. Smallhorn JF, Lukawa T, Benson L, et al. Noninvasive recognition of functional pulmonary atresia by echocardiography. Am J Cardiol 1984; 54: 925–6.

21. Newfeld EA, Cole RB, Paul MH. Ebstein's malformation of the tricuspid valve in the neonate: functional and anatomic pulmonary outflow tract obstruction. Am J Cardiol 1967; 19: 727–31.

22. Mangoni AA, DiSalvo TG, Vlahakes GJ, et al. Outcome following isolated tricuspid valve replacement. Eur J Cardiothoracic Surg 2001; 19: 68–73.

23. Misbach GA, Turley K, Ebert PA. Pulmonary valve replacement for regurgitation after repair of tetralogy of Fallot. Ann Thorac Surg 1983; 36: 684–91.

24. Kobayashi J, Kawashima Y, Matsuda H, et al. Prevalence and risk factors of tricuspid regurgitation after correction of tetralogy of Fallot. J Thorac Cardiovasc Surg 1991; 102: 611–16.

25. Kanter KR, Dooelling NR, Fyfe DA, et al. De Vega tricuspid annuloplasty for tricuspid regurgitation in children. Ann Thorac Surg 2001; 72: 1344–8.

26. Reddy VM, McElhinney DB, Brook MM, et al. Repair of congenital tricuspid valve abnormalities with artificial chordae tendinae. Ann Thorac Surg 1998; 66: 172–6.

27. Katogi T, Aeba R, Ito T, et al. Surgical management of isolated congenital tricuspid regurgitation. Ann Thorac Surg 1998; 66: 1571–4.

28. Freedom RM, Benson LN. Neonatal expression of Ebstein's anomaly. Prog Pediatr Cardiol 1993; 2: 22–7.

29. Freedom RM, Benson LN. Ebstein's malformation of the tricuspid valve. In: Freedom RM, Benson LN, Smallhorn JF (eds). Neonatal Heart Disease. London: Springer-Verlag, 1992; 471–83.

30. Fasoli G, Scognamiglio R, Daliento L. Uncommon pattern of tricuspid stenosis in Ebstein's anomaly Int J Cardiol 1985; 9: 488–92.

31. Celermajer DS, Cullen S, Sullivan ID, et al. Outcome in neonates with Ebstein's anomaly. J Am Coll Cardiol 1992; 19: 1041–6.

32. Yetman AT, Freedom RM, McCrindle BW. Outcome in cyanotic neonates with Ebstein's anomaly. Am J Cardiol 1998; 135: 1081–5.

33. Bialostoszky D, Horwitz S, Espino-Vela J. Ebstein's malformation of the tricuspid valve: a review of 65 cases. Am J Cardiol 1972; 29: 826–36.

34. Giuliani ER, Fuster V, Brandenburg RO, Mair DD. Ebstein's anomaly: the clinical features and natural history of Ebstein's anomaly of the tricuspid valve. Mayo Clin Proc 1979; 4:1 63–75.

35. McLellan-Tobert S, Driscoll D, Motram C, et al. Exercise tolerance in patients with Ebstein's anomaly. J Am Coll Cardiol 1997; 29: 1615–22.

36. Roberson DA, Silverman NH. Ebstein's anomaly: echocardiographic and clinical features in the fetus and neonate. J Am Coll Cardiol 1989; 13: 1300.

37. Celermajer DS Bull C, Till JA, et al. Ebstein's anomaly: presentation and outcome from fetus to adult. J Am Coll Cardiol 1994; 23; 170–6.

38. Shiina A, Seward JB, Tajik AJ, et al. Two-dimensional echocardiographic – surgical correlation in Ebstein's anomaly: preoperative determination of patients requiring tricuspid valve plication vs. replacement. Circulation 1983; 68: 534–44.

39. Rigby M, Mota C. Echocardiographic evaluation and diagnosis of Ebstein's malformation. In: The Right Heart in Congenital Heart Disease. London: Greenwich Medical Media, 1988.

40. Seward JB. Ebstein's anomaly: ultrasound imaging and hemodynamic evaluation. Echocardiography 1993; 1: 641.

41. Celermajer DS, Cullen S, Sullivan ID, et al. Outcome in neonates with Ebstein's anomaly. J Am Coll Cardol 1992; 19; 1041–6.

42. Saxena A, Fong LV, Tristam M, et al. Late non-invasive evaluation of cardiac performance in mildly symptomatic older patients with Ebstein's anomaly of tricuspid valve: role of radionuclide imaging. J Am Coll Cardiol 1991; 17: 182–6.

43. Benson LN, Child JS, Schwaiger M, et al. Left ventricular geometry and function in adults with Ebstein's anomaly of the tricuspid valve. Circulation 1987; 75: 353–9.

44. Starnes VA, Pitlick PT, Berstein D, et al. Ebstein's anomaly appearing in the neonate. A new surgical approach. J Thorac Cardiovasc Surg 1991; 101: 1082–7.

45. Endo M, Ohmi M, Sato K, et al. Tricuspid valve closure for neonatal Ebstein's anomaly. Ann Thorac Surg 1998; 65: 540–2.

46. Knott Craig CJ, Overholt ED Ward KE, Razook JD. Neonatal repair of Ebstein's anomaly: indications, surgical technique, and medium-term follow-up. Ann Thorac Surg 2000; 69: 1505–10.

47. Knott Craig CJ, Overholt ED Ward KE, et al. Repair of Ebstein's anomaly in the symptomatic neonate: an evolution of technique with 7-year follow-up. Ann Thorac Surg 2002; 73: 1786–93.

48. Di Russo GB, Gaynor JW. Ebstein's anomaly: indications for repair and surgical technique. Semin Thorac Cardiovasc Surg Pediatr Card Surg Annu 1999; 2: 35–50.

49. Carpentier A, Chauvaud S, Mace L, et al. A new reconstructive operation for Ebstein's anomaly of the tricuspid valve. J Thorac Cardiovasc Surg 1988; 96: 92–101.

50. Kupilik N, Simon P, Moidl R, et al. Valve-preserving treatment of Ebstein's anomaly: perioperative and follow-up results. Thorac Cardiovasc Surg 1999; 47: 229–34.

51. Marianeschi SM, McElhinney DB, Reddy VM, et al. Alternative approach to the repair of the Ebstein's malformation: intracardiac repair with ventricular unloading. Ann Thorac Surg 1998; 66: 1546–50.

52. Wu Q, Huang Z. Anatomic correction of Ebstein's anomaly. J Thorac Cardiovasc Surg 2001; 12: 1237–8.

53. Hetzer R, Nagdyman N, Ewert P, et al. A modified repair technique for tricuspid incompetence in Ebstein's anomaly. J Thorac Cardiovasc Surg 1998; 115: 857–68.

54. Quaegebeur JM, Sreeram N, Fraser AG, et al. Surgery for Ebstein's anomaly: the clinical and echocardiographic evaluation of a new technique. J Am Coll Cardiol 1991; 17: 722–8.

55. Moons P, Gewillig M, Sluysmans T, et al. Long-term outcome up to 30 years after the Mustard or Senning operation: a nationwide multicentre study in Belgium. Heart 2004; 90: 307–13 (discussion 314–15).

56. Rees S. Somerville J, Warnes C, et al. Comparison of magnetic resonance imaging with echocardiography and radionuclide angiography in assessing cardiac function and anatomy following Mustard's operation for transposition of the great arteries. Am J Cardiol 1988; 61: 1316–22.

57. Hornung TS, Anagnostopoulos C, Bharwaj P, et al. Comparison of equilibrium radionuclide ventriculography with cardiovascular magnetic resonance for assessing the systemic right ventricle after Mustard or Senning procedures for complete transposition of the great arteries. Am J Cardiol 2003; 92: 640–3.

58. Chung KJ, Simpson IA, Glass RF, et al. Cine magnetic resonance imaging after surgical repair in patients with transposition of the great arteries. Circulation 1988; 77: 104–9.

59. Theissen P, Kaemmerer H, Sechtem U, et al. Magnetic resonance imaging of cardiac function and morphology in patients with transposition of the great arteries following Mustard procedure. Thorac Cardiovasc Surg 1991; 39: 221–4.

60. Rebergen SA, Helbing WA, van der Wall EE, et al. MR velocity mapping of tricuspid flow in healthy children and in patients who have undergone Mustard or Senning repair. Radiology 1995; 194: 505–12.

61. Lidegran M, Odhner L, Jacobson LA, et al. Magnetic resonance imaging and echocardiography in assessment of ventricular function in atrially corrected transposition of the great arteries. Scand Cardiovasc J 2000; 34: 384–9.

62. Laffon E, Jimenez M, Latrabe V, et al. Quantitiative MRI comparison of systemic hemodynamics in Mustard/Senning repaired patients and healthy volunteers at rest. Eur Radiol 2004; 14: 875–80.

63. Carrel T, Pfammatter JP. Complete transposition of the great arteries: surgical concepts for patients with systemic right ventricular failure following intraatrial repair. Thorac Cardiovasc Surg 2000; 48: 224–7.

64. Lang P, Norwood WI. Hemodynamic assessment after palliative surgery for HLHS. Circulation 1983; 68: 1041–8.

65. Barber G, Helton JG, Aglira BA, et al. The significance of tricuspid regurgitation in hypoplastic left heart syndrome. Am Heart J 1988; 116: 1563–7.

66. Hawkins JA, Doty DB. Aortic atresia: morphologic characteristics affecting survival and operative palliation. J Thorac Cardiovasc Surg 1984; 88: 620–6.

67. Chang AC, Farrell PE Jr, Mundison KA, et al. Hypoplastic left heart syndrome: hemodynamic and angiographic assessment after initial reconstructive surgery and relevance to modified Fontan procedure. J Am Coll Cardiol 1991; 17: 1143–9.

68. Geva T. Echocardiography and Doppler ultrasound. In: Garson A Jr, Bricker JT, Fisher DJ, Neish SR (eds). The Science and Practice of Pediatric Cardiology, 2nd edn. Baltimore: Williams & Wilkins, 1998: 789–843.

69. Zhang J, Shiota T, Shandas R, et al. Effects of adjacent surfaces of different shapes on regurgitant jet sizes: an in vitro study using color Doppler imaging and laser-illuminated dye visualization. J Am Coll Cardiol 1993; 22: 1522–9.

70. Reyes A, Bove E, Mosca RS, et al. Tricuspid valve repair in children with hypoplastic left heart syndrome during stated surgical reconstruction. Circulation 1997; 96(Suppl II): II-341–II-343.

71. Ohye RG, Gomez CA, Goldberg CS, et al. Tricuspid valve repair in hypoplastic left heart syndrome. J Thorac Cardiovasc Surg 2004; 127; 465–72.

72. Kobayashi J, Matsuda H, Nakano S, et al. Hemodynamic effects of bidirectional cavopulmonary shunt with pulsatile pulmonary flow. Circulation 1991; 84(Suppl III): III-219–III-225.

73. Chang AC, Hanley FL, Wernovsky G, et al. Early bidirectional cavopulmonary shunt in young infants. Circulation 1993; 88: 149–58.

74. Lundstrom U, Bull C, Wyse RKH, Sommerville J. The natural and 'unnatural' history of congenitally corrected transposition. Am J Cardiol 1990; 65: 1222–9.

75. McGrath LB, Kirklin JW, Blackstone EH, et al. Death and other events after cardiac repair in discordant atrioventricular connection. J Thorac Cardiovasc Surg 1985; 90: 711–23.

76. Hwang B, Bowman F, Malm J, Krongrad B. Surgical repair of congenital corrected transposition of the great arteries: results and follow-up. Am J Cardiol 1982; 50: 781–5.

77. Metcalfe J, Somerville J. Surgical repair of lesions associated with corrected transposition: late results. Br Heart J 1983; 50: 476–82.

78. Prieto L, Hordof A, Secic M, et al. Progressive tricuspid valve disease in patients with congenitally corrected transposition of the great arteries. Circulation 1998; 98: 997–1005.

79. Lorenz CH, Walker ES, Morgan VL, et al. Normal human right and left ventricular mass, systolic function, and gender differences by cine magnetic resonance imaging. J Cardiovasc Magn Reson 1999; 1: 7–21.

80. Acar P, Sidi D, Bonnet D, et al. Maintaining tricuspid valve competence in double discordance: a challenge for the paediatric cardiologist. Heart 1998; 80: 479–83.

81. Huhta JC, Danielson GK, Ritter DG, Ilstrup DM. Survival in atrioventricular discordance. Pediatr Cardiol 1985; 6: 57–60.

82. Sano T, Riesenfeld T, Karl TR, Wilkinson JL. Intermediate-term outcome after intracardiac repair of associated cardiac defects in patients with atrio-ventricular and ventriculoarterial discordance. Circulation 1995; 92(9 Suppl): II272–8.

83. Termignon JL, Leca F, Vouhe PR, et al. 'Classic' repair of congenitally corrected transposition and ventricular septal defect. Ann Thorac Surg 1996; 62: 199–206.

84. Rutledge JM, Nihill MR, Fraser CD, et al. Outcome of 121 patients with congenitally corrected transposition of the great arteries. Pediatr Cardiol 2002; 23: 137–45.

31

Methods of tricuspid valve repair and replacement

Gil Bolotin, Valluvan Jeevanandam

Dysfunction of the tricuspid valve, sometimes neglected or referred to as a 'second-class' structure, may cause significant morbidity and mortality. It can be the primary site of pathology or can secondarily be involved in left heart and/or pulmonary pathology.

Anatomy

The tricuspid valve normally has three leaflets, (Figure 31.1). The septal leaflet is semicircular in

shape and is attached to the fibrous trigone of the heart. Hence, it cannot dilate or stretch. The anterior leaflet is quadrangular and is the largest. The posterior leaflet is nearly triangular and is the smallest; it is positioned rightward and lateral when the valve is viewed from the atrium. The tricuspid valve is similar to the mitral valve, but has three leaflets, is usually 2–3 mm larger in diameter, and has papillary muscle and chordal attachments to the ventricular septum. Of particular surgical significance is the location of the atrioventricular (AV) node, which lies posterior to

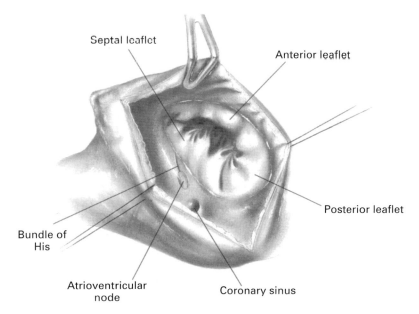

Septal leaflet

Anterior leaflet

Posterior leaflet

Bundle of His

Atrioventricular node

Coronary sinus

Figure 31.1

Normal anatomy of the tricuspid valve. (Reproduced from Doty DB. Cardiac Surgery: Operative Techniques. St Louis, MO: Mosby, 1997: 270–3 with permission from Elsevier.)

the commissure between the septal and anterior leaflets, and can be injured if sutures are placed in this area during annuloplasty or replacement.

Etiology

Tricuspid valve dysfunction is usually the result of annular dilatation and subsequent poor central coaptation of the leaflets. This leads to central regurgitation. Annular dilatation is usually secondary to right heart enlargement and/or failure. Less frequently, the leaflets may be involved with processes such as rheumatic fever, carcinoid tumor, or endocarditis. Injury may also result from previous cardiac surgery (especially congenital repairs), endomyocardial biopsies, indwelling pacemaker leads, or chest trauma. Some diet drugs may also cause a carcinoid type of leaflet dysfunction.

Indications for surgery

Surgery should be considered in primary tricuspid valve disease for medically refractory right heart failure, atrial enlargement causing atrial fibrillation, or progressive right ventricular dysfunction and dilatation. Persistent sepsis with vegetations or infected thrombus is another indication. Most commonly, tricuspid valve repairs are performed concomitant to repair of either aortic or mitral valve lesions.

Surgical exposure and cardiopulmonary bypass techniques

The surgical approach and exposure for tricuspid surgery is dependent upon the concomitant procedure and the preference of both patient and surgeon. For patients undergoing concomitant coronary artery bypass grafting (CABG) or aortic valve replacement, median sternotomy is usually the approach of choice. Minimally invasive approaches, such as partial lower sternotomy and right anterior thoracotomy, are used according to the preferences of patient and surgeon, mainly in isolated tricuspid valve surgery or when combined with mitral valve procedures.[1,2]

Median sternotomy

The traditional exposure of the tricuspid valve through median sternotomy includes arterial aortic cannulation. Bicaval venous cannulation with caval snares is essential to isolate the right atrium. The left-sided valve repair or replacement is performed under cardiac arrest with antegrade and/or retrograde cardioplegia, moderate systemic hypothermia, and topical cold saline surface cooling. The mitral valve can be exposed through a left atrial incision posterior to the intra-atrial septum or through a trans-septal incision. Similarly, the aortic valve can be exposed via a transverse aortotomy. A concomitant CABG can be performed on bypass with a similar cannulation technique, followed by right atrium incision to expose the tricuspid valve. Another option is to perform the tricuspid valve repair or replacement without cross-clamp while the heart is allowed to beat.

Right thoracotomy

The minimally invasive right anterior/lateral thoracotomy approach is widely used for mitral and/or tricuspid valve surgery, with direct vision, video-assisted, or robotically assisted surgery.[2–6] Cannulation is usually through the femoral vessels for both arterial and venous access. The venous cannulation can be with two separate cannulae – one from the groin to the inferior vena cava, and the second via the jugular vein or through the lateral thoracotomy directly to the superior vena cava. The full lateral thoracotomy approach can also be used for tricuspid valve surgery. Isolation of the right atrium can be established by means of conventional snaring done through the lateral thoracotomy or by using specially design transthoracic clamps.[7] Aortic cross-clamping is facilitated by using a single shaft instrument such as the Chitwood aortic clamp.[6]

Tricuspid resection

In the past, surgical resection of the tricuspid valve was an acceptable treatment for tricuspid endocarditis,[8] especially if there was a potential for continued intravenous drug abuse. Most patients tolerate the absence of the tricuspid valve well – at least for a while. However, 30% decompensate, especially with any increase in pulmonary vascular resistance or pulmonary valve insufficiency, and develop right heart failure.[9,10] Today, tricuspid vegetectomy or tricuspid repair or replacement are the surgical treatments of choice for tricuspid valve disease.[10,11]

Tricuspid annuloplasty

For tricuspid regurgitation due to a dilated or distorted annulus, several annuloplasty procedures can be applied. DeVega annuloplasty is widely used for mild to moderate tricuspid valve regurgitation, especially when performed concomitantly with other cardiac procedures. Ring and band annuloplasty are usually used for severe tricuspid valve regurgitation or for patients undergoing isolated tricuspid valve repair.[12–19]

Annular plication – DeVega

A double-armed 2-0 or 3-0 Prolene or Dacron polyester suture with Teflon felt pledget is used (Figure 31.2). The purse-string bites are placed at the junction of the annulus and right ventricular free wall, running around the anterior and posterior leaflets from the anterior septal commissure to the posterior septal commissure, avoiding the septal leaflet annulus. The second limb of the suture is placed through the pledget and runs parallel and 2–3 mm above the first suture line in the same clockwise direction in an alternative sequence. The suture depth is usually 2–3 mm and 10–12 bites are usually needed for each limb. Both needles are then passed through a second pledget at the posteroseptal commissure. The suture is tightened, producing a purse-string effect and reducing the length of the anterior and posterior annulus. A No. 27 valve sizer or equivalent is used to properly reduce the annular size, and several techniques are used for avoiding overtightening or postoperative loosening at a later stage.[12–14] Long-term hemodynamics at a mean period of 53 months after the operation were found to be maintained in patients with moderate to severe tricuspid regurgitation in the

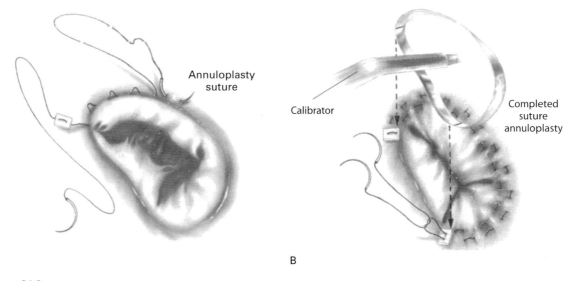

Annuloplasty suture

Calibrator

Completed suture annuloplasty

A

B

Figure 31.2

DeVega annuloplasty. (Reproduced from Doty DB. Cardiac Surgery: Operative Techniques. St Louis, MO: Mosby, 1997: 270–3 with permission from Elsevier.)

absence of an organically diseased or deformed valve.[14]

Ring and band annuloplasty

Ring or band annuloplasty is usually preferred for moderate or severe tricuspid regurgitation, especially if this is the main part of the operation. Rings and bands allow significant degrees of annular reduction with long-term durability. Several devices are available, including rigid rings (Carpentier–Edwards), flexible rings (i.e. Duran), or flexible bands (i.e. the Cosgrove annuloplasty system). The size of the ring or band is determined according to the length of the base of the septal leaflet. These devices are designed to avoid suture placement in the region of the AV node to preserve AV conduction.

The mattress sutures are placed circumferentially, with wider bites on the annulus and smaller corresponding bites through the ring or band, thus producing annular plication. The reduction in annular size is mainly along the annulus of the posterior leaflet. At the end of the procedure, the tricuspid valve orifice is primarily occluded by the leaflet tissue of the anterior and septal leaflets. Long-term results with ring or band annuloplasty were found to be excellent, and in some studies were superior when compared with DeVega annuloplasty.[15–19]

Annular plication – bicuspidization

A third and less used option is bicuspidization of the tricuspid valve. By plicating the annulus over the posterior tricuspid valve leaflet, this leaflet is excluded, thus converting the tricuspid valve into a bicuspid valve. Technically, a 2-0 or 3-0 Prolene suture with or without pledget is passed through the annulus at the anteroposterior commissure, through the annulus at the center of the posterior leaflet, and then through the annulus at the posteroseptal commissure. If a pledget is not used, another tricuspid valve stitch should be placed for reinforcement. The repair is not at the area of the AV node, and at the end of the repair the tricuspid valve should reach normal diameter.[20–23]

Tricuspid replacement

Tricuspid valve replacement is performed when the native valve is too deformed and not suitable for repair. Traditionally, the short- and long-term results after tricuspid replacement were poor; however, the reason is usually the poor medical status of the patient and the main underlying disease such as endocarditis or drug abuse. The results are better when the patient's comorbidities are less severe. There has been a long-standing debate regarding the decision between prosthetic and biological valves. In the past, the results were favorable with biological valves; however, since the introduction of the modern bileaflet mechanical valve, the results are similar, with some reports that long-term results with the mechanical valve are better. The decision should be made with regard to the patient's clinical condition and prognosis. Generally, the relatively young patient with possible long-term survival without contraindication for anticoagulation should receive a mechanical valve.[24–32]

Tricuspid replacement with a bioprosthesis

Exposure and connection to the heart–lung machine are similar to the procedures described above for tricuspid repair. If possible, the old valve should not be excised, in order that the subvalvular apparatus is maintained. If the valve is excised, a rim of cusp should be left, especially at the septal leaflet, to avoid damage to the conductive system while suturing. The technique for tricuspid valve implantation is with pledgeted mattress sutures, using an everting suture technique for either a supra-annular or an intra-annular implantation. The stitches through the septal area should be superficial and if possible through the leaflet rim at the area of the bundle of His. Beating heart suturing may help to detect conduction disturbances in real time, and the suture can be repositioned. Biological prostheses were initially considered ideal in the tricuspid position because they would not require anticoagulation and were expected to have a slower degeneration than in the mitral or aortic position. However, this belief was contradicted by the finding of limited durability of about 7–9 years. In some reports, the long-term valve dysfunction was due to panus formation on the mural cusp and not to structural degeneration. Generally, biological tricuspid valves are not exceptions to the rule that patients over 65–70 years of age obtain the greatest advantage from bioprostheses; however, the extent and the severity of cardiac disease might suggest, in some cases, a limited life expectancy and therefore might favor the use of biological prostheses in younger patients.[26–33]

Tricuspid replacement with a mechanical valve

Exposure and connection to the heart–lung machine are as described above for biological tricuspid valve replacement. If possible, the native leaflets are left in situ, and the pledgeted 2-0 Ethibond sutures are passed through the annulus and the edges of the leaflets. The subvalvular apparatus is visualized to ensure that there is no impingement of the prosthetic valve leaflets. The valve can be rotated if necessary to prevent leaflet contact with tissue. Permanent epicardial pacing electrodes should be placed during the operation. The incidence of permanent postoperative complete heart block ranges from 1% to 9% and it may be impossible to introduce transvenous pacemaker electrodes after tricuspid valve replacement. All mechanical valves in the tricuspid position require permanent anticoagulation with warfarin. The modern bileaflet mechanical valves have a low profile and the lowest thrombosis rate of the mechanical valves. The onset of valve thrombosis may be insidious and can be treated either with thrombolysis or with reoperation.[27–32]

Tricuspid repair during heart transplant

Tricuspid regurgitation has often been reported after orthotopic heart transplantation, with an incidence ranging from 47% to 98%. The cause of the regurgitation is multifactorial, including allograft dysfunction with right ventricular dilatation, pulmonary hypertension, severe donor–recipient size mismatch, and alterations in the geometry of the tricuspid valve and right atrium related to the technique of right atrial anastomosis. In several stud-

ies, moderate and greater levels of tricuspid regurgitation are associated with right-sided heart failure symptoms, renal and hepatic dysfunction, and decreased long-term survival. In a recent prospective randomized study, a preventive tricuspid valve annuloplasty of the donor heart before bicaval orthotopic heart transplantation was found to improve immediate donor heart function as demonstrated by better right ventricular performance, lower perioperative mortality, and shorter reperfusion times. At 1 year, there was less tricuspid valve regurgitation. The authors recommended that prophylactic DeVega annuloplasty should be performed as a routine adjunct with bicaval orthotopic heart transplantation.[34–40]

Removal of tricuspid vegetations/thrombus via inflow occlusion

Tricuspid valve endocarditis is often treated surgically by preserving the tricuspid valve while removing infected material.[7,8] Surgical intervention in the setting of sepsis carries the risk of worsening pulmonary function with exposure to cardiopulmonary bypass. In addition, bypass causes an inflammatory response, with activation of complement and a host of cytokines that can amplify a septic state.[5] For these reasons, the 'off-pump' route employing vena caval inflow occlusion is suggested.

The chest is opened through a median sternotomy. The superior and inferior venae cavae are dissected free and slings are placed around them. The body of the right atrium is brought into view and four stay sutures are placed. Ten thousand units of heparin are administered systemically. The superior and inferior venae cavae are then clamped and the body of the right atrium is opened vertically between the stay sutures. The tricuspid valve is visualized and the vegetation is excised. The right atrial cavity is washed out with antibiotic solution. At the end of the 'safe' 2-minute period, a partial occluding clamp with a long flat jaw is applied to the right atrium, incorporating the edges and the stay sutures, and the caval clamps are then released. If necessary, a second opening of the atrium for 2 minutes can be applied. The edges of the atrial incision are approximated within the clamp with 4/0 Prolene sutures. The pericardium is then closed. This procedure removes the septic focus while preserving the valve and avoids the downside of cardiopulmonary bypass. However, this technique would not be useful if there is significant destruction of the tricuspid valve, a significant patent foramen ovale, or significant involvement of left-sided heart valves.[41–44]

Results of tricuspid valve surgery

The durability of simple annuloplasty techniques such as bicuspidization and the DeVega procedure has been good when they have been employed only for mild to moderate degrees of functional tricuspid regurgitation. Tricuspid annuloplasty using Duran, Carpentier–Edwards, or Cosgrove rings or bands resulted in 85% freedom from moderate to severe tricuspid regurgitation at 6 years. The need for tricuspid reoperation is very low. Poor long-term results are usually due to persistent mitral disease and unrelenting pulmonary hypertension with right ventricular dilatation and dysfunction. Advanced right ventricular failure or arrhythmia cause late death. Patients who need valve replacement for endocarditis comprise a unique subgroup with the additional risk for death due to sepsis, reinfection, and the complications related to drug addiction.

Complete heart block may occur immediately postoperatively due to iatrogenic damage to the conduction system during tricuspid valve surgery. This complication can be minimized intraoperatively by performing the procedure on the perfused beating heart as described above. Late development of heart block rarely occurs after tricuspid annuloplasty. In the case of double valve replacement, the presence of two rigid prosthetic sewing rings can produce ongoing trauma and lead to AV node dysfunction over time.[28,27,30,45–47]

References

1. Doty DB, Flores JH, Doty JR. Cardiac valve operations using a partial sternotomy (lower half) technique. J Card Surg 2000; 15: 35–42.
2. Navia JL, Cosgrove DM 3rd. Minimally invasive mitral valve operations. Ann Thorac Surg 1996; 62: 1542–4.
3. Falk V, Walther T, Diegeler A, et al. Echocardiographic monitoring of minimally invasive mitral valve surgery using an endoaortic clamp. J Heart Valve Dis 1996; 5: 630–7.
4. Chitwood WR Jr, Elbeery JR, Chapman WH, et al. Video-assisted minimally invasive mitral valve surgery: the 'micro-mitral' operation. J Thorac Cardiovasc Surg 1997; 113: 413–14.
5. Vanermen H, Farhat F, Wellens F, et al. Minimally invasive video-assisted mitral valve surgery: from port-access towards a totally endoscopic procedure. J Card Surg 2000; 15: 51–60.
6. Kypson AP, Nifong LW, Chitwood WR Jr. Robotic mitral valve surgery. Semin Thorac Cardiovasc Surg 2003; 15: 121–9.
7. Kypson AP, Glower DD. Minimally invasive tricuspid operation using port access. Ann Thorac Surg 2002; 74: 43–5.
8. Wright JS, Glennie JS. Excision of tricuspid valve with later replacement in endocarditis of drug addiction. Thorax 1978; 33: 518–19.
9. Bernal JM, Gonzalez IM, Miralles PJ. Prophylactic resection of a tricuspid valve vegetation in infective endocarditis. Int J Cardiol 1986; 12: 255–7.
10. Stern HJ, Sisto DA, Strom JA, et al. Immediate tricuspid valve replacement for endocarditis. Indications and results. J Thorac Cardiovasc Surg 1986; 91: 163–7.
11. Lange R, De Simone R, Bauernschmitt R, et al. Tricuspid valve reconstruction, a treatment option in acute endocarditis. Eur J Cardiothorac Surg 1996; 10: 320–6.
12. Hashimoto K, Arai T, Kurosawa H. Technical considerations and intermediate-term results with modified DeVega tricuspid annuloplasty. Cardiovasc Surg 1993; 1: 573–6.
13. Meyer J, Bircks W. Predictable correction of tricuspid insufficiency by semicircular annuloplasty. Ann Thorac Surg 1977; 23: 574–5.
14. Chidambaram M, Abdulali SA, Baliga BG, Ionescu MI. Long-term results of DeVega tricuspid annuloplasty. Ann Thorac Surg 1987; 43: 185–8.
15. Grondin P, Meere C, Limet R, et al. Carpentier's annulus and De Vega's annuloplasty. The end of the tricuspid challenge. J Thorac Cardiovasc Surg 1975; 70: 852–61.
16. Brugger JJ, Egloff L, Rothlin M, et al. Tricuspidal annuloplasty. Results and complications. Thorac Cardiovasc Surg 1982; 30: 284–7.
17. Gatti G, Maffei G, Lusa AM, Puglise P. Tricuspid valve repair with the Cosgrave–Edwards annuloplasty system: early clinical and echocardiographic results. Ann Thorac Surg. 2001; 72: 764–7.
18. Revuelta JM, Garcia-Rinaldi R, Duran CM. Conservative repair of the mitral and tricuspid valves: eight years experience with Duran flexible ring annuloplasty. Bol Asoc Med P R 1984; 76: 429–41.

19. Matsuyama K, Matsumoto M, Sugita T, et al. De Vega annuloplasty and Carpentier–Edwards ring annuloplasty for secondary tricuspid regurgitation. J Heart Valve Dis 2001; 10: 520–4.

20. Kay JH, Mendez AM, Zubiate P. A further look at tricuspid annuloplasty. Ann Thorac Surg 1976; 22: 498–500.

21. Boyd AD, Engelman RM, Isom OW, et al. Tricuspid annuloplasty. Five and one-half years' experience with 78 patients. J Thorac Cardiovasc Surg. 1974; 68: 344–51.

22. Reed GE, Cortes LE. Measured tricuspid annuloplasty: a rapid and reproducible technique. Ann Thorac Surg 1976; 21: 168–9.

23. Reed GE, Boyd AD, Spencer FC, et al. Operative management of tricuspid regurgitation. Circulation 1976; 54(6 Suppl): III96–III98.

24. Solomon NA, Lim RC, Nand P, Graham KJ. Tricuspid valve replacement: bioprosthetic or mechanical valve? Asian Cardiovasc Thorac Ann 2004; 12: 143–8.

25. Carrier M, Hebert Y, Pellerin M, et al. Tricuspid valve replacement: an analysis of 25 years of experience at a single center. Ann Thorac Surg 2003; 75: 47–50.

26. Kaplan M, Kut MS, Demirtas MM, et al. Prosthetic replacement of tricuspid valve: bioprosthetic or mechanical? Ann Thorac Surg 2002; 73: 467–73.

27. Rizzoli G, Vendramin I, Nesseris G, et al. Biological or mechanical prostheses in tricuspid position? A meta-analysis of intra-institutional results. Ann Thorac Surg 2004; 77: 1607–14

28. Ratnatunga CP, Edwards MB, Dore CJ, Taylor KM. Tricuspid valve replacement. UK Heart Valve Registry mid-term results comparing mechanical and biological prostheses. Ann Thorac Surg 1998; 66: 1940–7

29. Rizzoli G, De Perini L, Bottio T, et al. Prosthetic replacement of the tricuspid valve: biological or mechanical? Ann Thorac Surg 1998; 66(Suppl): S62–S67.

30. Van Nooten GJ, Caes F, Taeymans Y, et al. Tricuspid valve replacement: postoperative and long-term results. J Thorac Cardiovasc Surg 1995; 110: 672–9.

31. Van Nooten GJ, Caes FL, Francois KJ, et al. The valve choice in tricuspid valve replacement: 25 years of experience. Eur J Cardiothorac Surg. 1995; 9: 441–6; discussion 446–7.

32. Dalrymple-Hay MJ, Leung Y, Ohri SK, et al. Tricuspid valve replacement: bioprostheses are preferable. J Heart Valve Dis 1999; 8: 644–8.

33. Nakano K, Eishi K, Kosakai Y, et al. Ten-year experience with the Carpentier–Edwards pericardial xenograft in the tricuspid position. J Thorac Cardiovasc Surg 1996; 111: 605–12.

34. Jeevanandam V, Russell H, Mather P, et al. A one-year comparison of prophylactic donor tricuspid annuloplasty in heart transplantation. Ann Thorac Surg 2004; 78: 759–66.

35. Sahar G, Stamler A, Erez E, et al. Etiological factors influencing the development of atrioventricular valve incompetence after heart transplantation. Transplant Proc 1997; 29: 2675–6.

36. Ichikawa S, Takeuchi Y, Suda Y, et al. Tricuspid valve replacement after cardiac transplantation. J Thorac Cardiovasc Surg 2000; 48: 659–62

37. Lewen M, Bryg R, Miller L, et al. Tricuspid regurgitation by Doppler echocardiography after orthotopic cardiac transplantation. Am J Cardiol 1987; 59: 1371–4.

38. Chan M, Giannetti N, Kornbluth M, et al. Severe tricuspid regurgitation after heart transplantation. J Heart Lung Transplant 2001; 20: 709–17.

39. Aziz T, Burgess M, Rahman A, et al. Risk factors for tricuspid valve regurgitation after orthotopic heart transplantation. Ann Thorac Surg 1999; 68: 1247–51.

40. De Simone R, Lange R, Sack F, et al. Atrioventricular valve insufficiency and atrial geometry after orthotopic heart transplantation. Ann Thorac Surg 1995; 60: 1683–6.

41. Raman J, Bellomo R, Shah P. Avoiding the pump in tricuspid valve endocarditis – vegetectomy under inflow occlusion. Ann Thorac Cardiovasc Surg 2002; 8: 350–3.

42. Lai DTM, Chard RB. Commissuroplasty: method of valve repair for mitral and tricuspid endocarditis. Ann Thorac Surg 1999; 68: 1727–30.

43. Allen MD, Slachman F, Eddy AC, et al. Tricuspid valve repair for tricuspid valve endocarditis: tricuspid valve 'recycling'. Ann Thorac Surg 1991; 51: 593–8.

44. Kirklin JK, Westaby S, Blackstone EH, et al. Complement and the damaging effects of cardiopulmonary bypass. J Thorac Cardiovasc Surg 1983; 86: 845–57.

45. Carozza A, Renzulli A, De Feo M, et al. Tricuspid repair for infective endocarditis: clinical and echocardiographic results. Tex Heart Inst J 2001; 28: 96–101.

46. Gatti G, Maffei G, Lusa AM, Pugliese P. Tricuspid valve repair with the Cosgrove–Edwards annuloplasty system: early clinical and echocardiographic results. Ann Thorac Surg 2001; 72: 764–7.

47. Nakano K, Ishibashi-Ueda H, Kobayashi J, et al. Tricuspid valve replacement with bioprostheses: long-term results and causes of valve dysfunction. Ann Thorac Surg 2001; 71: 105–9.

32

Available devices for percutaneous replacement of the tricuspid valve

Younes Boudjemline, Philipp Bonhoeffer

Introduction

Transcatheter valve replacement has become a possibility in the position of the pulmonary or aortic valves.[1–6] For the insertion of transcatheter valves in the atrioventricular (AV) position, a new series of considerations arise. First, the discrepancy between the size of the available percutaneous semilunar valves and the size of the annulus makes the use of current stent designs impossible. Surgeons using semilunar valves usually choose the diameter of the valve (with its surrounding fabric) as a function of the size of the annulus when it is in the range of available valve diameters. More rarely, they adapt the size of the annulus to the largest available valve, reducing the annulus.

Second, to prevent embolization, the valved device must be anchored to the annulus. This is done surgically by direct suturing of the prosthetic fabric surrounding the implanted valve.

Third, in the case of percutaneous reduction of annulus size, to avoid paravalvular leak, the device must have a way to anchor and assure the sealing of the gap between the true and reduced annulus diameters. Therefore, it is necessary to develop a specific device for this indication that will satisfy the above criteria.

Due to the more direct and easy catheter approach to the tricuspid valve, we have chosen this site as the first point of technical interest. Clearly, this is an important step in approaching the complexity of AV valve implantation. It is not, however, an attempt to resolve the clinical problem of tricuspid regurgitation in the human setting.

Non-surgical replacement of the tricuspid valve

Development of a specific device for transcatheter insertion of a semilunar valve in tricuspid position

In our previous work on transcatheter replacement of aortic and pulmonary valves, we developed balloon and self-expandable stents.[1–3] Following these developments, we designed and developed a self-expandable stent constructed from 0.22 mm nitinol wire. It is a symmetrical device formed by two disks separated by a tubular portion (AMF, Reuilly, France) (Figure 32.1). Mechanical fixation to the annulus was assured by trapping the annulus and the native valve between the two disks. The central part of the stent assured the downsizing of the annulus and acted as a supporting structure for the heterograft to be implanted. The overall length of the deployed device was 15 mm. The disks had a spontaneous diameter of 40 mm, which is slightly larger than the diameter of the tricuspid annulus of a 60 kg ewe. Since only 18 mm valves were available for these experiments, the tubular part of the stent was calibrated to shelter this valve. The diameter and length of this tubular portion were 18 and 15 mm, respectively, which is the approximate length of an 18 mm valve. A valved venous segment, harvested from the bovine jugular vein (Contegra, Medtronic Inc., Minneapolis, USA), was prepared as previously reported[1,2] and mounted into the tubular part of the self-expandable stent. To guarantee sealing of

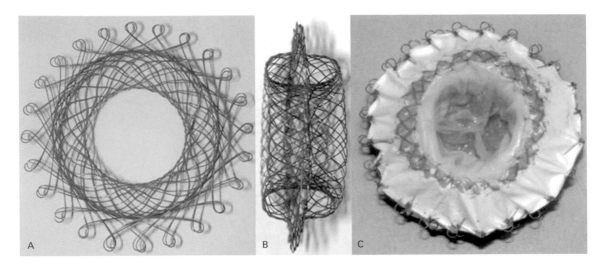

Figure 32.1

En-face and lateral views of the newly designed stent before its covering (A), after its covering with a PTFE membrane (B), and after suturing of the valve in the central tubular part (C). The stent is shown from the ventricular side, with the valve in the closed position.

this device, we finally sutured a PTFE membrane, usually used for covered stents, on the outside of the disks. The delivery system consisted of a 'home-made' front-loading long sheath. The distal tip of a dilator was cut off. A catheter was fixed to this part to free a 5.5 cm long space for valved stent placement. At the tip of the catheter, a 1 cm long dilator was attached to allow for a smooth transition between the tip and the sheath, and to facilitate the tracking of the delivery system during its course. Since the stent was made of memory-shape alloy, no balloons were necessary to deploy the device, which was delivered by simply retracting the sheath.

Animal experience: study design

Ten ewes weighing 60–70 kg were included in the study. We intended to implant a device sheltering an 18 mm valve as a one-step procedure in all animals. The device was considered to be perfectly functioning if the following criteria were met: (1) successful delivery; (2) appropriate position and alignment; (3) absence of valvular regurgitation; (4) absence of paravalvular leakage; (5) absence of significant modifications of right atrial pressure, end-diastolic right ventricular pressure,

and/or right ventricular function. The function of the device was considered deficient if any one of these factors was present. Animals were divided into two groups of four according to the sacrifice time points. Animals from groups 1 and 2 were sacrificed 1 hour and 1 month, respectively, after implantation. Two animals were sacrificed later at 2 months. The procedure was carried out under general anesthesia. Through the right jugular vein, a 5 Fr right Judkins coronary catheter was advanced in the distal right pulmonary artery and exchanged for an Amplatz 0.035 inch extrastiff guidewire. The valved device was loaded into the delivery system and inserted over the previously positioned wire. The device was advanced into the right ventricle. The distal disk was deployed first in the right ventricle by simply pulling on the external sheath. This disk was then applied to the tricuspid annulus, and the tubular part containing the valve and the second disk was delivered similarly in the right atrium. The two disks 'sandwiched' the annulus, with one disk laying into the right ventricle and the proximal one into the right atrium, assuring anchoring of the device (Figures 32.2 and 32.3). The delivery was followed using fluoroscopy and echocardiography performed epicardially through a left thoracotomy to enhance imaging of the area of interest. To evaluate the function of the device, hemodynamic (i.e.

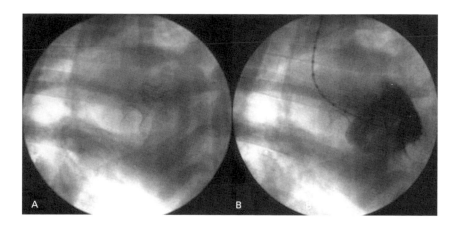

Figure 32.2

Angiograms: (A) the satisfactory opening of the device and its alignment with the tricuspid annulus; (B) the sealing of the disk.

right ventricular and right atrial pressures) and angiographic data were recorded before, after device implantation, and at the time of sacrifice.

Animal experience: study results

The implantation of these newly designed stents was feasible in 9 out of 10 ewes. Successfully implanted valves were competent. In one animal, it was impossible to completely deploy the valve, despite several attempts to dilate the device with a balloon catheter. In this animal, on fluoroscopy and echocardiography, the device was not aligned with the tricuspid annulus. Angiographic and echocardiographic evaluations showed a severe paravalvular leak secondary to a non-apposition of the ventricular disk on the superior margin of the right ventricle. At autopsy, the ventricular disk of the device was trapped in the tricuspid chordae, explaining the incomplete deployment. No migration occurred early or during the follow-up. One animal had a mild paravalvular leak superiorly due to a downsized device as compared with annulus size (35 mm for a 40 mm disk). This leak was noticed just after the procedure and persisted without clinical repercussion until the animal was electively sacrificed at 2 months. In one animal, a significant paravalvular leak was found at 1-month follow-up. In this case, despite a favorable acute evaluation,

the animal lost 2 kg in weight. At autopsy, a pericardial effusion was found and the PTFE was torn just beside a weld fracture.

The implantation of this newly designed device permitted the reduction of the annulus diameter to the desired diameter with no clinically significant increase in right atrial pressure in any implanted animals (from 5 mmHg to 7 mmHg). Excluding the animal with a significant paravalvular leak, this hemodynamic finding did not change in any animal with 'late' sacrifice time points (from 7 mmHg to 7.3 mmHg).

At autopsy, valve leaflets were thin and perfectly mobile in all animals. All devices were sitting perfectly aligned in the area of the tricuspid annulus. The nitinol wires were partially covered by fibrous tissue (Figure 32.4), making the devices impossible to retrieve. No macroscopic damage was noted when inspecting the right atrium and right ventricle. As expected, the proximal and distal disks were in the atrium and the ventricle, respectively. The tricuspid native valve was completely inactivated by the stent and was partially retracted.

Animal experience: study limitations and unanswered questions

In the present study, only animals with normal tricuspid valves were evaluated. Therefore, the

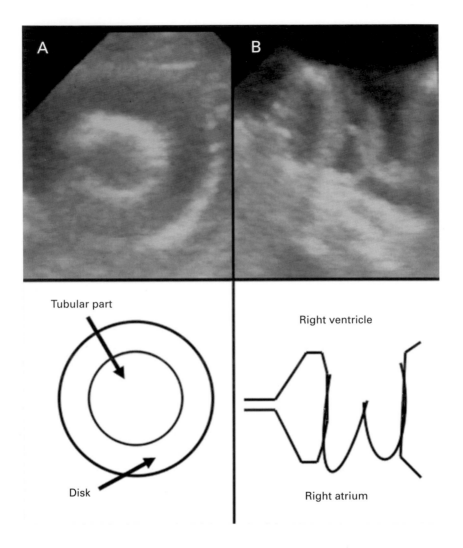

Figure 32.3

Echocardiographic and schematic views showing the profile of the implanted device on long (A) and short (B) axes.

design of our device would most likely not be adapted to the range of human pathology of the tricuspid valve.

Further developments are needed to encompass these difficulties, particularly in situations where no clear annulus exists (e.g. in Ebstein's anomaly). Another concern is myocardial trauma or reaction to the presence of the stent with regard with cyclic contraction of the heart. The stent is also submitted to high stress during the cardiac cycle, which can lead to stent fracture more frequently than in the vascular position. During the overall study, no myocardial complication occurred; however, weld

fractures were noticed at 1-month evaluation in one animal. This fracture led to tear of the PTFE membrane, which further led to a clinically relevant paravalvular leak. The sewing of a second PTFE membrane on the atrial disk should have prevented the leak, but the occurrence of such an early stent fracture is alarming. Bench tests different from those realized for 'standard' stents implanted in the vascular position should be applied to this particular device to address these concerns more accurately. Another serious concern is entrapment of the device in the tricuspid chordae. In one animal, this led to incomplete

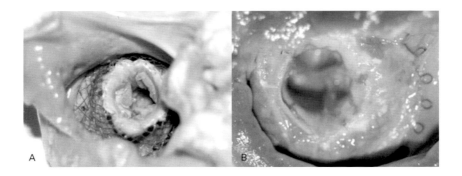

Figure 32.4

Macroscopic views showing the newly designed valved nitinol stent explanted 1 month after implantation: (A) ventricular side; (B) atrial side. Note the partial fibrous covering of the nitinol wires and the thin valve inside the stent.

opening of the device, with a severe paravalvular leak followed by the acute death of the animal. This complication, which was not predicted by the imaging, was encountered once and should be avoidable in the future by the use of balloon flow catheters to get through the tricuspid valve as well as by more careful echocardiographic assessment before complete release of the device. Although it has not appeared to be necessary to time the delivery of the device in coordination with a specific phase of the cardiac cycle, this could be important with regard to this particular problem. Techniques of rapid ventricular pacing or vagal stimulation also need to be further investigated.

Despite these limitations, we have successfully inserted a semilunar valve in the tricuspid position through a transcatheter technique. Long-term studies are obviously needed before considering the use of such a device in humans. However, these results open a new perspective on transcatheter replacement of the atrioventricular valve.

Acknowledgments

We thank the Fondation de l'Avenir (Paris, France) for financial support and Philippe Marx (AMF, Reuilly, France), who designed the device in collaboration with Younes Boudjemline. We also acknowledge Medtronic Inc. for providing us with Contegra conduits.

References

1. Bonhoeffer P, Boudjemline Y, Saliba Z, et al. Transcatheter implantation of a bovine valve in pulmonary position: a lamb study. Circulation 2000; 102: 813–16.
2. Boudjemline Y, Bonhoeffer P. Percutaneous implantation of a valve in the descending aorta in lambs. Eur Heart J 2002; 23: 1045–9.
3. Boudjemline Y, Bonhoeffer P. Steps toward percutaneous aortic valve replacement. Circulation 2002; 105: 775–8.
4. Bonhoeffer P, Boudjemline Y, Saliba Z, et al. Percutaneous replacement of pulmonary valve in a right-ventricle to pulmonary-artory prosthetic conduit with valve dysfunction. Lancet 2000; 356: 1403–5.
5. Bonhoeffer P, Boudjemline Y, Qureshi SA, et al. Percutaneous insertion of the pulmonary valve. J Am Coll Cardiol 2002; 39: 1664–9.
6. Cribier A, Eltchaninoff H, Bash A, et al. Percutaneous transcatheter implantation of an aortic valve prosthesis for calcific aortic stenosis: first human case description. Circulation 2002; 106: 3006–8.

Section 5

Tissue engineering

33

Heart valve tissue engineering: Choosing the right cell source

Dörthe Schmidt, Simon P Hoerstrup

Introduction

Progress in valve technology for the repair of heart valve disease has been significant in recent decades, providing a lifesaving surgical treatment for numerous patients each year. Today, heart valve replacements by either mechanical or biological prostheses remain the most common treatment for advanced valvular heart disease, with an increasing use of biological prostheses.[1] However, this therapy is still associated with a number of problems resulting in a significant morbidity and mortality. Being inherently different from the tissue they replace, both manufactured mechanical and biological valve replacements are often associated with shortcomings such as material failure, increased rate of infections, thromboembolism, and immunologic reactions against the foreign material. In addition, with the exception of the Ross principle, all contemporary heart valve replacement procedures involve non-living structures lacking the capacity for self-repair, remodeling, or growth.

In particular, in today's congenital heart surgery, there is a substantial need for appropriate, growing replacement materials for the repair of infant heart valve defects. This surgical treatment is commonly based on non-autologous valves or conduits,[1,2] with disadvantages including obstructive tissue ingrowth and calcification of the replacement.[3] These limitations and the lack of growth typically necessitate various reoperations on pediatric patients with cardiovascular defects, which are associated with increased morbidity and mortality each time. Heart valve tissue engineering, focusing on the fabrication of autologous, living tissues with the potential for regeneration, is a promising scientific field, addressing the so far unmet medical need for growing replacements in congenital heart surgery.

Principle of heart valve tissue engineering

Ideal heart valve tissue replacements would be a copy of their native counterparts, exhibiting adequate mechanical function, durability, and adequate hemodynamic performance, as well as the absence of immunogenic, thrombogenic, and/or inflammatory reactions. Such goals were first outlined by Harken et al[4] in 1962 for artificial heart valve prostheses, but also represent requirements for cardiovascular replacements in general.

Tissue engineering aims to match these requirements by in vitro fabrication of living, autologous tissue replacements. Autologous cells are obtained and isolated from the patient's tissue. After isolation, the cells are expanded using in vitro culturing technology and are seeded onto biodegradable three-dimensional matrices, which can be of biological or synthetic origin. For the seeding procedure, a sufficient initial number of cells is necessary in order to enable appropriate maturation of the neo-tissue. The success of this tissue engineering procedure depends on three main components: (1) the biodegradable matrix (scaffold) that determines the three-dimensional shape and serves as an initial guiding structure for cell attachment and tissue development; (2) the cell source from which the living tissue is grown; and (3) the in vitro culture conditions of the living construct before implantation.

In heart valve tissue engineering, these three components have to be chosen and controlled in a highly orchestrated manner to meet the stringent mechanical requirements on the neo-tissue at the time of implantation. In order to create a functional heart valve with the mechanical properties of the native counterpart, rapid development of the extracellular matrix is crucial. Therefore, the choice of cells responsible for production of the extracellular matrix is an important factor. Two cell types are routinely used for the fabrication of heart valve tissues: cells with the capacity to form extracellular matrix, commonly myofibroblasts, and endothelial cells with antithrombogenic characteristics. The seeding procedure onto three-dimensional scaffolds is mostly performed sequentially: first by seeding of the myofibroblasts, followed by the endothelial cells.[5] The seeded scaffolds can be cultured either in static or dynamic systems, aiming at optimal tissue development in vitro. It has been shown that mechanical preconditioning accelerates the production of viable, functional tissues, making them appropriate for implantation.[6,7]

This concept of heart valve tissue engineering, summarized in Figure 33.1, has already been validated in large-animal studies.[8–10] Completely autologous, living trileaflet heart valves have been successfully implanted in a growing sheep model for up to 20 weeks. These valves showed good functional performance as well as structural and biomechanical characteristics strongly resembling those of native semilunar heart valves[8] (Figure 33.2). The first clinical application of a tissue-engineered pulmonary artery graft in a pediatric patient was reported by Shinoka et al.[11] However, long-term results have not been presented so far.

The three pillars of heart valve tissue engineering

Regarding the three pillars of tissue engineering, the related interdisciplinary technologies have already reached an advanced standard. Scaffolds with adjustable biodegradation properties are available and can be fabricated into three-dimensional matrices. The technology of in vitro cell culture has made significant progress and allows the control of tissue growth conditions. The cell source is the least controlled factor, yet is the most important for the quality of the living replacement. Cell quality, for instance, is influenced by the individual conditions of the patient's tissue, including systemic comorbidities such as atherosclerosis, which in many cases have led to the underlying cardiovascular disease. Thus, the choice of the right cell source is of major importance to the success of heart valve tissue engineering.

The scaffold

Currently, two principal types of scaffold materials have been used in the tissue engineering approach: synthetic and biological. Several synthetic biodegradable polymers, such as poly-

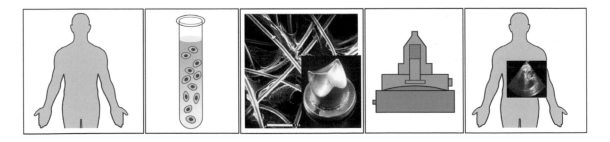

Figure 33.1

The concept of tissue engineering. Autologous cells are harvested from the patient and cultured. After expansion, cells are seeded onto scaffold material and preconditioned in a bioreactor. After tissue development, the autologous replacement is implanted into the patient.

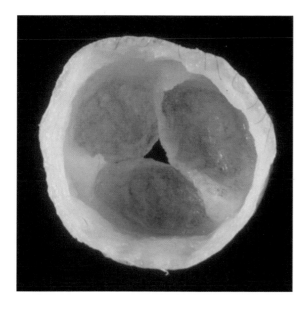

Figure 33.2

An autologous living tissue engineered heart valve in a sheep model, based on vascular-derived myofibroblasts and endothelial cells. (Reproduced from Hoerstrup SP, Sodian R, Daebritz S, et al. Circulation 2000; 102: II144–II149[8] with permission from Lippincott Williams & Wilkins.)

Table 33.1 Scaffold materials for heart valve tissue engineering

	Synthetic matrix	Biological matrix
Source	Biocompatible biodegradable polymers	• Xenogenic • Homogenic
Pretreatment	• Fabrication into three-dimensional structures • Sterilization	Fixation with: • Glutaraldehyde • Alternative fixation procedures (e.g. photofixation, cryopreservation) • Decellularization
Cells	Seeded with autologous cells	• Acellular • Seeded with autologous cells
Growth	+	−

galactin,[9] polyglycolic acid (PGA),[10] polylactic acid (PLA), and a copolymer of PGA and PLA (PGLA),[12] have been investigated. Another approach for fabricating complete, trileaflet heart valves is the use of PGA coated with poly-4-hydroxybutyrate (P4HB).[8,13] This biologically derived rapidly absorbable copolymer is strong and pliable. Due to its thermoplasticity, it can be molded into almost any shape, and is completely degraded 8 weeks after implantation.[8]

Other studies in heart valve tissue engineering have been based on biological scaffolds such as xenogenic or allogeneic decellularized fixed heart valves. Removing the extracellular components results in a material composed essentially of extracellular matrix proteins that serves as an intrinsic template for cell attachment.[14] When non-fixed decellularized valve leaflets were used in an animal model, recellularization by the host was demonstrated.[15] When implanted in children, severe foreign body-type reactions were detected and were associated with a mortality rate of 75%[16]. A summary of the currently used scaffold materials is presented in Table 33.1.

The cells

In contrast to the highly standardized and industrially fabricated scaffolds, the quality of cells varies from patient to patient, depending on the individual tissue characteristics and comorbidities. In order to create a functional, living tissue replacement, the choice of cell source is critical. Besides cell growth and expansion capacity, an important issue is the possibility to develop a cell phenotype that matches the native counterpart. This is expected to have a major impact on the long-term functionality of replacements.[17] Using cells originating from the tissue to be replaced would be the safest approach. In the case of heart valve tissue engineering, the usage of valvular interstitial cells obtained by biopsy has been shown to be feasible.[18] However, with respect to clinical applications, these cells are difficult to obtain and the approach carries substantial risks. Therefore, several alternative human cell sources have been investigated for their use in heart valve tissue engineering (Table 33.2). Among the most promising are vascular-derived cells, bone marrow-derived cells, blood-derived cells, and umbilical cord-derived cells, particularly for pediatric applications.

Table 33.2   Cell sources for heart valve tissue engineering

Human cell source	Construct	Refs
Human dermal fibroblasts (covered with bovine endothelial cells)	Valve leaflets	9,10
Human foreskin fibroblasts (covered with human endothelial cells)	Patch	12
Human marrow cells	Trileaflet heart valve	13
Human aortic myofibroblasts	Patch/trileaflet heart valve	55,56
Human aortic myofibroblasts and human venous cells	Patch	19,57
Human venous myofibroblasts	Valve leaflets	52
Human umbilical cord myofibroblasts from vein	Pulmonary artery conduits	40
Human umbilical cord myofibroblasts covered with human endothelial cells derived from umbilical cord blood endothelial progenitor cells	Patch	36

Vascular-derived cells

In most cardiovascular tissue engineering approaches, cells are harvested from vascular structures. With regard to clinical application, several human vascular cell sources have been investigated, including mammary, radial artery, and saphenous vein.[19] The obtained mixed cell populations, consisting of myofibroblasts and endothelial cells, were sorted by fluorescence-activated cell sorting (FACS) and the pure cell populations were cultivated and used for the fabrication of the replacements.[20] Alternatively, in order to detach the endothelium from the luminal layer of the vessel, biopsies were digested with collagenase and the endothelial cells were harvested. Afterwards, the tissue was minced into small pieces and outgrowing myofibroblasts were cultured. Unfortunately, harvesting cells from a vascular cell source necessitates the sacrifice of intact vascular donor tissue. Particularly in children, obtaining cells in an invasive procedure can result in dysfunction and disturbance of the growth and development of the harmed structures. Additionally, cardiovascular risk factors

and comorbidities such as atherosclerosis and diabetes can influence the quality of vessel tissue. In order to avoid damage to tissue and ensure high quality of the cells, alternative cell sources have been investigated.

Bone marrow-derived cells

With regard to future clinical applications, bone marrow represents an attractive alternative heterogeneous cell source. Apart from progenitor cells for red blood cells, platelets, monocytes, granulocytes, and lymphocytes,[21] non-hematopoietic stem cells are also present. These adult stem cells have the ability to differentiate into cells with features of mesenchymal or marrow stromal cells because they arise from the complex array of supporting structures found in the marrow.[22] Recently, human marrow stromal cells have been used successfully for the generation of living trileaflet heart valves (Figure 33.3). Flow-cytometric characterization of the marrow-derived cells prior to seeding confirmed a myofibroblast-like phenotype. The cells expressed alpha-smooth muscle action (α-SMA) and vimentin, while there was no uptake of low-density lipoprotein (LDL) and the expression of desmin, CD31, and CD14 was negative. Upon seeding on the biodegradable scaffold and preconditioning in a biomimetic environment, the cells showed adequate production of extracellular matrix proteins. Additionally, mechanical properties comparable to those of native tissue were demonstrated.[13] The bone marrow is also a cell source for endothelial progenitor cells[23] that could be used to create an antithrombogenic surface on the tissue engineered constructs, underlying the potential of this promising cell source.

Blood-derived cells

Endothelial progenitor cells (EPC) can be isolated from peripheral and umbilical cord blood.[24–26] They represent a rare heterogeneous population of mononuclear blood cells. Their origin and phenotype are still not fully understood and are a matter of controversy. Several possible sources for EPC exist: hematoipoetic stem cells, myeloid cells, circulating progenitor cells, and circulating mature endothelial cells shed from vessel walls.[27] EPC have the potential to differentiate into mature endothelial cells and show regenerative features. They have been used successfully for the repair of injured vessels, neovascularization, or regeneration of ischemic tissue,[28–31] as well as for coating of synthetic vascular grafts.[32] Recently, animal-derived EPC have been used for endothelialization of decellularized grafts in animal models[33] and for seeding of hybrid grafts.[34] Furthermore, the feasibility of using human umbilical cord blood-derived EPC for tissue engineering of cardiovascular replacements for pediatric application has recently been demonstrated[35,36] (Figure 33.4). When differentiated EPC were cocultured with non-endothelial cells as well as when they were exposed to mechanical stimuli, they showed stabile phenotypes.[35,36] The extracellular matrix production of undifferentiated EPC was demonstrated to be insufficient, whereas the differentiation into endothelial cells on biodegradable scaffolds was observed.[37] In the overall tissue engineering concept, EPC represents a promising cell source for the endothelialization of heart valves. Since EPC are easily accessible, current research aims at their transdifferentiation into myofibroblast cells in

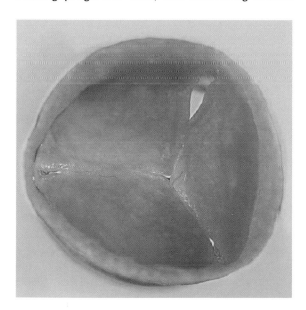

Figure 33.3

Tissue-engineered functional trileaflet heart valves from human marrow stromal cells. (Hoerstrup et al. Circulation 2002; 106 (12 Suppl): I143–I150[13] with permission from Lippincott Williams & Wilkins.)

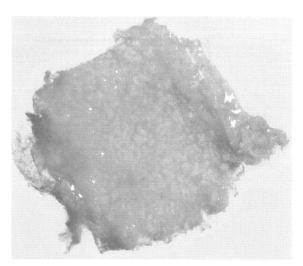

Figure 33.4

Living tissue-engineered patch material based on umbilical cord myofibroblast from Wharton`s jelly and umbilical cord blood-derived endothelial progenitor cells. (Reproduced from Schmidt D, Mol A, Neuenschwander S, et al. Eur J Cardiothorac Surg 2005; 27: 795–800.[36])

order to enable the use of blood as a sole cell source for pediatric applications.

Umbilical cord-derived cells

With regard to pediatric heart valve tissue engineering, the umbilical cord may serve as an optimal perinatal cell source. It is composed of two arteries and one vein transporting the blood of the embryonic circulation. The vessels are imbedded in Wharton's jelly, an embryonic connective tissue.[38] Due to its anatomic structure, the umbilical cord is rich in different cell types: myofibroblasts, endothelial cells, and progenitor cells, harvested from different parts of the tissue (Figure 33.5).

Currently, there is little experience with umbilical cord-derived cells for pediatric cardiovascular tissue engineering. In 1996, Sipehia et al[39] described the use of human umbilical cord vein-derived endothelial cells. In 2002, human umbilical cord-derived myofibroblasts were established as a new cell source for pediatric cardiovascular tissue engineering and were used for pulmonary conduits.[40,41] In 2004, Koike et al[42] created long-lasting blood vessels with endothelial cells from umbilical cord vein in a three-dimensional fibronectin–type I collagen gel connected to the mouse circulatory system. Recently, the fabrication of cardiovascular replacements based on Wharton's jelly-derived myofibroblasts and endothelial cells derived from umbilical cord blood endothelial progenitors has been demonstrated.[36] Despite these achievements, the engineering of autologous pediatric cardiovascular tissue from umbilical cord is still in an early stage of development and a number of issues remain to be investigated. Of particular importance is cell harvesting at the early perinatal stage, for example by ultrasound-guided cordocentesis of umbilical cord blood, which allows the tissue-engineered replacement to be ready for implantation at the birth of the patient.

In vitro culture conditions

The refinement of in vitro culture conditions for the living tissue-engineered construct prior to implantation is another key focus of research in heart valve tissue engineering. In general, neotissue formation is stimulated by chemical and/or mechanical conditioning.

The strategy of chemical conditioning includes the addition of cytokines, either directly into the growth medium or by indirect incorporation into the scaffold structure, enabling targeted promotion of specific tissue growth.[43,44] Cytokines are a group of regulatory molecules mediating cell communication and exerting multiple biological functions by interactions with specific cell surface receptors. They include interleukins, hematopoietic growth factors, interferons, tumor necrosis

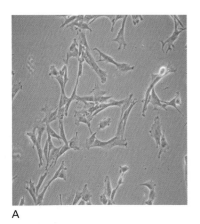
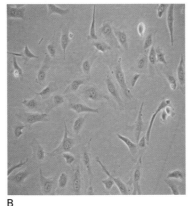
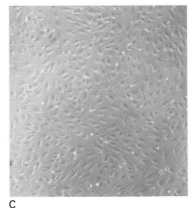

A   B   C

Figure 33.5

Different cells for cardiovascular tissue engineering derived from umbilical cord: (A) Wharton's jelly-derived myofibroblasts; (B) endothelial cells derived from umbilical cord vein; (C) differentiated endothelial progenitor cells from umbilical cord blood.

factors, and growth factors.[45] Well-known cytokines influencing vascular cell behavior are fibroblast growth factor (FGF), platelet derived growth factor (PDGF), transforming growth factor β (TGF-β), and vascular endothelial growth factor (VEGF).[46,47] Apart from cytokines, matrix metalloproteinases (MMPs) play an important role in tissue development and subsequent remodeling.[48] When cytokines are applied directly to the growth medium, the effect is short term and has to be repeated several times. When incorporated into a biodegradable scaffold material, slow cytokine release can be achieved by coupling with the polymer degradation rate.

Mechanical conditioning involves the utilization of mechanical stimuli in in vitro bioreactors, such as flow, shear stress, and strain applied to the developing tissue. For heart valve tissue engineering, the most commonly used bioreactor is a pulse duplicator system mimicking the biological environment and facilitating the opening and closing behavior of the valve.[8,49] A schematic of a bioreactor is shown in Figure 33.6. In order to improve tissue formation and strength, the tissue is exposed to increasing flow rates and pressures. Recently, new bioreactors have been developed for heart valve tissue engineering in which the exact physiological conditions of a heart valve in vivo can be applied,[50,51] enabling mechanical properties of neo-tissues approximating those of native aortic tissues.[52]

Chemical and mechanical stimuli interact with the regulation of tissue development. On the one hand, the production of cytokines can be stimulated mechanically, and on the other hand, the effect of mechanical conditioning can be increased by the addition of cytokines.[53] The meticulous orchestration of these components is still under investigation in an attempt to optimize in vitro tissue maturation, enabling fully functional, autologous heart valves also for systemic pressure applications.

Summary: Choosing the right cell source

Various cell sources have been investigated for heart valve tissue engineering. Vascular-derived cells have been widely used, but as far as clinical applications are concerned, they are burdened with the disadvantage of harming intact donor structures. Alternatively, bone marrow cells can be obtained easily by biopsy, avoiding the sacrifice of intact donor tissue,[54] and have shown good production of extracellular matrix when used for heart

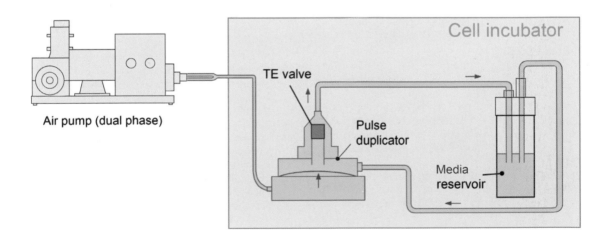

Figure 33.6

Schematic of an in vitro pulse duplicator.

valve tissue engineering.[13] Differentiation of EPC into endothelial cells on biodegradable scaffolds has been observed,[37] and differentiated EPC kept their phenotype when cultured on living tissue-engineered matrices, as well as when exposed to mechanical stimuli.[35,36] However, sufficient extra-cellular matrix production of undifferentiated EPC has not yet been shown. Nevertheless, EPC represent a promising cell source for the endothelialization of heart valves. As EPC can be obtained not only from bone marrow but also from peripheral or umbilical cord blood, they represent a valuable cell source with respect to easy accessibility, which is important for pediatric applications. In addition, future studies have to elucidate whether EPC can also produce extracellular matrix, enabling the clinical realization of the tissue-engineering concept based on a sole cell source.

In conclusion, the optimal cell source still remains to be defined. It must be chosen with regard to the individual clinical profile of the patient and his or her individual requirements. However, heart valve tissue engineering is a promising approach for living, functional autologous replacements. In particular, pediatric patients will benefit from growing replacement materials for the repair of congenital heart defects. However, before clinical application of the tissue-engineered heart valve concept becomes routine, several issues will have to be addressed. The search for the optimal cell source has to continue, as does the improvement of in vitro conditioning technology.

References

1. Schoen FJ, Levy RJ. Tissue heart valves: current challenges and future research perspectives. J Biomed Mater Res 1999; 47: 439–65.
2. Mayer, J. Uses of homograft conduits for right ventricle to pulmonary artery connections in the neonatal period. Semin Thorac Cardiovasc Surg 1995; 7: 130–2.
3. Endo S, Saito N, Misawa Y, et al. Late pericarditis secondary to pericardial patch implantation 25 years prior. Eur J Cardiothorac Surg 2001; 20: 1059–60.
4. Harken DF, Taylor WJ, Le Femine AA, et al. Aortic valve replacement with a caged ball valve. Am J Cardiol 1962; 9: 292–9.
5. Zund G, Hoerstrup SP, Schoeberlein A, et al. Tissue engineering: a new approach in cardiovascular surgery; seeding of human fibroblasts followed by human endothelial cells on resorbable mesh. Eur J Cardiothorac Surg 1998; 13: 160–4.
6. Hoerstrup SP, Sodian R, Sperling JS, et al. New pulsatile bioreactor for in vitro formation of tissue engineered heart valves. Tissue Eng 2000; 6: 75–9.
7. Niklason LE, Gao J, Abbott WM, et al. Functional arteries grown in vitro. Science 1999; 284: 489–93.
8. Hoerstrup SP, Sodian R, Daebritz S, et al. Functional living trileaflet heart valves grown in vitro. Circulation 2000; 102: II144–II149.
9. Shinoka T, Breuer CK, Tanel RE, et al. Tissue engineering heart valves: valve leaflets replacement study in a lamb model. Ann Thorac Surg 1995; 60(6 Suppl): 513–16.
10. Shinoka T, Ma PX, Shum-Tim D, et al. Tissue engineered heart valves. Autologous valve leaflet replacement study in a lamb model. Circulation 1996; 94(9 Suppl): I164–I168.
11. Shinoka T, Shum-Tim D, Ma PX, et al. Creation of viable pulmonary artery autografts through tissue engineering. J Thorac Cardiovasc Surg 1998; 115: 536–46.
12. Zund G, Breuer CK, Shinoka T, et al. The in vitro construction of a tissue engineered bioprosthetic heart valve. Eur J Cardiothorac Surg 1997; 11: 493–7.
13. Hoerstrup SP, Kadner A, Melnitchouk S, et al. Tissue engineering of functional trileaflet heart valves from human marrow stromal cells. Circulation 2002; 106(12 Suppl): I143–I150.
14. Samouillan V, Dandurand-Lods J, Lamure A, et al. Thermal analysis characterization of aortic tissues for cardiac valve bioprosthesis. J Biomed Mater Res 1999; 46: 531–8.
15. Wilson GJ, Courtman DW, Klement P, et al. Acellular matrix: a biomaterials approach for coronary artery bypass and heart valve replacement. Ann Thorac Surg 1995; 60: 353–8.
16. Simon P, Kasimir MT, Seebacher G, et al. Early failure of the tissue engineered porcine heart valve synergraft in pediatric patients. Eur J Cardiothorac Surg 2003; 23: 1002–6.
17. Butcher JT, Nerem RM. Porcine aortic valve interstitial cells in three-dimensional culture: comparison of phenotype with aortic smooth muscle cells. J Heart Valve Dis 2004; 13: 478–86.
18. Maish MS, Hoffman-Kim D, Krueger PM, et al. Tricuspid valve biopsy: a potential source of cardiac myofibroblasts cells for tissue-engineered cardiac valves. J Heart Valve Dis 2003; 12: 264–9.
19. Schnell AM, Hoerstrup SP, Zund G, et al. Optimal cell source for cardiovascular tissue engineering: venous vs. aortic human myofibroblasts. Thorac Cardiovasc Surg 2001; 49: 221–5.
20. Hoerstrup SP, Zund G, Schoeberlein A, et al.

Fluorescence activated cell sorting: a reliable method in tissue engineering of a bioprosthetic heart valve. Ann Thorac Surg 1998; 66: 1653–7.

21. Hay E. Regeneration. New York: Holt, Rinehart and Winston, 1966.

22. Prockop DJ. Marrow stromal cells as stem cells for nonhematopoietic tissues. Science 1997; 276: 71–4.

23. Reyes M, Dudeck A, Jahagirdar B, et al. Origin of endothelial progenitors in human postnatal bone marrow. J Clin Invest 2002; 109: 337–46.

24. Asahara T, Murohara T, Sullivan A, et al. Isolation of putative progenitor endothelial cells for angiogenesis. Science 1997; 275: 964–7.

25. Dimmeler S, Aicher A, Vasa M, et al. HMG-CoA reductase inhibitors (statins) increase endothelial progenitor cells via the PI 3-kinase/Akt pathway. J Clin Invest 2001; 108: 391–7.

26. Vasa M, Fichtlscherer S, Adler K, et al. Increase in circulating endothelial progenitor cells by statin therapy in patients with stable coronary artery disease. Circulation 2001; 103: 2885–90.

27. Urbich C, Dimmeler S. Endothelial progenitor cells: characterization and role in vascular biology. Circ Res 2004; 95: 343–53.

28. Kocher AA, Schuster MD, Szabolcs MJ, et al. Neovascularization of ischemic myocardium by human bone-marrow-derived angioblasts prevents cardiomyocyte apoptosis, reduces remodeling and improves cardiac function. Nat Med 2001; 7: 430–6.

29. Kawamoto A, Gwon HC, Iwaguro H, et al. Therapeutic potential of ex vivo expanded endothelial progenitor cells for myocardial ischemia. Circulation 2001; 103: 634–7.

30. Assmus B, Schachinger V, Teupe C, et al. Transplantation of progenitor cells and regeneration enhancement in acute myocardial infarction (TOPCARE-AMI). Circulation 2002; 106: 3009–17.

31. Pesce M, Orlandi A, Iachininoto MG, et al. Myoendothelial differentiation of human umbilical cord blood-derived stem cells in ischemic limb tissues. Circ Res 2003; 93: e51–e62.

32. Shirota T, Yasui H, Shimokawa H, et al. Fabrication of endothelial progenitor cell (EPC)-seeded intravascular stent devices and in vitro endothelialization on hybrid vascular tissue. Biomaterials 2003; 24: 2295–302.

33. Kaushal S, Amiel GE, Guleserian KJ, et al. Functional small-diameter neovessels created using endothelial progenitor cells expanded ex vivo. Nat Med 2001; 7: 1035–40.

34. Shirota T, He H, Yasui H, et al. Human endothelial progenitor cell-seeded hybrid graft: proliferative and antithrombogenic potentials in vitro and fabrication processing. Tissue Eng 2003; 9: 127–36.

35. Schmidt D, Breymann C, Weber A, et al. Umbilical cord blood derived endothelial progenitor cells for

tissue engineering of vascular grafts. Ann Thorac Surg 2004; 78: 2094–8.

36. Schmidt D, Mol A, Neuenschwander S, et al. Living patches engineered from human umbilical cord derived fibroblasts and endothelial progenitor cells. Eur J Cardiothorac Surg 2005; 27: 795–800.

37. Dvorin EL, Wylie-Sears J, Kaushal S, et al. Quantitative evaluation of endothelial progenitors and cardiac valve endothelial cells: proliferation and differentiation on poly-glycolic acid/poly-4-hydroxybutyrate scaffold in response to vascular endothelial growth factor and transforming growth factor beta1. Tissue Eng 2003; 9: 487–93.

38. Schoenberg MD, Moore RD. Studies on connective tissue III: enzymatic studies on the formation and nature of carbohydrate umbilical cord. Arch Pathol 1958; 65: 115–24.

39. Sipehia R, Martucci G, Lipscombe J. Enhanced attachment and growth of human endothelial cells derived from umbilical veins on ammonia plasma modified surfaces of PTFE and ePTFE synthetic vascular graft biomaterials. Artif Cells Blood Substit Immobil Biotechnol 1996; 24: 51–63.

40. Hoerstrup SP, Kadner A, Breymann C, et al. Pulmonary conduits tissue engineered from umbilical cord cells. Ann Thorac Surg 2002; 74: 46–52.

41. Kadner A, Hoerstrup SP, Tracy J, et al. Human umbilical cord cells: a new cell source for cardiovascular tissue engineering. Ann Thorac Surg 2002; 74: 1422–8.

42. Koike N, Fukumura D, Gralla O, et al. Tissue engineering: creation of long-lasting blood vessels. Nature 2004; 428: 138–9.

43. Hubbell JA, Massia SP, Desai NP, et al. Endothelial cell-selective materials for tissue engineering in the vascular graft via a new receptor. Biotechnology 1991; 9: 568–72.

44. Zisch AH, Lutholf MP, Ehrbar M, et al. Cell-demand release of VEGF from synthetic, biointeractive cell-ingrowth matrices of vascularized tissue growth. FASEB J 2003; 17: 2260–2.

45. Takehara K. Growth regulation of skin fibroblasts. J Dermatol Sci 2000; 24: 70–7.

46. Ziegler T, Alexander RW, Nerem RM. An endothelial cell–smooth muscle cell co-culture model for the use in the investigation of flow effects on vascular biology. Ann Biomed Eng 1995; 23: 216–25.

47. Bos GW, Scharenborg NM, Poot AA, et al. Proliferation of endothelial cells on surfaces-immobilized albumin-heparin conjugate loaded with basic fibroblast growth factor. J Biomed Mater Res 1999; 44: 340–50.

48. Streuli C. Extracellular matrix remodelling and cellular differentiation. Curr Opin Cell Biol 1999; 11: 634–40.

49. Sodian R, Hoerstrup SP, Sperling JS, et al. Early in vivo experience with tissue engineered trileaflet heart valves. Circulation 2000; 102(Suppl 3): III-22–III-29.

50. Dumont K, Yperman J, Verbeken E, et al. Design of a new pulsative bioreactor for tissue engineered aortic heart valve formation. Artif Org 2002; 26: 710–14.

51. Hildebrandt DK, Wu ZJ, Mayer JE et al. Design and hemodynamic evaluation of a novel pulsatile bioreactor for biologically active heart valves. Ann Biomed Eng 2004; 31: 1039–49.

52. Mol A, Bouten CVC, Zund G et al. The relevance of large strains in functional tissue engineering of heart valves. Thorac Cardiovasc Surg 2003; 51: 78–83.

53. O'Callahagan CJ, Williams B. Mechanical strain induced extracellular matrix production by human vascular smooth muscle cells: role of TGF-β. Hypertension 2000; 36: 319–24.

54. Kadner A, Hoerstrup SP, Zund G et al. A new cell source for cardiovascular tissue engineering: human marrow stromal cells. Eur J Cardiothorac Surg 2002; 21: 635–41.

55. Ye Q, Zund G, Benedikt P, et al. Fibrin gel as a three dimensional maxtrix in cardiovascular tissue engineering. Eur J Cardiothorac Surg 17 2000; 17: 587–91.

56. Jockenhoevel S, Zund G, Hoerstrup SP, et al. Fibrin gel – advantages of a new scaffold in cardiovascular tissue engineering. Eur J Cardiothorac Surg 2001; 19: 424–30.

57. Zund G, Cheng S, et al. A new approach to completely autologous cardiovascular tissue in humans. ASAIO J 2002; 48: 234–8.

Section 6

Valve testing

34

Valve testing: Durability and beyond

Jack D Lemmon

Introduction

Replacement heart valve device design and physician use have advanced over the past 50 years from the first implant of the Hufnagel valve in the descending thoracic aorta without cardiopulmonary bypass in 1952[1] to recent transcatheter implantation of pulmonary valves by Bonhoeffer et al[2] and aortic valves by Cribier et al[3] reported in 2000 and 2002, respectively. Along with the evolution of heart valve designs (Figure 34.1) and materials, the preclinical testing of devices has also improved over the past quarter-century, providing data critical to the initiation of clinical investigations. During this time, test

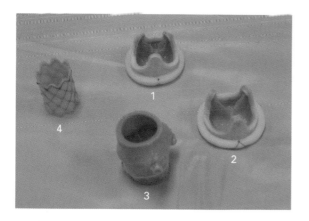

Figure 34.1

Evolution of replacement heart valve design during the past three decades. 1, Hancock I stented bioprosthesis (1970s); 2, Hancock II stented bioprosthesis (1980s); 3, Freestyle stentless porcine bioprosthesis (1990s); 4, transcatheter pulmonary valve (2000s).

method development for replacement heart valves has progressed because of advances in measurement techniques and systems, lessons learned from previous clinical device failures,[4] unanticipated clinical complications not discovered during preclinical testing,[5] and the introduction of new types of replacement heart valves, such as stentless bioprostheses.[6] Preclinical evaluation of transcatheter heart valves will again necessitate the development of testing methods based on specific device design and intended use, but can also utilize many of the methods already developed for existing replacement heart valve designs and catheter-based interventional devices.

In many ways, transcatheter heart valves offer unique challenges in preclinical and clinical evaluation. However, for preclinical testing, viewing current transcatheter heart valve designs as stented valve conduits delivered by non-traditional methods could simplify some challenges with regard to performance evaluation. This view of transcatheter valves suggests that preclinical evaluation of these devices is covered by the existing preclinical test methodologies outlined in the International Standards Organization (ISO) and US Food and Drug Administration (FDA) documents developed in the 1980s and revised during the 1990s.[7,8] The uniqueness of the expandable–collapsible supporting structure used to deliver and secure the valve to the implant site necessitates additional testing for evaluation and characterization of these features. For preclinical testing, the delivery of these devices (i.e. collapsed to a small diameter for navigating the vasculature and then expanded into position) requires special steps for deployment prior to testing and the development of new fixtures to hold the device in test systems that approximate the intended clinical implant environment.

The ISO and FDA documents can provide a starting point for preclinical testing of transcatheter heart valves. These documents reference developed evaluation methods for replacement heart valves that are based on an extensive clinical history and provide an outline for the areas of evaluation that should be considered in testing transcatheter heart valve device designs. Other standards from the area of vascular stents and balloon catheters[9] may be useful in providing some of the areas of investigation that are not addressed in heart valve guidance documents. These guidelines can provide a reference for device evaluation, but the valve should be assessed in relation to the outcome of risk management activities based on device design and intended use.

The preclinical testing performed on replacement heart valves is rooted in the results of project risk management activities according to ISO 14971.[10] The risk management activities allow for the identification of clinical complications/hazards, severity of identified hazards, potential failure modes, effects on device and patients, methods to detect failure modes, and controls to mitigate the risks associated with identified hazards. These activities examine the failure modes and effects associated with both device design and manufacturing processes, effects of specific failures on patients, and potential failure modes induced by the operator. Preclinical testing is one of the methods used for risk reduction in evaluating the identified failure modes. Risk assessment for the product and its intended use is updated continuously during the product development cycle, adding information to the analysis as it is gathered from qualification and validation testing.

The combination of available regulatory standards based on previous clinical experience and risk management activities based on identified hazards for the specific device design and intended use provide an outline for preclinical testing of transcatheter heart valve substitutes. This evaluation includes component and device level testing to assure proper function and durability. Many of the replacement heart valve test methodologies are available in the published literature and can provide valuable information on

lessons learned for test set-up and data gathering/interpretation. Preclinical testing of transcatheter heart valve substitute can be separated into three main areas: evaluation of device hydrodynamic function, device durability/life cycle, and device biocompatibility/host response.

Preclinical testing

Preclinical testing is used to evaluate the replacement heart valve produced under its final design and manufacturing specifications. The testing assesses the performance of the device under a range of proposed physiologic conditions based on the intended implant site and clinical patient population. The testing addresses valve hydrodynamics, structural durability, and biological response. No single test methodology or area of investigation can predict the clinical safety and efficacy of the device, so each test is used to address specific hazards identified in the risk analysis. During the product development cycle, device testing progresses from benchtop, in vitro tests for general functional characterization into long-term durability evaluation, and finally through in vivo testing in animals prior to final release for clinical evaluation. Iterations in device design may occur at any stage in the product development cycle as determined by results of testing based on specific pass/fail criteria.

Hydrodynamics

Hydrodynamic testing is used to evaluate the function of replacement heart valves under a range of physiologic conditions. It uses a mock circulatory loop[11,12] that can be operated over a range of heart rates (typically 45–150 beats/min) and cardiac outputs (typically 2–10 l/min). The replacement heart valve is placed in the flow loop with a mounting fixture that is intended to simulate the implant configuration (Figure 34.2), which in some transcatheter valve cases would be balloon-expanded into a compliant fixture. The mock circulatory loop is operated over a range of flow conditions by changes in heart rate and cardiac output to obtain measurements of pressure drop (Figure 34.3), effective orifice area (Figure 34.3), and regurgitant flow volume

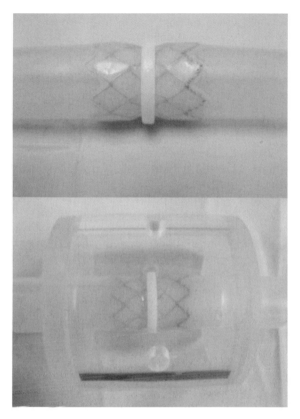

Figure 34.2

A transcatheter stented valve conduit mounted in the test fixture for insertion into a mock circulatory flow system.

(Figure 34.4). The valves can also be evaluated for regurgitant flow under increasing systemic pressure to relate valve competence to back-pressure (Figure 34.5), simulating conditions ranging from normal to hypertensive. Figures 34.3–34.5 provide examples of the data obtained from hydrodynamic testing to assess how a replacement heart valve functions over the range of physiologic flow conditions.

Measurements of flow rate, pressure drop, and effective orifice area give an overall view of valve function by measuring bulk flow properties. Other measurement techniques are needed to determine more precisely the flow field patterns and level of fluid velocity through the valve. This additional information can provide assessment of laminar and turbulent flow regions, as well as identifying areas of stagnant flow that could lead to complications such as thrombus formation.

Flow visualization studies in a pulsatile flow system can be performed using a laser light sheet illuminating a test solution seeded with small glass or plastic particles.[13] This test provides excellent reconstruction of the flow patterns through the valve by using particles that are neutrally buoyant so that they outline the pulsatile flow fields when illuminated by the laser light sheet. Recording these flow patterns via video or still images provides visualization of streaklines (Figure 34.6) that detail how the flow passes through the valve.

The flow visualization study can provide only qualitative information about the flow fields, so other methods are required to obtain quantitative data. Velocities through the valve can be measured utilizing either clinical techniques such as color Doppler echocardiography or laboratory techniques such as hot-film anemometry, particle image velocimetry, or laser Doppler velocimetry.[14–16] These techniques can provide the time course of velocity at a point in the flow field with a high level of accuracy and frequency response. The laboratory techniques have the added benefit of permitting advanced analysis on the datasets to calculate the turbulent shear stresses in the flow field,[16] and thus evaluate potential damage to blood elements that could lead to clinical complications.

Hydrodynamic test methods are also used for verification of clinical measurement techniques for replacement heart valves. Since Doppler ultrasound is primarily used during patient follow-up, verification of the Bernoulli relationship is required and can be performed in a pulse duplicator system.[17] For this evaluation, the peak velocity of the flow through the replacement heart valve is measured by continuous-wave Doppler ultrasound and this velocity is used to calculate the pressure drop via the Bernoulli equation ($\Delta p = 4V^2$). For comparison, the pressure drop is also measured directly using pressure transducers under identical test conditions. These measurements are compared in order to find out whether the Bernoulli relationship to calculate pressure drop using continuous-wave velocity measurements and the coefficient 4 in the equation is accurate. This determines how accurate the Bernoulli relationship is for calculating pressure drop measurements by clinical methods, but caution is warranted in the clinical setting, since other factors may influence this measurement during follow-up examinations.

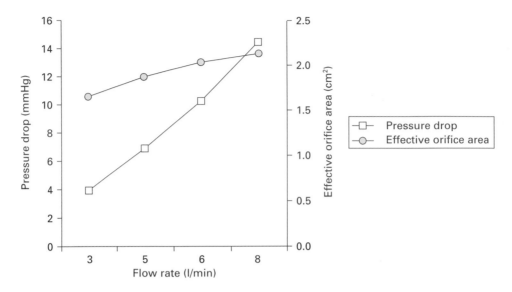

Figure 34.3

Pressure drop and effective orifice area versus flow rate for a stented valve.

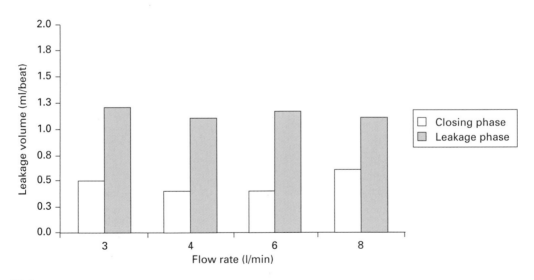

Figure 34.4

Regurgitant flow per beat versus cardiac output of a stented valve. The regurgitant volume is separated into the closing (back-flow as leaflets close) and leakage (back-flow while leaflets are closed) phases.

Device durability

Evaluation of the structural integrity of the transcatheter heart valve must give consideration to the potential damage induced during operation, initiation of sites of damage, ultimate failure modes of the device, and the fatigue life of the materials used in manufacturing. Each piece of information feeds into the overall assessment of the structural performance of the transcatheter

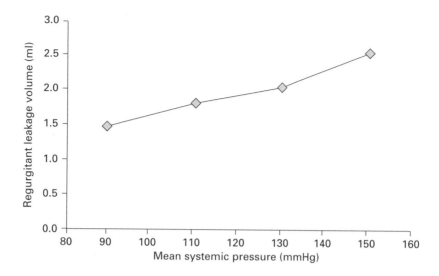

Figure 34.5

Regurgitant leakage volume per beat as a function of mean systemic back-pressure.

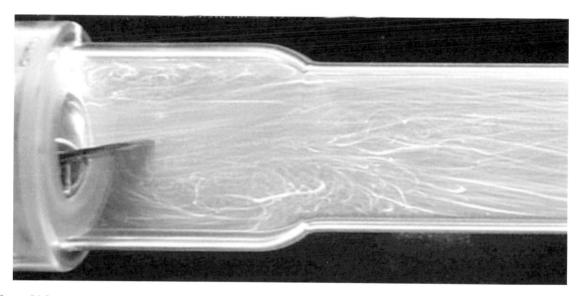

Figure 34.6

Example of streaklines for a mechanical bioprosthesis, outlining the forward and recirculation flow regions.

heart valve, ensuring proper function of the device under the intended operating conditions. Areas of testing can include failure mode analysis, accelerated wear, stent evaluation, computational analysis, stent fatigue testing, and fatigue lifetime analysis.

Failure mode analysis

Failure mode analysis is a test methodology that examines the exact nature of how the transcatheter heart valve fails during operation. Its purpose is to determine if the failure mode is catastrophic or degenerative. The initiation of replacement heart valve failure modes under in vitro conditions is best observed through changes to parameters governed by the intended implant environment of the device. In particular, failure modes can be induced by acceleration of the cycle rate and/or elevation of the loading to which the device is subjected. A change in operation variables is required, since real-time observation of failures is neither reasonable nor expected in the time frame of a product development cycle. An increase in cycle rate will apply a great number of cycles to the materials in a short period of time to produce damage on the valve, but may not produce ultimate failure. Testing replacement valves under elevated loads will produce device failures by overloading the device in order to break its components. By testing under increased loading, the weakest components of the device are identified, along with the manner of the device failure. Biological transcatheter heart valves can fail by valve incompetence via leaflet prolapse, leaflet tears, or valve dehiscence from the stent. Other failure modes include leaflet abrasion, stent migration, and stent fracture. The identification of failure modes along with accelerated wear findings provide details into the areas of highest stress and the areas of greatest damage during operation, respectively.

Accelerated wear testing

As previously noted, real-time testing to determine the damage induced during the operational life of a transcatheter heart valve is not feasible during the product development cycle. Historically, accelerated wear testing of heart valves has provided adequate information to indicate which regions of the device exhibit contact and how that contact induces damage to the device. Several authors have documented methodologies and types of equipment used previously.[18,19] In some cases, the amount of wear observed during accelerated wear testing has been shown to be much worse than the wear measured on explanted devices.[20,21]

Accelerated wear testing is performed under conditions that are 10–20 times physiologic cycle rates, allowing the equivalent number of cycles seen clinically in 5 years to be achieved in 5–6 months in the laboratory. For this testing, the valves are cycled under normal pressures based on the intended implant site. The acceleration of the device cycling allows for evaluation of the wear patterns on either the tissue or the stent if performed properly. To obtain meaningful results from this type of test, two main requirements are that the opening and closing of the leaflets should be full and complete, as seen under physiologic conditions in a pulse duplicator, and that a sustained pressure should be developed upon closing to hold the leaflets closed for a portion of the cycle. These conditions should be monitored at the start of testing to help in the set-up of the accelerated wear test equipment and then checked periodically during testing to ensure that valve opening and closing are properly maintained throughout the duration of the test. In addition to the ongoing test monitoring, the devices are examined periodically for damage to record its type, location, and progression over time. The function of the device is also evaluated to record any changes over time. Some types of wear that could be observed include leaflet tears, abrasions, material removal on the stent, and stent fracture. For polymeric or metallic elements, the wear can be measured directly to determine its depth during the cycling of the valve.

For biological valves, guidance documents indicate evaluation of the device for 200 million cycles, representing 5 years of clinical implantation. The testing duration may be shorter if the implant is not intended as a permanent replacement and/or the duration meets the needs outlined in the risk analysis. Accelerated wear testing provides information about the progressive nature of damage that can occur to the transcatheter heart valve during years of clinical service.

Stent testing

Failure mode analysis and accelerated wear testing target device level evaluation, and in particular concentrate on the valve leaflets for biological valves since they are typically the weakest components of the replacement heart valve. This testing does provide some information about the frame to which the valve leaflets are attached, but specific component testing is better suited for complete evaluation of these elements. Currently, manufacturers have utilized metal stents for the delivery of the transcatheter heart valves, so that is the type of frame discussed here. There is some history for metal stent testing methodologies, and regulatory bodies have outlined recommended testing and evaluation for preclinical assessment of intravascular stents.[9] The testing and analysis called for in the documents covering intravascular stents overlap with the testing described in the heart valve guidance because test/analysis methodologies for a stented heart valve replacement are covered in the heart valve guidance.

Stent testing is required to address hazards outlined during the risk analysis activities. In general, the stent must be characterized for mechanical properties, radial strength, recoil, foreshortening, deployment uniformity, and stent-to-balloon pressure dimensional verification. These elements identify general characteristics of the stents prior to rigorous testing under normal and worst-case use conditions. Since the stents provide the structure to the device, it is essential that fatigue testing and analysis be utilized in addition to the accelerated wear testing to ensure that no failures will occur over the life cycle of the device. The fatigue analysis should include computational analysis, structural fatigue life testing, and fatigue lifetime analysis.

Computational analysis

In order to perform a fatigue analysis for the device, the stresses on the structural components must be calculated based on the loading conditions that will be experienced in its intended use. Finite element analysis provides a means to calculate these stresses for comparison with the material and fatigue properties. The analysis should consider the steps involved in manufacturing, handling of the device during implant, and intended operating conditions to calculate induced stresses on the device during each step. For intravascular stents, a cyclic loading can be employed to simulate the pulsatile blood flow in an artery, producing a radial load on the device. In the case of the transcatheter valve, consideration must also be given to the loading of the stent by the closed leaflets. The loading to be considered should be the worst-case conditions for the intended implant site.

Advanced modeling with fluid–structure interaction[22–24] has advanced over the past decade and could be useful in simulating the interaction of the flexible leaflets and rigid stent frame under flow conditions, but rigorous validation of models will be needed to ensure accuracy of calculated stresses. To reduce the complexity of the simulation, models are often simplified by neglecting the tissue and fluid components to concentrate on simulating only the structural members during the loading and unloading of the device. Either assumptions of physiologic parameters (pressure or deflection) based on implant site conditions or experimentally measured data from the laboratory are employed in the analysis to supply the loading conditions for the model to calculate the maximum stress and deformation. Several different loading conditions may need to be considered for the analysis, depending on the totality of clinically relevant loading conditions. As will be discussed later in this chapter, the peak stresses are used in the fatigue life analysis to determine whether the device design is robust enough to function in the intended implant environment.

Fatigue life testing

While accelerated wear testing does apply loads to the stent for a prescribed number of cycles, the testing is carried out under normal pressure levels. To ensure that the stent does not fail over the life of the implant, fatigue testing of the stent is performed under more rigorous conditions and for a higher number of cycles. The loading conditions of the stent used in the fatigue testing can come from several sources, including the aforementioned finite element analysis. One approach is to use the finite element analysis results under hypertensive conditions to provide the strain on the device during loading, and to use that strain level to control the testing of the device for fatigue life. Once the loading levels have been determined, testing can be performed using pulsatile pressure in a mock circulatory system with the stent deployed to maximum size. Monitoring of the test system is performed throughout testing to make sure that the stent is being loaded at the proper strain levels. At the end of the test, the stents are examined visually to determine if any types of failures have occurred – for example, strut fractures or cracks on the stent due to the cyclic loading.

Depending on the intended life cycle of the device, the stent testing is carried out for a period 2–3 times longer than the accelerated wear testing. Per the FDA guidance, traditional stented valves are tested to 200 million cycles (5 years of operational use), while stents are tested to 600 million cycles (15 years) to ensure that no structural failures will occur. In comparison, the guidance for intravascular stents requires only 400 million cycles (10 years) of testing. Again, the risk management activities for the project aid in determining the acceptable level of testing based on the intended implant length of the device and the severity of the potential failure modes.

Fatigue life analysis

Although the fatigue testing previously described provides a pass/fail test for the stent, a conservative fatigue analysis is needed in order to predict the expected fatigue life of the device. What the pass/fail testing does not provide is a factor of safety determination for the device design operating under worst-case loading conditions. The fatigue analysis can be performed in several ways, including methodologies that fall under stress/life principles or damage tolerance analysis.[25,26] For stents, the traditional stress/life analysis (S–n) has been used to experimentally obtain the endurance limit of the device. Experiments are performed, loading devices at different alternating stress levels to determine the number of cycles to failure, evaluating both low-cycle and high-cycle fatigue. The data are plotted as stress versus number of cycles to failure (Figure 34.7) to approximate the endurance limit. The alternating stress-versus-cycles to failure curve shows that at very high stresses the number of cycles to failure is low (<100 000) and that as the stresses decrease, the number of cycles to failure increases. The knee of the solid curve, beyond which no failures are anticipated, identifies the endurance limit. For a device design, the stresses when operating under hypertensive conditions, as shown by the dashed line, should be below the endurance limit and the amount below provides the factor of safety for the application.

Durability analysis

The assessment of device durability combines the results from the failure mode analysis, accelerated wear testing, computational analysis, fatigue life testing, and fatigue life analysis to determine if the design is robust enough for the intended application. No single test from this list

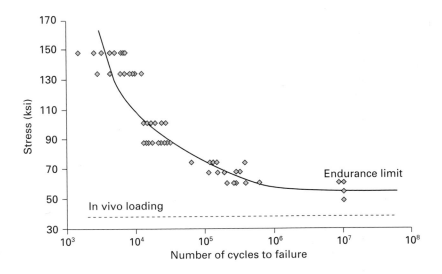

Figure 34.7

Alternating stress versus number of cycles until failure, showing a curve fit and determination of endurance limit for the device. The level of the in vivo loading condition is also provided for comparison with the endurance limit.

can be used to determine device durability. The failure mode and accelerated wear testing provide data on the weakest components and areas of contact during device operation. The computational results and fatigue life analysis provide quantitative data on the level of operating stresses for the device and where that level is in relation to the inherent fatigue properties of the device. The durability testing of the individual structural components provides a pass/fail examination of the device when functioning under worst-case in vivo conditions. In total, the durability testing and analysis provide the data to evaluate valve performance in the proposed fatigue environment.

Biological testing

The testing discussed above provides the in vitro evaluation of the device and its components. Preclinical animal studies provide the final verification testing prior to clinical trials to determine the host response to the implant. This testing evaluates the transcatheter heart valve for biocompatibility and chronic implantation.[27] Biocompatibility testing provides data on inflammation, cytotoxicity, sensitization, irritation, thrombogenicity, and pyrogenicity of the device. Chronic animal studies are used to test the host response at the implant site, device histology, and hemodynamic function of the valve. If a non-orthotopic position is required for chronic study implantation because of differences between the animal model and human anatomy, hemodynamics can be assessed by acute implantation and monitoring of the device. These studies provide the final piece of data to address potential failure modes prior to start of a clinical trial.

Summary

During the product development cycle, preclinical tests are utilized to help understand how the transcatheter heart valve may operate clinically. Preclinical in vitro testing allows for accurate assessment under controlled conditions to determine the functionality and durability of the device. Preclinical in vivo testing provides a biological environment for device evaluation to provide further proof that the device will perform as intended. In total, the preclinical testing is used to address the risks identified with regard to implantation and operation of the device during clinical use. A well-designed, controlled clinical trial provides the ultimate evaluation of the device in the intended implant population and for treatment of the indicated pathologies.

References

1. Hufnagel CA, Harvey WP. Aortic plastic valvular prosthesis. Bull Georgetown U Med Cent 1952; 4: 1.
2. Bonhoeffer P, Boudjemline Y, Saliba Z, et al. Percutaneous replacement of pulmonary valve in a right-ventricle to pulmonary-artery prosthetic conduit with valve dysfunction. Lancet 2000; 356: 1403–5.
3. Cribier A, Eltchaninoff H, Bash A, et al. Percutaneous transcatheter implantation of an aortic valve prosthesis for calcific aortic stenosis: first human case description. Circulation 2002; 106: 3006–8.
4. Kumar N, Balasundaram S, Rickard M, et al. Leaflet embolisation from Duromedics valves: a report of two cases. Thorac Cardiovasc Surg 1991; 39: 382–3.
5. Bodnar E. The Medtronic Parallel valve and the lessons learned. J Heart Valve Dis 1996; 5: 572–3.
6. Yoganathan AP, Eberhardt CE, Walker PG. Hydrodynamic performance of the Medtronic Freestyle Aortic Root Bioprosthesis. J Heart Valve Dis 1994; 3: 571–80.
7. ISO 5840: 1996. Cardiovascular Implants – Cardiac Valve Prostheses. April 8, 1996.
8. FDA Draft Replacement Heart Valve Guidance. October 14, 1994.
9. FDA Draft Guidance for the Submission of Research and Marketing Applications for Interventional Cardiology Devices: PTCA Catheters, Atherectomy Catheters, Lasers, Intravascular Stents. May 1995.
10. ISO 14971: 2000. Medical devices – Application of Risk Management to Medical Devices. March 23, 2001.
11. Yoganathan AP, Woo YR, Sung HW, et al. In vitro hemodynamic characteristics of tissue bioprostheses in the aortic position. J Thorac Cardiovasc Surg 1986; 92: 198–209.
12. Scotten LN, Walker DK. New laboratory technique measures projected dynamic area of prosthetic heart valves. J Heart Valve Dis 2004; 13: 120–32.
13. Gross JM, Shermer CD, Hwang NH. Vortex shedding in bileaflet heart valve prostheses. ASAIO Trans 1988; 34: 845–50.

14. Hasenkam JM, Westphal D, Reul H, et al. Three-dimensional visualization of axial velocity profiles downstream of six different mechanical aortic valve prostheses, measured with a hot-film anemometer in a steady state flow model. J Biomech 1987; 20: 353–64.

15. Lim WL, Chew YT, Chew TC, Low HT. Particle image velocimetry in the investigation of flow past artificial heart valves. Ann Biomed Eng 1994; 22: 307–18.

16. Woo YR, Yoganathan AP. Two-component laser Doppler anemometer for measurement of velocity and turbulent shear stress near prosthetic heart valves. Med Instrum 1985; 19: 224–31.

17. Stewart SF, Nast EP, Arabia FA, et al. Errors in pressure gradient measurement by continuous wave Doppler ultrasound: type, size and age effects in bioprosthetic aortic valves. J Am Coll Cardiol 1991; 18: 769–79.

18. Reul H, Potthast K. Durability/wear testing of heart valve substitutes. J Heart Valve Dis 1998; 7: 151–7.

19. Campbell A, Baldwin T, Peterson G, et al. Pitfalls and outcomes from accelerated wear testing of mechanical heart valves. J Heart Valve Dis 1996; 5(Suppl 1): S124–S132.

20. Hasenkam JM, Pasquino E, Stacchino C, et al. Wear patterns in the Sorin Bicarbon mechanical heart valve: a clinical explant study. J Heart Valve Dis 1997; 6:105–14.

21. More RB, Chang BC, Hong YS, et al. Wear analysis of retrieved mitral bileaflet mechanical heart valve explants. In: Proceedings of Society for Heart Valve Disease, First Biennial Meeting, London, UK, 2001: 284 (abst).

22. Peskin CS, McQueen DM. A general method for the computer simulation of biological systems interacting with fluids. Symp Soc Exp Biol 1995; 49: 265–76.

23. Lemmon JD, Yoganathan AP. Three-dimensional computational model of left heart diastolic function with fluid–structure interaction. J Biomech Eng 2000; 122: 109–17.

24. Nicosia MA, Cochran RP, Einstein DR, et al. A coupled fluid–structure finite element model of the aortic valve and root. J Heart Valve Dis 2003; 12: 781–9.

25. Ritchie RO, Lubock P. Fatigue life estimation procedures for the endurance of a cardiac valve prosthesis: stress/life and damage-tolerant analyses. Biomech Eng 1986; 108: 153–60.

26. Ryder JK, Cao H. Structural integrity assessment of heart valve prostheses: a damage tolerance analysis of the CarboMedics Prosthetic Heart Valve. J Heart Valve Dis 1996; 5(Suppl 1): S86–S96.

27. ISO 10993–1: 2003. Biological Evaluation of Medical Devices – Part 1: Evaluation and Testing. August 1, 2003.

Index